T0299904

Brain Tumor and Nanotechnology

RIVER PUBLISHERS SERIES IN BIOTECHNOLOGY AND MEDICAL RESEARCH

Editors-in-Chief:

PAOLO DI NARDO
University of Rome Tor Vergata,
Italy

PRANELA RAMESHWAR
Rutgers University,
USA

ALAIN VERTES
London Business School,
UK and NxR Biotechnologies,
Switzerland

Aiming primarily at providing detailed snapshots of critical issues in biotechnology and medicine that are reaching a tipping point in financial investment or industrial deployment, the scope of the series encompasses various specialty areas including pharmaceutical sciences and healthcare, industrial biotechnology, and biomaterials. Areas of primary interest comprise immunology, virology, microbiology, molecular biology, stem cells, hematopoiesis, oncology, regenerative medicine, biologics, polymer science, formulation and drug delivery, renewable chemicals, manufacturing, and biorefineries.

Each volume presents comprehensive review and opinion articles covering all fundamental aspect of the focus topic. The editors/authors of each volume are experts in their respective fields and publications are peer-reviewed.

For a list of other books in this series, visit www.riverpublishers.com

Brain Tumor and Nanotechnology

Rishabha Malviya

School of Medical and Allied Sciences, Galgotias University,
Greater Noida, India

Arun Kumar Singh

School of Medical and Allied Sciences, Galgotias University,
Greater Noida, India

Sonali Sundram

School of Medical and Allied Sciences, Galgotias University,
Greater Noida, India

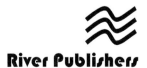

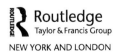

NEW YORK AND LONDON

Published 2024 by River Publishers
River Publishers
Alsbjergvej 10, 9260 Gistrup, Denmark
www.riverpublishers.com

Distributed exclusively by Routledge
605 Third Avenue, New York, NY 10017, USA
4 Park Square, Milton Park, Abingdon, Oxon OX14 4RN

Brain Tumor and Nanotechnology / Rishabha Malviya, Arun Kumar Singh and Sonali Sundram.

Routledge is an imprint of the Taylor & Francis Group, an informa business

ISBN 978-87-7004-088-4 (hardback)
ISBN 978-87-7004-180-5 (paperback)
ISBN 978-10-4012-082-8 (online)
ISBN 978-1-003-51579-1 (ebook master)

While every effort is made to provide dependable information, the publisher, authors, and editors cannot be held responsible for any errors or omissions.

Contents

Preface   ix

Foreword   xi

List of Figures   xiii

List of Tables   xv

List of Abbreviations   xvii

About the Book   xxiii

1   Anatomy of the Brain and Nervous System   1
   1.1   Introduction   1
   1.2   Component of CNS   2
       1.2.1   The neuronal cell   2
       1.2.2   Glial cells   3
   1.3   The Human Brain: Anatomy   5
       1.3.1   Spinal cord.   5
       1.3.2   Brainstem   6
       1.3.3   Diencephalon   7
       1.3.4   Cerebellum   9
       1.3.5   Hemispheres.   9
       1.3.6   Ventricle system   12
   1.4   CNS Hurdles.   12
       1.4.1   Blood–brain barrier (BBB)   12
       1.4.2   Blood–CSF barrier   13
   1.5   Brain Cancer.   14
       1.5.1   Incidence-specific tumors   14
       1.5.2   Non-geographically specified malignant tumors . . .   15
   1.6   Melanocytic Tumors.   18
       1.6.1   Lymphomas   18

1.6.2   Whole-brain or stereotactic radiosurgery   18
1.6.3   Chemotherapy: hydroxyurea, bevacizumab,
        or temozolomide.   19
1.6.4   Alternative treatment for tumor-treating fields   20
1.7   Conclusion.   20
References   21

2   The Role of Angiogenesis in Neuronal Tumors   **27**
2.1   Introduction   27
2.2   The Central Nervous System and Angiogenesis   28
2.3   Brain Cancer Angiogenesis: Cellular or Molecular
      Mechanism of Action   29
2.4   BBB, Hypoxia, BBB, or Brain Tumor Vessel   32
2.5   Anti-angiogenic Factors   34
2.6   Angiogenic: Transition and Homeostasis   34
2.7   Primary Brain Tumors and Glioblastoma Angiogenesis . . .   35
2.8   Angiogenesis in Glioblastoma.   36
2.9   Conclusion.   38
References   38

**3   Methods of Transduction and the Physiology of the
    Blood−Brain Barrier**   **51**
3.1   Introduction   51
3.2   BBB's Advancement   54
3.3   The BBB's Physiology   54
3.3.1   Transcellular diffusion.   55
3.3.2   Ion transportation   57
3.3.3   Carrier-mediated transportation   58
3.3.4   Receptor-mediated transcytosis   59
3.3.5   Transcytosis via adsorptive means   63
3.4   Conclusion.   64
References   65

**4   Specific Brain Tumor Treatments Supplied using Active
    Nanotechnology Delivery Systems**   **77**
4.1   Introduction   77
4.2   Transcending the Blood−Brain Barriers via
      Transcytosis Mediated by Receptors   78
4.3   Based on Transferrin Targeting   83
4.4   Targeting Relying on Lactoferrin   85
4.5   Based on Folic Acid Targeting   86

4.6	Targeting using Antibodies	87
	4.6.1 Delivery of drugs	87
	4.6.2 Tumor imaging	90
	4.6.3 Gene delivery	93
	4.6.4 Radiotherapy	93
4.7	Peptide-based Targeting	94
	4.7.1 Delivery of drugs	94
4.8	Conclusion	95
	References	96

5 Solid-core Lipid Nanoparticles as a Vehicle for Brain Drug Delivery

5 Solid-core Lipid Nanoparticles as a Vehicle for Brain Drug Delivery		**105**
5.1	Introduction	105
	5.1.1 Physiological and anatomical dissection of the BBB	105
	5.1.2 Statistics on brain tumors	109
5.2	Novel Drug Delivery System Approach: Nanoparticles	111
	5.2.1 Definition and structural characteristics	111
	5.2.2 Comparative advantages of SLNs vs. polymeric nanoparticles (other delivery systems like liposomal drug delivery)	113
	5.2.3 The downside of SLNs	114
	5.2.4 Factors to be considered in the formulation of SLNs	114
	5.2.5 Method of preparation of SLNs	118
5.3	Conclusion	123
	References	125
6 Clinical Studies on the Efficacy and Safety of Nano-enabled Carriers for the Treatment of Brain Tumors		**137**
6.1	Introduction	137
6.2	Nanoparticle Delivery and Glioma Targeting	138
6.3	Lipid-based Nanomedicines	140
	6.3.1 Liposomes	140
	6.3.2 Exosomes	145
6.4	Polymeric Nanomedicines	147
6.5	Dendrimers	148
6.6	Nanomedicines Constructed from Amino Acids and Nucleic Acids	150
	6.6.1 Spherical nucleic acids	150
	6.6.2 Nanomedicines that rely on amino acids	152
6.7	Drug Conjugates	154

   6.8   Conclusion.   157
   References   158

**7 Degenerative Diseases Treated with Brain-directed
    Lipid/Polymeric (Hybrid) Nanoparticles   171**
   7.1   Introduction   171
   7.2   Blood–Brain Barrier Crossing with Brain Targeting   173
         7.2.1   Anatomy and role of the BBB.   173
         7.2.2   The improvement of brain drug delivery   176
   7.3   Nano-engineered Colloid Drug Delivery Systems   177
         7.3.1   Liposomes.   179
         7.3.2   Nanoparticles of polymeric materials   179
         7.3.3   Solid nanoparticles   180
         7.3.4   Ligands   180
   7.4   Neurodegenerative Diseases: New Advances in
         Nanomedicine.   181
         7.4.1   Alzheimer's disease   181
         7.4.2   Parkinson's disorder.   182
         7.4.3   Huntington's disease.   182
         7.4.4   Multiple sclerosis   183
   7.5   Conclusion.   184
   References   185

**8 Challenges and Intellectual Property Rights Prospects
    Particular to Nanotechnology in Treating Brain Tumors   197**
   8.1   Introduction   197
   8.2   Obstacles in Delivering Drugs to the Brain   199
   8.3   Perils of the Blood–Brain Barrier and Blood–Brain
         Tumor Barrier   201
   8.4   Overcoming BBB's Obstacles.   203
         8.4.1   Convection-enhanced delivery (CED).   203
         8.4.2   Gene therapy and virotherapy.   205
         8.4.3   The carmustine wafer   205
         8.4.4   Ultrasound and brain tumors   207
   8.5   Laws Protecting the Use of Nanomedicine to Treat
         Brain Tumors as a Protected Invention   209
   8.6   Conclusion.   209
   References   212

Index   223

About the Editors   227

Preface

The diagnosis and treatment of brain tumors have long been an alarming challenge in the field of medical science. Medical practitioners and academics working to develop efficient treatments have faced considerable obstacles because of the complexity of the human brain with the restrictive behavior of the blood–brain barriers. However, in recent years, the development of nanotechnology has offered new prospects for resolving challenging issues.

The book *Brain Tumors and Nanotechnology* is an offering to both the amazing advancements made in the study of brain tumors and the innovative possibilities of nanotechnology.

The chapters in this book cover a wide range of subjects, from a fundamental knowledge of the components of the central nervous system and the anatomy of the brain to the complex mechanisms of angiogenesis in neuronal tumors. The physiological complexities of the blood–brain barrier will be examined in depth, and readers will learn about the transduction mechanisms that enable the administration of medications to the brain. The book also investigates the unique therapies offered by active nanotechnology delivery systems and the promise of solid-core lipid nanoparticles as delivery systems for drugs intended for the brain.

This book's focus on clinical research that looks into the effectiveness and safety of nano-enabled carriers for the treatment of brain tumors is one of its highlights. The book provides insightful information about the real-world uses of nanomedicine, highlighting its potential to transform the treatment of brain tumors and enhance patient outcomes.

Although nanotechnology offers a promising future, the book also discusses the difficulties and hurdles that still need to be overcome. Readers can gain a thorough knowledge of the field's larger background and ethical considerations by reading about intellectual property rights and the legal prospects surrounding nanotechnology in the treatment of brain tumors.

We, as the authors of this book, have worked hard to produce an extensive source that provides encouraging additional investigation and advancement in the field of brain tumor treatment. We want to give academics, medical professionals, and students a thorough and current assessment of the developments in this quickly changing subject.

We anticipate that *Brain Tumors and Nanotechnology* will act as a catalyst for additional investigation and cooperation among scientists and medical experts. Together, we can keep pushing the limits of medical knowledge and work toward the ultimate goal of enhancing the lives of people with brain tumors.

Author

Foreword

In the world of medical science, developments and findings consistently pave the way for innovative therapies and improved outcomes for patients. The field of treating brain tumors is receiving a lot of attention and investigation. Medical practitioners and researchers have long faced substantial challenges as a result of the complexity of brain tumors and the difficulties in administering medicines to the complex structure of the brain.

In *Brain Tumors and Nanotechnology*, the author takes readers on an amazing journey through the most recent advances in the detection and treatment of brain tumors. This comprehensive book sheds light on the ground-breaking role of nanotechnology in redefining brain tumor therapies.

Dr. Rishabha Malviya, the author, organized the effortless integration of numerous perspectives and research findings into a comprehensive and unique resource. Dr. Malviya's dedication and expertise in the field are evident throughout the book, providing readers with a comprehensive and up-to-date account of the advancements in brain tumor treatment.

This book's chapters explore several aspects of brain tumor treatment, providing a multifaceted viewpoint on the topic. The book offers a strong basis for understanding the complexity of brain tumors and their treatment by revealing the intricate anatomy of the brain and nervous system and investigating the difficulties presented by the blood–brain barrier.

One of the book's standout features is its emphasis on nanotechnology and how it can be used to deliver treatments to the brain. With their distinctive qualities and abilities, nanoparticles have become effective tools for overcoming the challenges posed by the complex structural makeup of the brain. The chapters on nanoparticle-based drug delivery methods offer insightful information on the conception, production, and effectiveness of these novel strategies.

In addition, *Brain Tumors and Nanotechnology* analyzes the physiology of the blood–brain barrier, looks into the function of angiogenesis in neural tumors, and includes clinical trials demonstrating the effectiveness and safety of nano-enabled carriers. In addition, the book discusses the potential applications of nanotechnology for the treatment of brain tumors and the issues surrounding intellectual property rights, providing a thorough understanding of the legal and moral issues involved.

I am confident that the book *Brain Tumors and Nanotechnology* will be a stepping stone for scientists, doctors, and students who want to acquire more knowledge about brain tumors and explore the potential of nanotechnology in transforming their diagnosis and treatment. The valuable information presented in this book will certainly get us one step closer to conquering the difficulties posed by brain tumor therapy and ultimately enhancing the lives of patients all around the world.

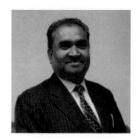

Dr. Sharad Wakode
Professor
Delhi Pharmaceutical Sciences and Research University
New Delhi, India

List of Figures

Figure 1.1   Spinal column anatomy..   6
Figure 1.2   A sagittal image of the brainstem and its related
components..   8
Figure 1.3   Cerebral lobes.   10
Figure 2.1   The creation of vessels and the interactions between
biological mediators.   29
Figure 2.2   The angiogenic inducers and inhibitors are displayed
by angiogenic balance.   35
Figure 2.3   Illustration of brain tumor anticancer drugs that target
the angiogenic process (bottom panel) and molecular
targets utilized to decrease tumor angiogenesis (upper
panel)..   37
Figure 3.1   Schematic representations of cerebral capillaries or
the link between the neurovascular component depict
the blood–brain barrier..   53
Figure 4.1   Blood–brain barrier transportation..   83
Figure 5.1   Receptor-specific ligands used to transport drugs over
the BBB.   107
Figure 5.2   (A) Drug-enriched cell model, (B) a drug-enriched
core model, and (C) a homogeneous matrix model
of drug inclusion in solid lipid nanoparticles (solid
solution).   112
Figure 5.3   Solid lipid nanoparticle production by high
homogenization processes.   121
Figure 5.4   Solid lipid nanoparticles are generated by
microemulsion and emulsification evaporation. . . .   123
Figure 6.1   Nanoparticles used in glioma targeting.   142
Figure 7.1   The BBB in normal and abnormal states..   174

List of Tables

Table 4.1   Nanoscale therapeutic or imaging agents for brain
tumors can be produced by conjugating a variety
of ligands, including peptides, aptamers, folic acid
antibodies, transferrin, and lactoferrin.   79

Table 5.1   Mechanisms, benefits, and drawbacks of lipid
nanoparticle preparation techniques.   119

Table 6.1   The characteristics of nanoparticles and their
observed effect on tumor location.   139

Table 6.2   Trials of liposomal nanomedicines in the treatment of
GBM.   141

Table 6.3   Investigation of nanomedicines for glioma in
preclinical studies.   143

Table 6.4   Studies on peptide-based nanomedicines for glioma
in preclinical studies.   153

Table 6.5   Research on glioma drug conjugates in preclinical
and clinical settings.   155

Table 8.1   WHO tumor grading system.   199

Table 8.2   Brain-expressed drug transporter associated with
drug-resistance in brain tumors.   202

Table 8.3   Various formulation patents for brain targeted
delivery of drug..   211

List of Abbreviations

AB	Antibody
ABC	ATP-binding cassette
AD	Alzheimer's disease
AJ	Adherent junction
AMT	Adsorption-mediated transcytosis
API	Active pharmaceutical ingredient
ATP	Adenosine triphosphate
AUC	Area under the curve
Aβ	Amyloid-β
BBB	Blood–brain barrier
BBTB	Blood–brain tumor barrier
BCNU	Carmustine
BCRP	Breast cancer resistance protein
BCSFB	Blood-cerebrospinal fluid barrier
BDNF	Brain-derived neurotrophic factor
BEV	Bevacizumab
Bfgf	Basic fibroblast growth factor
BIF	Brain interstitial fluid
BMEC	Brain microvascular endothelial cell
BRB	Blood–retinal barrier
BSA	Bovine serum albumin
BTB	Blood–tumor barrier
CAG	Cytosine–adenine–guanine
CASK	Ca^{2+}-dependent serine protein kinases
CED	Convection-enhanced delivery
cMOAT	Canalicular multispecific organic anion transporter 1
CNS	Central nervous system
cRGD	Cyclic RGD
CSF	Cerebrospinal fluid
CUR	Curcumin
CVO	Circumventricular organ
CVS	Cerebrovascular system

Dll4	Delta-like ligand 4
DOX	Doxorubicin
DTX	Docetaxel
EAE	Experimental autoimmune encephalomyelitis
EBP	Enhancer-binding protein
EC	Endothelial cell
ECM	Extracellular matrix
EDTA	Ethylenediaminetetraacetic acid
EGFR	Epidermal growth factor receptor
EMF	Electromagnetic field
EPR	Enhanced permeability and retention
ESAM	Endothelial cell specific adhesion molecule
ETP	Etoposide
EV	Extracellular vesicle
FA	Folic acid
GB	Glioblastomas
GBM	Glioblastoma multiforme
GLUT	Glucose transporters
GMS	Glyceryl monostearate
GnRH	Gonadotropin-releasing hormone
GRAS	Generally regarded as safe
GSC	Glioblastoma stem cell
GSH	Glutathione
HA	Hyaluronic acid
HBMEC	Human brain microvascular endothelial cell
HD	Huntington's disease
HGF	Hepatocyte growth factor
HIF	Hypoxia-inducible factor
HIR	Human insulin receptor
HIV	Human immunodeficiency virus
HLB	Hydrophilic–lipophilic balance
HPC	Hypoxic postconditioning
HPH	High-pressure homogenization
HSA	Human serum albumin
HSPG	Heparan sulfate proteoglycans
HU	Hydroxyurea
HUVEC	Human umbilical vein endothelial cells
IDO	Indoleamine 2,3-dioxygenase
IFN	Interferon
IGF	Insulin-like growth factor

IKVAV	Peptide sequence Ile-Lys-Val-Ala-Val
IL8	Interleukin-8
IONP	Iron oxide nanoparticle
IQR	Interquartile range
JAM	Junctional adhesion molecule
JAM-1	Junctional adhesion molecule-1
LDC	Lipid drug conjugate
LDL	Low-density lipoprotein
LDLR	Low-density lipoprotein receptor
LfR	Lactoferrin
LM	Liposomal formulations of methylprednisolone
LRP	Lipoprotein receptor-related protein
LV	Lipid vesicle
MA	Melanotransferrin antibody
MAPK	Mitogen-activated protein kinases
MB	Microbubble
MDR	Multidrug resistance
MDR1	Multidrug resistance protein 1
MGMT	O(6)-methylguanine-DNA methyltransferase
MMP	Matrix metalloproteinase
MRI	Magnetic resonance imaging
MRP	Multidrug resistance associated protein
MRPAP	Mean resting pulmonary artery pressure
MS	Multiple sclerosis
MSN	Moderately spiny neurons
NAA	N-amino acid
NAC	N-acetylcysteine
NAchR	Nicotinic Acetylcholine Receptor
NDDS	Nano drug delivery system
NF	Neurofilament
NGF	Nerve growth factor
NIA	Nanoscale imaging agent
NIR	Near-infrared
NLC	Nanostructured lipid carrier
NP	Nanoparticle
NVU	Neurovascular unit
OAT	Organic anion transporter
OVLT	Organum Vasculosum of the Lamina Terminalis
PaH	Para hippocampal gyrus

PASA	Poly(aspartic acid)
PCD	Passive cavitation detection
PCL	Pro-cationic liposome
PD	Parkinson's disease
PDA	Patent ductus arteriosus
PDB	Protein Data Bank
PDC	Peptide–drug conjugates
PEG	Poly(ethylene glycol)
PGF	Placental growth factor
PGK	Phosphoglycerate Kinase
P-gp	Permeability glycoprotein
PL	Polylactide
PLA	Polylactic acid
PLGA	Poly-lactic acid-glycolic acid copolymer
PLL	Polylysine
PNS	Peripheral nervous system
PSA	Polar surface area
PTEN	Phosphatase and TENsin homolog deleted on chromosome 10
PTX	Paclitaxel
RES	Reticuloendothelial system
RGD	Arginylglycylaspartic acid
RMT	Receptor-mediated transcytosis
RNW	RGD-DM1 loaded nanoscaled wormlike micelles
ROS	Reactive oxygen species
RVG	Rabies virus glycoprotein
SA	Stearic acid
SCF	Supercritical fluid
SERS	Surface-enhanced Raman scattering
SFT	Solitary fibrous tumor
siRNA	Small interfering RNA
SLN	Solid lipid nanoparticle
SM	Stria medullaris
SPION	Superparamagnetic iron oxide nanoparticle
TAT	Trans-activating transcriptor
Tf	Transferrin
TfR	Transferrin receptor
TfR1	Transferrin receptor 1
TJ	Tight junction
TKI	Tyrosine kinase inhibitor

TMN	Tempamine
TMZ	Temozolomide
TPGS	D-α-tocopheryl poly(ethylene glycol)1000 succinate
TPM	Transferrin-modified polyphosphoester hybrid micelles
TUNEL	Terminal deoxynucleotidyl transferase biotin-dUTP nick end labeling
TX	Tamoxifen
VEGF	Vascular endothelial growth factor
VEGF-A	Vascular endothelial growth factor A
VEGFR	VEGF receptor
VHL	Von Hippel–Lindau
VM	Venous malformations
WBRT	Whole brain radiation therapy
WGA	Wheat germ agglutinin
WHO	World Health Organization

About the Book

The book *Brain Tumors and Nanotechnology* explores the complex world of brain tumors and the ground-breaking role that nanotechnology plays in both detection and treatment. This comprehensive book offers an in-depth analysis of the anatomy of the brain and nervous system, highlighting the constituents of the central nervous system (CNS) such as neurons and glial cells. It offers a thorough understanding of the intricate structure of the human brain, including the hemispheres, brainstem, diencephalon, and ventricular system. The CNS presents challenges for treating brain tumors, including the blood–brain barrier, blood–cerebrospinal-fluid barrier, and CSF–brain barrier, which are explored in the book.

By examining the complex anatomy and functioning of the brain, Chapter 1, "Anatomy of the Brain and Nervous System," lays the groundwork for the rest of the book. It provides a thorough grasp of the CNS by examining various brain regions and the ventricular system. Chapter 2, "The Role of Angiogenesis in Neuronal Tumors," explores the process of angiogenesis and its importance in brain tumors. With a special emphasis on glioblastoma, it investigates the cellular and molecular principles of brain tumor angiogenesis and sheds light on its pathological features. Chapter 3, "Methods of Transduction and the Physiology of the Blood–Brain Barrier," delves into the progress made in overcoming the difficulties presented by the blood–brain barrier. It discusses the physiology of the blood–brain barrier and various transduction methods that have been explored to enhance drug delivery to the brain.

The use of active nanotechnology delivery systems for the treatment of brain tumors is explored in Chapter 4, "Specific Brain Tumor Treatments Supplied using Active Nanotechnology Delivery Systems." It discusses different targeting strategies, including transferrin, lactoferrin, folic acid, antibodies, peptides, and gene delivery, highlighting their potential in enhancing drug delivery efficacy. Chapter 5, "Solid-Core Lipid Nanoparticles as a Vehicle for Brain Drug Delivery," introduces the idea of nanoparticles as a brand-new method of brain drug administration. It focuses on the benefits of solid-core lipid nanoparticles (SLNs) over other delivery systems. The chapter covers the creation of SLNs for better therapeutic benefits. Chapter 6, "Clinical Studies on the Efficacy and Safety of Nano-enabled Carriers for the Treatment of Brain Tumors," is a summary of clinical research on various nanomedicines used to treat brain tumors. It examines dendrimers, polymeric nanomedicines, exosomes, liposomes, and nucleic-acid-based and amino-acid-based nanodrug delivery systems.

By exploring how brain-directed lipid/polymeric (hybrid) nanoparticles can be used to treat degenerative disorders, Chapter 7, "Degenerative Diseases Treated with Brain-directed Lipid/Polymeric (Hybrid) Nanoparticles," broadens the field of nanomedicine. It showcases nanoengineered colloid drug delivery technologies and explores the difficulties in overcoming the blood–brain barrier.

Specifically addressing the risks of the blood–brain barrier, Chapter 8, "Challenges and Intellectual Property Rights Prospects Particularly to Nanotechnology in Treating Brain Tumor," discusses the difficulties and barriers associated with delivering medications to the brain. It also explores different approaches to overcome these challenges, by utilizing convection-enhanced delivery systems, gene therapy, and ultrasound-controlled delivery system.

As a result, *Brain Tumors and Nanotechnology* offers comprehensive and up-to-date strategies in the treatment of brain tumors, with a special emphasis on the revolutionary impact of nanotechnology. It reveals the understanding of the complicated nature of brain tumors and the potential for nanotechnology to revolutionize their diagnosis and treatment, making it a valuable resource for researchers, medical professionals, and students in the field.

1

Anatomy of the Brain and Nervous System

Abstract

Central nervous system (CNS) consists of brain and spinal cord, which is an intricate network of tissues and systems. It plays an important part in the regulation and coordination of bodily activities such as sensory perception, motor control, and mental processes. Tumors in the CNS may either originate in the CNS (primary tumors), such as in the brain or spinal cord, or spread from elsewhere in the body (secondary tumors, also known as metastatic tumors). The majority of malignant tumors develop from cells inside the central nervous system (CNS), with possible origins including glial cells, brain cells, and even the CNS's underneath connective tissues. CNS tumors are considered among the most lethal cancers due to their potential to disrupt vital brain functions and the challenges associated with their treatment. In this chapter, the author discusses the basic anatomical interactions within the CNS. In this chapter, readers will also learn about current therapeutic methods and the role of nanoparticles in the treatment of CNS tumors. By understanding these fundamental aspects, readers will gain valuable knowledge about how CNS tumors behave based on their anatomical location within the CNS. This understanding will lay down the basic concept or foundation of the topic.

1.1 Introduction

According to the statistics provided, in 2014, there were 162,341 people in the United States of America who were diagnosed with cancer of the central nervous system. In 2017, there were around 23,800 new cases of brain tumors [1]. At first glance, the reality is that CNS tumors are quite uncommon, ranking as the 16th most prevalent kind of cancer. Central nervous system neoplasms have a very poor survival rate, having a death rate of about 70%, which makes them one of the most lethal types of solid tumors. It is challenging to do research on pediatric central nervous system malignancies due to the low survival rate (33% of children survive five years following diagnosis) and the difficulty in obtaining samples from these uncommon CNS tumors [2]. Because of this, researchers continuously look into novel fields of inquiry in their search for a therapy that is more effective and a cure for cancers that affect the central and peripheral nervous system (PNS). Adjuvant treatment approaches, such as nanotechnology-based therapy, show that it is possible to reach this objective. Cancer that develops in the central nervous system (CNS) has the potential to manifest itself in a wide variety of distinct forms and to spread to a wide assortment of different parts of the brain. These four parts will provide a general review of CNS tumors, including their causes, types, and locations. They also include current or possible curative therapies that are being used or considered as well as a quick look at nanoparticle (NP) applications and their function in CNS tumors. By at the end of this chapter, the reader should understand CNS malignancies and their treatment. Armed with this knowledge, they can now critically evaluate whether the nanoparticle therapy holds promise as a viable approach in the fight against CNS malignancies.

1.2 Component of CNS

1.2.1 The neuronal cell

In the neurological system, the neuron is the basic building block. Even though there are many different kinds of neurons in the nervous system, they all share the same fundamental structure. This structure consists of cellular mass, a nucleus, and connecting points such as single axons or nerve cells that are joined together. The neuron's huge and spherical nucleus, known as the soma, and the cytoplasmic ring that surrounds it, known as the perikaryon. Perikaryon consists of the cell body, or soma, of the neuron. An elongated extension of the cell body of a neuron, called a nerve fiber, receives electrical impulses and transmits them anterogradely, or backward, to the cell body. The axon conical projection seems to be a specialized area of a nerve cell that has a responsibility to integrate and collect impulses received from the soma just before transmitting them down the axon. This region is found at the point where the axon and the body of the cell meet. At the distal end of an axon, one or more terminal buttons, also known as swellings, may be visible. These terminal buttons are used to transmit chemical signals to other neurons or organs in the human body.

Dendrites are outgrowths that originate at the opposite pole of the neuron. Dendrons are non-axonal body extensions that either receive action potential from other nerve cells or the environment or then transfer it back to the body or transmit action potential from the environment to the body. Dendrites are indeed important structures in neurons that play a crucial role in receiving and transmitting neural signals. They are branch-like extensions that project from the cell body of a neuron. The primary function of dendrites is to receive incoming signals from other neurons or sensory receptors. These signals are typically transmitted in the form of electrical impulses called action potentials. Dendrites are covered in numerous small protrusions called dendritic spines, which greatly increase their surface area and allow for a larger number of connections with other neurons. When a neighboring neuron or sensory receptor releases neurotransmitters, these chemical messengers bind to specialized receptor molecules on the dendritic spines or dendritic membranes. This binding triggers a series of electrical and chemical changes in the dendrite, generating an electrical signal known as a postsynaptic potential. If the postsynaptic potential is strong enough, it can propagate toward the cell body of the neuron and potentially trigger an action potential, which is the fundamental unit of neural communication.

1.2.2 Glial cells

Glia, which are non-synaptic support cells, keep the parenchymal milieu within the nervous system at its ideal state for neuronal activation [3]. The most common type of a nerve cell is the glial cell, and this cell is composed of nerve tissues. Ependymal cells, astrocytes, microglia, and oligodendrocytes are all examples of cells that belong to the neuroglial cell type. Neuroglial cells, which have the ability to proliferate, are the most common factor in the development of tumors in the nervous system. Astrocytes provide protection to neurons in the brain and spinal cord on a number of fronts, including the structural, functional, mechanical, and cellular levels [3]. The astrocytes that line the brain and spinal cord are connected at their proximal ends to form a glial limitans that provides structural support [4]. These projections protect the brain and spinal cord. Astrocytic end feet, which line every blood vessel in the central nervous system (CNS), also have an effect on the formation of the blood–brain barrier (BBB), which further separates the brain from the rest of the body [5]. In addition, astrocytes play an essential role in the recovery process after damage to the CNS. After a lesion or the resultant loss of vulnerable nerve tissues, they proliferate and build a permanent scar. This scar protects the adjacent living tissues from the inflammatory as well as the poisonous environment [6]. They play an important role in the control of the electrolyte and neurotransmitter metabolisms as well as in the storage of energy in the body. Among the several types of neurological cancer, glioblastoma (GBM) is the most lethal because it begins in astrocytes and affects the brain and spinal cord. Oligodendrocytes are a special kind of neuroglial cell. Oligodendrocytes, which derive from the neuroectoderm, are the cells that are responsible for myelinating the axons of neurons found in the central nervous system. Oligodendrocytes are the most common type of substantia alba; therefore, they are the beginning site of "oligodendrogliomas" within the temporal and frontal lobes [7, 8]. That is why oligodendrocytes are the starting point for oligodendrogliomas. Microglia are primarily responsible for mediating inflammatory reactions in the brain. Microglia are formed from egg white granulocytes or monocytes that are neural stem cells. They operate in a manner that is similar to that of marginal neutrophils. Microglial cells have lengthy, widely twisted channels that radiate from their cellular bodies, which allow them to retain scavenger or watchdog activity in the absence of brain injuries. Microglia "stimulate," changing morphologically or reproducing rapidly in response to infections and neurodegenerative diseases, and migrate to the site of neuronal damage to defend the central nervous system (CNS) immunologically [9]. Despite the fact that microglial cells are essential for the protection of the central nervous system (CNS), excessive activation of these cells may have harmful impacts on the body. Examples include the etiology of diseases like senile dementia, which may be influenced by the inflammatory and toxic actions of microglia [9]. Endometrial cells are the latest type of glial cell to be found in the brain and spinal cord. This is true for both regions. Ependymal cells, which develop from neural ectoderm, line the surfaces of the ventricular and central canals of the brain and spinal cord, respectively. Desmosomes connect the ependymal cells of the ventricular system, which in turn causes the formation of a simple cuboidal epithelium that has microvilli at the microscale and cilia at the apex [10]. The choroid plexus is an epithelial layer of cells that is highly vascularized and villous, and it is responsible for producing CSF in the ventricular system [10]. The term "encephaloma" refers to a tumor that originates in the ependymal cells of the brain. Ependymomas are common types of childhood malignancies that may result in deadly CSF barriers and severe catastrophic effects [10]. Tumors in this region of the brain are referred to as "choroid plexus tumors" [11]. Auxiliary cells of the PNS are known as satellite cells or Schwann cells [3]. Although their specific role in the PNS ganglion remains unclear, it is known that satellite cells operate as a protective sheath for the neuronal bodies. In addition to this, it has been shown that PNS cells are essential for the functioning of Schwann cells. Schwann cells are responsible for providing structurally and functionally supportive myelinated PNS neurons. Neurilemma cells offer intrinsic support for PNS fibers, giving them a greater chance of mending and regenerating following brain damage [12]. The implications of disorders that affect the functioning of neurilemma cells or the process of myelinization draw attention to the relevance of Schwann cells. The vestibulocochlear schwannoma, which develops close to the cerebellopontine angle, is one of the Schwann cell tumors that are most well-known to the general public [13].

1.3 The Human Brain: Anatomy

The human nervous system has two primary parts: the central nervous system (CNS) and the peripheral nervous system (PNS). Anatomical and cellular barriers prevent the most common and malignant neurological system cancers from spreading beyond the central nervous system (CNS). They are able to design the most effective nanoparticle treatments that are now accessible, thanks to their prior expertise with the structure of the central nervous system (CNS) as well as with these problems.

1.3.1 Spinal cord

The spinal cord acts as the principal channel for the transmission of afferent and exogenous impulses to and from the brain. These impulses originate from the main body of the spinal card, that is located in the vertebral canals of the spinal column. The cervical, thoracic, lumbar, and sacrum vertebrae are the ones that are responsible for separating the spinal cord into its four portions, which run from the top to the bottom of the body (Figure 1.1) [3]. The medulla is one of the organs that cannot be used because of these limitations. The superior and inferior ends of the spinal column's filum terminal are often the sites of ependymomas [3, 14]. The meninges are made up of three layers of tissue that surround and protect the spinal column. These layers also serve as storage areas for the cerebrospinal fluid (CSF). The outer covering of the spinal cord consists of three distinct layers, such as dura mater, pia mater, and arachnoid. Out of the three, the subarachnoid space is located between the arachnoid and the pia mater, and it is the location where the CSF surrounds the CNS as well as the vascular systems. Meningiomas (meningeal tumors) are common in the brain and spinal cord (CNS) [3, 15]. Vertebral arteries or the medullary branches of the aorta are the principal routes of blood flow to the spinal cord [16].

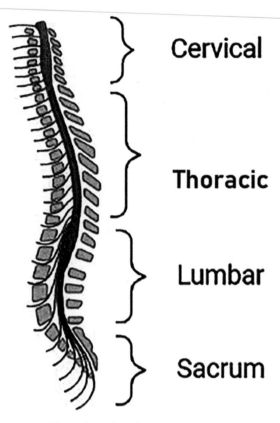

Figure 1.1   Spinal column anatomy.

1.3.2 Brainstem

The myelencephalon, metencephalon, and mesencephalon are the three parts of the brainstem that are arranged in a caudal-to-rostral pattern. The brainstem is responsible for processing, relaying, and integrating data from the sensory, motor, and autonomic nervous systems. In addition to the nucleus of cranial nerves III–XII, it has a variety of sensory or motor channels that proceed in both an ascending and descending direction. The most caudal section of the brainstem is called the medulla, and it is derived from the myelencephalon. The foramen magnum is an opening that connects the medulla to the spinal column. The central part of the spinal column is composed of the posterior medulla oblongata, which is also a part of the floor of the fourth ventricle (IV ventricle), which decreases dorsally. Melanocytic tumors have been identified in this particular region of the brainstem [17]. Blood flows to this region through multiple arteries, including the ventral spinal arteries, the dorsal lower cerebellar arteries, and the vertebral blood vessel branch [16]. The region of the brainstem that may be found extending above and behind the medulla is referred to as the pons. There are various cranial nerve nuclei that may be found in this area, which can be found anteriorly between the medulla oblongata and the mesencephalon. The telencephalon and the tiny brain are connected by the pons-Varolii, which acts as a connecting point. The cerebellum enables the departure of the seventh (facial) and eighth (vestibulocochlear) cranial nerves of the central nervous system (CNS) by means of the cerebellopontine position, which forms between the pons and the cerebellum. Toxic tumors in this area, especially vestibular schwannomas, may induce unique and revealing clinical symptoms such as hearing impairment, ringing in the ears, or unsteady walking as a result of cranial nerve VIII degeneration and mass effect on the cerebellum. Other symptoms include tinnitus (a sensation of a buzzing or humming sound in the ear) and vertigo. The rhomboid fossa, which is composed of the pons and the medulla [3], serves as the foundation for the base of the fourth ventricle. The pontine branches of the basilar artery and the superior cerebellar artery are responsible for the majority of the blood supply to the pons [16]. The pons gives rise to the rostral extension of the midbrain. The midbrain, which is located in the most rostral part of the brainstem, is derived from the mesencephalon. Along the axial axis, the posterior tectum, the dorsal region of the midbrain, and the anterior crus cerebri are all capable of being dissected into three distinct sections: the processing of both sound and vision is handled by the lower and upper colliculi, which are two sets of projections located on either sides of the dorsal tectum [3]. The pontine and ventral tegments combine and extend rostrally to the tectum. The cerebral aqueduct, commonly known as ventricular tube, joins the third and fourth ventricles and extends ventrally between the tectum and tegmentum. This passage connects the tertiary and lateral ventricles. The posterior connecting arteries, such as anterior choroidal, the rear cerebral, and the anterior cerebral, are in rich supply of blood vessels that provide oxygen and nutrients to the midbrain (Figure 1.2) [16].

1.3.3 Diencephalon

The diencephalon is divided into four sections: the thalamus, the hypothalamus, the epithalamus, and the pons [3, 4]. The diencephalon serves as the principal integrative center for the vast majority of sensory, limbic, and motor impulses [3]. It possesses extensive connections to the cortex and subcortical regions of the brain, and it operates in this capacity since it is the region that is responsible for the majority of these connections. The third ventricular foramen of Monroe separates the diencephalon into two equal halves, which are connected to the lateral ventricles through the cerebral aqueduct and

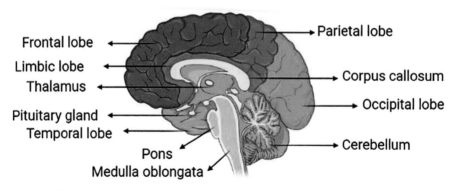

Figure 1.2   A sagittal image of the brainstem and its related components.

interventricular foramen. The arteries in the posterior cerebral region provide the majority of the diencephalon's blood supply [16]. The diencephalon is a part of the brain and plays a crucial role in many physiological processes, such as information processing, homeostasis maintenance, and endocrine system function. The thalamus is a key node in the nervous system because it mediates between the sensory and motor systems and the sensory and cognitive systems. Each thalamic nucleus consists of efferent and afferent neurons that target specific regions of the cerebral cortex, rendering the thalamus the biggest diencephalic component of the brain [17]. The thalamus may also function as a transmitter, passing along messages from the various motor, limbic, sensory, and cerebellar channels to the proper region of the cerebral cortex or it can function as a receiver, taking in these signals and processing them locally. As a consequence of this, the dorsal thalamus of the brain acts as a liaison between the cerebral cortex and the rest of the mind. In contrast to the somatic functions that the thalamus is responsible for, the hypothalamus acts as the body's neural control center for maintaining homeostasis and endocrine regulation. Changes in temperature, hunger, and sleep patterns, along with other biological processes that are precisely regulated, are monitored and responded to by sensory neurons located in the hypothalamus. The hypothalamus also plays a crucial role in regulating the pituitary gland (neurohypophysis) that is found in the pituitary fossa (*Sella turcica*) of the bone [3]. It has been shown that the activities of histiocytic tumors have a considerable effect on hypothalamus function [18]. The ventral thalamus is the succeeding component of the diencephalon and comes next to the subthalamus in a series of diencephalic structures. The ventral thalamus receives information from the motor-controlling cerebral cortex and the dorsal pallidum. After receiving these signals or information, the ventral thalamus then transmits them back to either the pallidus or the substantia nigra. Therefore, the anterior thalamus plays an essential function in the coordination and performance of movement. The diencephalon cannot be complete without the epithalamus, which might be composed of the epiphysis cerebri, the habenular nuclei, or the stria medullaris (SM) thalami. The epiphysis cerebri is a very small organ that has the form of a cone and is extensively vascularized. It may be found just above and directly above the superior colliculi, close to the midline of the third ventricle [3]. Pinacocytes are responsible for the production of melatonin, which controls the circadian rhythm of the body. This starts when the suprachiasmatic nucleus of the hypothalamus is stimulated in a manner that is not directly related to the retina. Melatonin is synthesized from the pineal gland, and these glands play a crucial role in maintaining the biological clock, i.e., the circadian rhythm cycle. If the cancerous cells originate in this region, they have the potential to cause obstructive hydrocephalus [19, 20].

1.3.4 Cerebellum

The cerebellum lies inferior to the tentorium cerebelli in the posterior fossa of the skull. It is placed behind the brain stem. Its origin may be traced back to the metencephalon. This structure is made up of two halves, and each of those halves has two sides that together form a wedge. The upper edge, which links to the cerebellar tentorium, and the lower edge, which preserves the shape of the occipital bone, are the two sides that make up the wedge. Anatomically, the cerebellum may be split into three lobes: the dorsal, the ventral, and the floccule-nodular lobes. A posterolateral groove serves as a barrier between the flocculonodular lobe and the ventral or ventral lobes. The main groove serves as a barrier between the ventral and dorsal lobes. The cerebellum controls motor outputs through its broad efferent connections to the cerebral cortex, thalamus, and spinal cord [20]. This allows the cerebellum to maintain a consistent movement or posture. The presence of certain cancers, such as hemangioblastomas [21], ultimately contributes to the development of the Von Hippel–Lindau syndrome. The superior cerebellar artery is responsible for not only delivering oxygenated blood to the upper portion of the cerebellum, but it also distributes blood flow to the inferior surface of the cerebellum [16].

1.3.5 Hemispheres

The cerebrum is the most significant part of the human brain and is present on the outer part of the brain. In the outermost layer of the brain, there

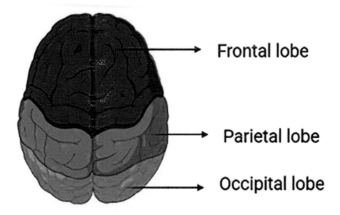

Figure 1.3   Cerebral lobes.

are depressions known as sulci. Rising ridges known as gyri separate these depressions. The brain consists of five lobes: frontal, temporal, parietal, limbic, and occipital. Out of these, only the insular segment is exposed to the outside world; it is separated from the other five lobes by the midline cerebral groove (Figure 1.3). Anatomically, the two lobes may be separated in two different ways: by a substantial cortical sulcus or by an unseen system that links certain anatomic sites. The corpus callosum is the largest bundle of nerve fibers in the brain, and it connects the cortical parts of one hemisphere to their mirror or functionally equivalent regions in the other. There are several arteries supplying blood to the bulk of the cortex; however, each individual area of the cortex has its own unique blood supply. The frontal region of the brain is the most extensive of the six lobes, and it may be located inside the lower part of the cranial cavity. The frontal region from the parietal lobes is separated by the central fisher, whereas the Sylvian fissure acts as a lateral groove in the brain, which separates it from the neocortex. When considering the frontal area, it is vital to keep in mind that it is divided from the limbic lobe by two unique sulci. One of these sulci may be found on the medial or sagittal side of this part of the brain. In the image, the reader can see that the bulbous olfactory system and the olfactory tract are positioned in the olfactory sulcus, which is on the underside of the frontal lobe. In a general sense, the frontal lobe is connected with executive function and the processes involved in higher-level decision-making. The ventral or central cranial arteries, in addition to their extensions, are responsible for supplying the frontal lobe with the majority of the blood flow that is delivered to this region of the brain. The parietal region of the brain is situated in the middle of the occipital and frontal areas, and it is more caudal to the frontal region than it is to the occipital region. A central sulcus separates the frontal and parietal lobes. The parietal and occipital areas are separated from one another by sulci located in the parieto-occipital region as well as by an imaginary line formed between that region and the occipital notch. It is the responsibility of the parietal lobe to receive and process afferents from the body, which are sent through the primary and secondary somatosensory cortices. Some examples of these afferents are pain, temperature, and proprioception. The region of the parietal lobe receives its blood supply from either the ventral, central, or dorsal cerebral vessels, as well as from the extensions of those veins. The occipital lobe's cortex has the least area. An imaginary line between the occipital notch and the end of the parietal–occipital sulcus separates the occipital lobe from the parietal and temporal lobes. These two classifications can be made on the dorsal axis. The posterior cerebral artery acts as the major pathway for the supply of blood to the occipital region [16]. The occipital notch or the distal extremities of the parieto-occipital fissure may be used to identify the caudal limit of the temporal lobe. Both of these landmarks are located at the back of the head. The central fossa of the skull is responsible for forming both the inferior and superior margins of the temporal lobe of the brain [3]. Speech, the processing of auditory information, and the maintenance of long-term memory are controlled and regulated by the temporal lobe. There have been multiple instances of neuronal tumors in this area, and every one of them caused the patients to exhibit signs and symptoms of receptive aphasia [3, 4]. The cerebral artery transports majority of blood to the temporal lobe [16]. It is the only part of the brain that is not visible on the surface. The insular lobe may be hidden deep inside the lateral fissure. Each gyrus of the insular lobe is separated by a central insular sulcus. The only part of the cortex is the operculum, which is not visible on the surface, and may be removed to get access to this area. The main functions of this lobe are to either improve the processing of auditory data or enhance the integration of sensory inputs from the senses of taste and smell. Insula originates from the branches of the middle cerebral artery and these arteries responsible for blood supply, as shown in [16]. The para hippocampal gyrus (PaH), the cingulate gyrus (Cingula), and the uncus are all examples of different parts that make up the limbic system. The limbic cortex is not limited to a single purpose; rather, it participates in a wide range of intricate and lengthy activities, including learning, memory, emotion regulation, and the expression of behavior. Learning and memory are two functions that fall into this category. Blood may be delivered to the limbic lobe through the dorsal or ventral cerebral arteries, in addition to the ventral choroidal artery [16]. Alternatively, the ventral choroidal artery can also be used.

1.3.6 Ventricle system

These systems are the primary route for the transportation of CSF through the central nervous system. The ventral system consists of choroid plexus, and these plexuses consist of seven segments, such as the two lateral ventricles, fourth ventricle, the cerebral aqueduct, and the central canal of the spinal column. The choroid plexus' epithelial cells are the first to produce CSF. The choroid plexus may be seen in all of the ventricles of the brain, with the exception of the occipital and frontal horns. The choroid plexus is located on the roof of the third and fourth ventricles of the central nervous system. Some researchers assumed that CSF is produced on the lateral side of ventricles. The two intraventricular foramina (foramen of Munro) carried CSF from the lateral ventricles to the third ventricle. The cerebral sulcus transports CSF between the third and fourth ventricles. The foramina of Luschka, Magendie, and a middle foraminal orifice carried cerebral spinal fluid (CSF) from the skull's fourth ventricle to the brain and spinal cord. The central canal of the spinal column connects the fourth and final ventricles, concluding the ventricular system. It is possible for a tumor in the fourth ventricle, such as an ependymoma, medulloblastoma, or choroid plexus tumor, to create issues with the flow of CSF, which may then develop to a condition known as obstructive or communicative hydrocephalus. Complications with CSF reabsorption are the most prevalent cause of hydrocephalus, and the most common kind of hydrocephalus is known as non-obstructive or communicative hydrocephalus.

1.4 CNS Hurdles

There are a number of different barriers preventing the central nervous system from coming into direct contact with other physiological systems. These barriers serve as compartments to protect both CNS hurdles such as the brain and the spinal cord. In the process of developing therapies that have the potential to circumvent these challenges, one must first have a solid understanding of what those challenges are.

1.4.1 Blood–brain barrier (BBB)

The blood–brain barrier (BBB) is a membrane that separates the cerebrovascular system (CVS) from the brain parenchyma. The adherens junction and the tight junction are two kinds of specialized junctions that impede a direct fluid passage but allow for selective fluid diffusion. These junctions make up the core of the blood–brain barrier (BBB). Other cell types other than astrocytes and pericytes reside in this region. The involvement of astrocytes in the formation of the blood–brain barrier is highly controversial. Despite this, evidence of communication between endothelial cells and astrocytes has been uncovered [5]. It is thought that calcium-dependent signaling regulates aortic dilation, which might be a potential target for medication delivery. Tight-junction development is also thought to be governed by this transmission. The most common location to find pericytes is at the intersection of different micro-vessels [22]. The engagement of these cells is necessary for angiogenesis as well as the development of micro-vessel cells [22]. As a result of their fenestrated nature, the capillaries that develop near the choroids of the plexus do not possess the firmly connected endothelium that is seen in the BBB. The epithelial cells at the top of the plexus choroids develop the necessary tight junctions to form this barrier. The meningeal arachnoid membrane is also in this group since it separates CSF from blood vessels and modifies its composition [5]. Perchlorate acts as a competitive inhibitor of active transport pathways involved in the efflux of certain solute molecules, such as I2 or thiocyanate, from cells [5]. These delivery methods are essential when selecting how to provide medication to a patient.

1.4.2 Blood–CSF barrier

These barriers regulate the movement of blood between the cerebrospinal fluid (CSF) and the tissue of brain. These barriers play a significant role in maintaining the homeostasis and protection of the brain and spinal cord.

There are two main barriers that regulated the exchange of substance between the cerebrospinal fluid and the brain.

Blood–brain barrier (BBB): Brain blood arteries are lined by specialized endothelial cells that comprise the BBB. Tight connections between endothelial cells block most molecules, especially big and hydrophilic ones, from entering the brain.

Blood–cerebrospinal-fluid barrier: These barriers found in the choroid plexus, which is responsible for the production of CSF. Choroid plexus epithelial cells are responsible for the formation of endothelial cell. The tight junction present between blood and cerebrospinal fluid and these junctions prevent the diffusion of big molecules across it. The BCSFB plays a significant role to maintain the composition of CSF by actively transporting certain substances, such as ions, into the CSF and limiting the entry of other substances.

1.5 Brain Cancer

Tumors that begin in certain regions of the human brain, like the hippocampus, are among the most common types of brain tumors. The hippocampus is one of these areas of the brain. These consist of two sections:

1.   Tumors that have a non-specific or specialized localization of incidence, respectively.

2.   Tumors that are caused by the spread of malignant cells from another part of the human body into the brain and spinal cord are known as metastatic tumors, and they are not the same as primary tumors. In the last, but not least, part of this section, we will examine conventional and alternative therapies for brain tumors.

1.5.1 Incidence-specific tumors

Some of these cancers are linked to specific parts of the CNS.

1.5.1.1 Choroid plexus tumors

These tumors are originated from cells in the choroid plexus, which are important for the formation of cerebrospinal fluid (CSF). Choroid plexus tumors can affect both adults as well as children. The cerebral aqueduct, frontal horn, and occipital horn are the three ventricular structures that do not include the choroid plexus [11]. Choroid plexus papillomas usually remain localized to the ventricles of the brain where the choroid plexus is located. Choroid plexus carcinomas are less common than papillomas and are more aggressive in nature [23].

1.5.1.2 Lesions of the pineal gland

Lesions of pineal gland tumors act as an uncommon kind of neoplasm that grows in the pineal gland, which is a tiny gland found deep inside the brain. Pineal gland tumors may affect both adults and children. Melatonin is a hormone produced by the pineal gland that controls sleep and wake cycles. This gland is located in the brain and plays a significant role in the biological-cycle-maintaining activities.

Tumors that originate in the pineal gland may be classified as either benign (non-cancerous) or malignant (cancerous), depending on their severity. The following categories make up the majority of pineal gland tumors:

1.5.1.2.1 Pineocytoma

Pineocytoma is a benign tumor with a slow growth rate that originates from pinacocytes, which are the normal cells that make up the pineal gland. Pineocytomas are generally low-grade tumors that have a very favorable prognosis. Pineocytomas may occur anywhere in the pineal gland.

1.5.1.2.2 Pineal Parenchymal tumors
Pineal parenchymal tumors are broken down into their two primary kinds, pineocytomas and pine blastomas. Pine blastomas are types of malignant tumors that, in comparison to pineocytomas, have a tendency to grow more quickly and have a less favorable prognosis. Both children and adults are susceptible to developing these tumors.

1.5.1.2.3 Germ cell tumors
Germ cell tumors are found in different parts of the body, such as the pineal gland. Germ cell tumors of the pineal gland are often cancerous and develop from cells that would ordinarily give birth to sperm or eggs. These tumors may affect either the pineal gland or the pineal lobe. They are more prevalent in young people and often need a treatment regimen that includes surgery, radiation therapy, and chemotherapy all in conjunction with one another.

1.5.1.3 Embryonal tumors
This type of tumor is most common in infants and children and is caused by embryonic stem cells that have survived birth and is now used in developing in a mitotic fashion. These cells may be found in the brain tissue. These embryonic cells may also be transported by the CSF to various parts of the brain [24]. Medulloblastomas originate from cells in the cerebellum or are present in the fourth ventricle of the brain (CNS) [24]. The most common place for these malignancies to begin is in the brain, specifically in areas that are not associated with medulloblastoma. Despite the fact that it is more challenging to localize them, the cluster of symptoms that they exhibit may be used in order to obtain a notion of where the tumor is located.

1.5.1.4 Sellar area cancer
The basement of the brain includes the pituitary gland. The location of the third ventricle is dorsal and opposite the optic chiasma [3]. Craniopharyngioma is a separate tumor subtype in this region [25], and it is an extension of the hypophysis into the mind [25]. It is believed that tumors of this kind have their roots in the embryonic development of the pituitary gland since they arise during the process of gland development. However, unlike other types of embryological tumors, it does not metastasize [25].

1.5.2 Non-geographically specified malignant tumors

1.5.2.1 Gliomas
The most initial tumors are gliomas seen in the central nervous system, accounting for more than one-third of all cases. Gliomas (ependymal

cells) come in a variety of types, the most frequent of which are astrocytoma, oligodendrogliomas (oligodendrocytes), and ependymomas. Glial brain tumors, such as astrocytoma, are the most common type, and they are further classified into four different levels such as (1) benign pilocytic astrocytoma (WHO level I), diffuse astrocytoma (WHO level 2), anaplastic astrocytoma (WHO level 3), and glioblastoma multiforme (GBM) (WHO level IV) [26]. The cerebellum, the posterior brainstem, or the optic systems are the most common locations in which to find tumors of this kind [27]. Oligodendroglioma, a kind of cancer that is uncommon but potentially fatal, is the most common type of glioma. This kind of tumor develops slowly over the course of several years before reaching full maturity [28]. They have a tendency to cluster near the pia mater, neurons, and micro-vessels due to the diffusing nature of their invasion [28]. Because of the particular nature of their calcification, they are able to conduct accurate radiological detection [29]. Although tumors may develop everywhere in the body, their precise location is often not understood [26]. These tumors are classified using a grading system that is comparable to the one that is used for astrocytoma. Ependymal cells, which are responsible for the formation of ependymomas [10], are also responsible for the formation of the CSF–brain barrier. Even though they may be discovered everywhere in the ventricular system, the most common places for them to be found are the filum terminale, the central canal, and the fourth ventricle [14].

1.5.2.2 Neural or combined neuroglial cancer

Gangliocytoma is the medical word for a tumour that develops solely from neurons; this type of tumour is also known as a pure neuronal cell tumour [4]. The presence of glial cells in a tumor prevents it from progressing to a malignant state, despite the neoplastic nature of the tumor. It is possible for tumors of this kind to develop anywhere along the cervicothoracic or cerebral spinal column. These areas of the brain are most often located in the temporal lobes of the two hemispheres of the brain, although they may also be found in the anterior and posterior parts of both hemispheres as well as in the cortex of the brain. The seller area, cerebellum, pineal region, and hypothalamus also participate [4]. The development of a cancer in the central nervous system that is simultaneously a glioma and a neuronal tumor is highly unusual. The temporal lobe is a typical location for the development of these cancers. Because neuroglia cells exhibit a wide variety of neural plasticity, this form of tumor is notoriously difficult to distinguish from pure neuronal tumors [4].

1.5.2.3 Cranial or paraspinal nerve cancer

These particular malignancies originate from components of the PNS, namely the peripheral nerve sheath, which serves as the major origination point for these tumors. These tumors are the most common kind of cancer. Some examples of tumors that fall into subgroups include neurofibromas, perineurium's, and malignancies of the nerve sheath. The medical word for nerve sheath tumors is neurinomas. It may be difficult to identify this kind of tumor, and most of the time, it is either misdiagnosed as a different type of tumor or its severity is exaggerated beyond what it really is.

1.5.2.4 Meningiomas

Meningiomas intracranial brain tumor is originated from the membranes that cover the central nervous system. As a result of the histopathological pattern of these carcinomas, the World Health Organization, or WHO, has classified tumors as being of category III severity. There are now 15 histologic sub-types, of which 9 fall into the grade I category, 3 into the grade II category, and 3 into the grade III category [15]. When assessing these cancers, a num-ber of characteristics, including tissue invasion, mitotic activity, cell density, and necrosis, are taken into consideration. It is feasible to pinpoint precisely where a tumor is situated inside the meninges based on the clinical symptoms that are manifested.

1.5.2.5 Mesenchymal–nonmeningothelial cancer

Cancers that originate from mesenchymal stromal cells but are not associ-ated with the "meningeal epithelia" are referred to as mesenchymal, non-meningothelial tumors. The most common categorization for these tumors is sarcomas since they are not connected to the epithelium but rather to the connective tissue and non-epithelial tissues that lie underneath it. Sarcomas are the most common kind of tumor. The types of tumors known as heman-gioblastoma and hemangiopericytoma (SFTs and HPCs, respectively) are two that have received a lot of attention recently. It is believed that SFTs are the kind of mesenchymal tumor that occurs most often inside the body [30]. Clinically, nonmeningeal SFT includes pleural SFT and soft-tissue SFT [30]. The category of pleural SFTs, which is reserved for actual HPCs, includes tumors that have differentiated into myoid or pericytic cell types. Certain HPC-like lesions are seen in soft tissue tumors; however, this is not always the case. As a direct result of this, an incorrect diagnosis is a distinct possi-bility. According to WHO criteria [30], a tumor is considered malignant if it exhibits hypercellularity and mitotic activity. There has been no research done to pinpoint the precise location of the species. Hemangioblastomas are forms of mesenchymal cancer that begin in the blood vessels of the brain and spinal cord. These tumors can multiply very quickly. Von Hippel–Lindau tumors and spinal cord tumors are the most common types of this cancer. It has also been shown that the peripheral nerves, the supratentorial compartment, and the optic nerve are all affected [21].

1.6 Melanocytic Tumors

Inherited mutations in melanocytes lead to melanocytic tumors. Skin, mucous membranes, the urogenital tract, and the leptomeninges are all impacted by these cells. Melanocytes are abundant in the ventrolateral medulla and cervical spinal cord leptomeninges [17]. Primary melanocytic tumors, which range from the most benign, the melanocytotic, to the deadlier and more lethal melanocytoma, as well as melanocytotic (most malignant), are common in today's world [26].

1.6.1 Lymphomas

Non-Hodgkin lymphoma may also manifest as primary CNS lymphoma. It has the potential to harm any part of the brain or spinal cord. This cancer is more likely in immunocompromised people. Immunocompetent people constitute about 90% of widespread big B-cell cases, which are characterized by centroblasts and immunoblasts (antigen-activated lymphocytes ready for clonal development). It is possible that it might cause damage to any portion of the brain or spinal cord [31]. These two types of stem cells have a propensity to congregate close to cerebral blood vessels. Lymphoid cells seen in tumors may originate from the late-germinal center and have a "neurotropism" that has not yet been characterized [31].

1.6.2 Whole-brain or stereotactic radiosurgery

The most common radiation treatments for brain cancer are stereotactic radiosurgery and whole-brain irradiation. Brain metastases are treated by whole brain radiation therapy (WBRT) [32]. However, this medication does come with certain unwanted side effects that might be harmful. Acute toxicity often presents itself many days to several weeks after medication has been discontinued. Some of the adverse reactions include hair loss, rashes, sickness, and vomiting. These unwanted consequences may be treated medically [32]. Early delayed toxicity is defined as harmful effects seen during the first several weeks or months of therapy. Among the many negative consequences are drowsiness, forgetfulness, and fatigue [32]. Toxicity that occurs 90 days or later after treatment has stopped is considered late. Radiation necrosis, leuko-encephalopathy, neurodegeneration, and mental decline are all frequent and permanent adverse consequences [32]. However, whole-brain radiation is recommended for long-term neuro-behavioral improvement since the repercussions of allowing the tumor to spread are now more severe. It has also been demonstrated that a whole-brain radiation may be an effective adjunct to resection surgery [32]. Since SRS focuses and localizes radiation to specific parts of the brain, it is an effective adjuvant to WBRT [33]. To treat small brain lesions with precise and ablative radiation, stereotactic radiosurgery was developed as a less invasive option. With image-guided SRS, both with and without a fixed frame, many metastases may be treated in a single session. Due to its greater patient safety and reduced radiation dose, SRS is quickly replacing WBRT as the treatment of choice for people with malignant tumors [33].

1.6.3 Chemotherapy: hydroxyurea, bevacizumab, or temozolomide

Another strategy for retarding tumor growth is chemotherapy based on toxicity. Brain tumors are often treated with bevacizumab (BEV) and hydroxyurea (HU). It is an oral anticancer medication that has been shown to inhibit the growth of brain tumors [34]. In the treatment of specific cancers, such as skin cancer, brain tumors, lymphoma, and glioblastoma multiforme, TMZ has demonstrated potential when used in conjunction with chemotherapy and radiation therapy [35]. Despite the vast majority of other medications that are delivered orally, TMZ has the potential to penetrate the BBB and attain therapeutic levels throughout the CNS [36]. The apoptosis of tumor cells is induced by the methylation of guanine residues in their DNA. Although it has not been shown to boost overall survival [36], this medication has been shown to effectively limit brain metastases from primary tumors, therefore improving patients' prognoses. Bevacizumab (BEV), an angiogenesis inhibitor, has been demonstrated to significantly reduce tumor angiogenesis [37]. GBMs are among the most fatal primary brain tumors, as shown by their frequent recurrence and new diagnoses. Because GBM cells grow and divide, the tumor needs a steady supply of oxygen to maintain its size and pace of expansion. The process of angiogenesis is often used to meet these needs. Therefore, GBMs produce pro-angiogenic characteristics, such as VEGF [38], and are among the most heavily vascularized tumors. The human monoclonal antibody BEV is effective against all forms of VEGF. BEV blocks VEGF's downstream activities by sterically inhibiting

VEGF Receptor-1 and VEGF Receptor-2. Additional research has demonstrated that BEV is useful in regular therapy for radiation necrosis and reducing edema related to GBMs [38]. The proliferation antagonist hydroxyurea is effective against glioblastomas, medulloblastomas, and meningiomas [39, 40, 41]. It achieves its effect by inhibiting S-phase ribonucleoside diphosphate reductase [39]. This decrease in ribonucleotide-to-deoxyribonucleotide conversion prevents de novo DNA synthesis [39]. As an additive to 5-fluorouracil, it has the potential to block DNA polymerase. Surgical method is not a treatment approach for the patients suffering from recurrent neoplasms [39, 42]. Meningioma progression may be halted by HU [39]. Radiation therapy has been used to treat primary gliomas since the 1970s; therefore, the effectiveness of this medicine still remains relevant.

1.6.4 Alternative treatment for tumor-treating fields

There are often few therapeutic choices available to patients who have been diagnosed with GBM. The most effective form of therapy at the moment is surgical excision followed by radiation and temozolomide combined. Alternating electric fields (TTFields) delivered by electrodes connected to the head were authorized for use by the Food and Drug Administration in 2011 for the treatment of recurrent GBM as well as newly diagnosed GBM [43]. Despite this, this treatment approach has not yet been integrated into the standard of care [44]. TTFields increased the duration of progression-free survival by three months and life expectancy by five months in the EF-14 clinical study [45, 46]. This is the most important result in chemotherapy since the release of temozolomide in 2005 [44]. Multiple anti-mitotic treatments are now available. Disrupting normal tubulin polymerization, as TTFields do, leads to incorrect chromosomal partitioning during mitosis, which in turn lowers tumor cell development [47].

1.7 Conclusion

Patients with CNS cancers have a poor chance of surviving and quality of life, no matter how strongly they are treated with surgery, chemotherapy, or radiation. Patients with localized tumors have a 75% survival rate, whereas those with regional tumors (those that have spread to lymph nodes in close proximity to the primary tumor) have a 21.4% survival rate, patients with metastatic illness have a 33.9% survival rate, and patients with undetected malignancies have a 25% survival rate. Drugs must be successful in overcoming natural CNS barriers like the BBB in order to treat cancer. These barriers include diffusion, vascular access, pressure gradients, vascular access, and hypoxia. Nanoparticle therapy is needed to overcome these obstacles and improve CNS malignancy survival rates. Brain tumors have been shown to alter the particular selective characteristics of the BBB, leading to increased mobility. For instance, NPs may be employed to obtain access to these tumors because of the diseased environment in which they thrive. The BBB allows for the passage of NPs and certain chemotherapeutic drugs, although hydrophobic drugs have trouble doing so. The solubility and transport of these hydrophobic medications across the BBB may be enhanced by using NPs. As a consequence, NPs encase the medicine in a hydrophilic capsule that is not covalently bonded. However, this method has not yet been optimized, which creates serious challenges for NP-dependent drug delivery due to the hydrophobic nature of endothelial cell membranes. Efforts are being made to create NPs with theranostics and multifunctional properties. That is to say, NPs may have a role in both diagnosis and treatment.

References

[1] Howlader N., Noone A., Krapcho M., Miller D.; Bishop K., Kosary C.L., Yu M., Cronin K.A. *SEER Cancer Statistics Review*, **2017**. Retrieved from: https://seer.cancer.gov/csr/1975_2014/

[2] Bondy, M.L., Scheurer, M.E., Malmer, B., Barnholtz-Sloan, J.S., Davis, F.G., Il'yasova, D., Buffler, P.A. (2008). Brain tumor epidemiology: Consensus from the brain tumor epidemiology consortium (BTEC). *Cancer*, **2008**, *113*(7), 1953–1968. Available from https://doi.org/10.1002/cncr.23741.

[3] Bear, F.C.B., & Paradiso, M. Lippincott Williams & Wilkins, Neurons and glia, *Neuroscience- exploring the brain*, **2007**, *3*, 28

[4] Shin, J.H., Lee, H.K., Khang, S.K., Kim, D.W., Jeong, A.K., Ahn, K.J., ... Suh, D.C. Neuronal tumors of the central nervous system: Radiologic findings and pathologic correlation. *Radiographics*, **2002**, *22*(5), 1177–1189. Available from https://doi.org/10.1148/radiographics.22.5.g02se051177.

[5] Engelhardt, B., & Sorokin, L. The blood-brain and the blood-cerebrospinal fluid barriers: Function and dysfunction. *Seminars in Immunopathology*, **2009**, *31*(4), 497-511. Available from https://doi.org/10.1007/s00281-009- 0177-0.

[6] Sofroniew, M.V., & Vinters, H.V. Astrocytes: Biology and pathology. *Acta Neuropathologica*, **2010**, *119*(1), 7–35. Available from https://doi.org/10.1007/s00401-009-0619-8.

[7] Gladson, C.L., Prayson, R.A., & Liu, W.M. The pathobiology of glioma tumors. *Annual Review of Pathology*, **2010**, *5*, 33–50. Available from https://doi.org/10.1146/annurev-pathol-121808-102109

[8] Van den Bent, M.J., Reni, M., Gatta, G., & Vecht, C. Oligodendroglioma. *Critical Reviews in Oncology/ Hematology*, **2008**, *66*(3), 262–272. Available from https://doi.org/10.1016/j.critrevonc.2007.11.007.

[9] Lull, M.E., & Block, M.L. Microglial activation and chronic neurodegeneration. *Neurotherapeutics*, **2010**, *7*(4), 354–365. Available from https://doi.org/10.1016/j.nurt.2010.05.014.

[10] Del Bigio, M.R. Ependymal cells: Biology and pathology. *Acta Neuropathology*, **2010**, *119*(1), 55–73. Available from https://doi.org/10.1007/s00401-009-0624-y.

[11] Jaiswal, S., Vij, M., Mehrotra, A., Kumar, B., Nair, A., Jaiswal, A.K., ... Jain, V.K. Choroid plexus tumors: A clinicopathological and neuroradiological study of 23 cases. *Asian Journal of Neurosurgery*, **2013**, *8*(1), 29–35. Available from https://doi.org/10.4103/1793-5482.110277.

[12] Catala, M., & Kubis, N. Gross anatomy and development of the peripheral nervous system. *Handbook of Clinical Neurology*, **2013**, *115*, 29–41. Available from https://doi.org/10.1016/b978-0-444-52902-2.00003-5

[13] Kurtkaya-Yapicier, O., Scheithauer, B., & Woodruff, J.M. The pathobiologic spectrum of Schwannomas. *Histology & Histopathology*, **2003**, *18*(3), 925–934. Available from https://doi.org/10.14670/hh-18.925.

[14] Yao, Y., Mack, S.C., & Taylor, M.D. Molecular genetics of ependymoma. *Chinese Journal of Cancer*, **2011**, *30*(10), 669–681. Available from https://doi.org/10.5732/cjc.011.10129

[15] Alahmadi, H., & Croul, S.E. Pathology and genetics of meningiomas. *Seminars in Diagnostic Pathology*, **2011**, *28* (4), 314–324.

[16] Purves, D.A.G., & Fitzpatrick, D. (Eds.). Sunderland, MA: Sinauer Associates. Olfactory Perception in Humans, *Neuroscience*, **2001**, *2*, 15–20.

[17] Kusters-Vandevelde, H.V., Kusters, B., van Engen-van Grunsven, A.C., Groenen, P.J., Wesseling, P., & Blokx, W.A. Primary melanocytic tumors of the central nervous system: A review with a focus on molecular aspects. *Brain Pathology*, **2015**, *25*(2), 209–226. Available from https://doi.org/10.1111/bpa.12241.

[18] Grois, N., Prayer, D., Prosch, H., & Lassmann, H. Neuropathology of CNS disease in Langerhans cell histiocytosis. *Brain*, **2005**, *128*(Pt 4), 829–838. Available from https://doi.org/10.1093/brain/awh40

[19] Fang, A.S., & Meyers, S.P. Magnetic resonance imaging of pineal region Tumors. *Insights into Imaging*, **2013**, *4*(3), 369–382. Available from https://doi.org/10.1007/s13244-013-0248-6.

[20] Mandera, M., Bazowski, P., Wencel, T., & Dec, R. Melatonin secretion in patients with pineal region tumors-preliminary report. *Neuro Endocrinology Letters*, **1999**, *20*(3-4), 167–170

[21] Wanebo, J.E., Lonser, R.R., Glenn, G.M., & Oldfield, E.H. The natural history of hemangioblastomas of the central nervous system in patients with von Hippel-Lindau disease. *Journal of Neurosurgery*, **2003**, *98*(1), 82–94. Available from https://doi.org/10.3171/jns.2003.98.1.0082.

[22] Ballabh, P., Braun, A., & Nedergaard, M. The blood-brain barrier: An overview: Structure, regulation, and clinical implications. *Neurobiology of Disease*, **2004**, *16*(1), 1–13. Available from https://doi.org/10.1016/j.nbd.2003.12.016.

[23] Whish, S., Dziegielewska, K.M., Mollgard, K., Noor, N.M., Liddelow, S.A., Habgood, M.D., ... Saunders, N.R. The inner CSF-brain barrier: Developmentally controlled access to the brain via intercellular junctions. *Frontiers in Neuroscience*, **2015**, *9*, 16. Available from https://doi.org/10.3389/fnins.2015.00016.

[24] Board, P.P.T.E. (2017, 01/27/2017). PDQ Childhood Central Nervous System Embryonal Tumor Treatment. Retrieved from https://www.cancer.gov/types/brain/hp/child-cns-embryonal-treatment-pdq.

[25] Jagannathan, J., Kanter, A.S., Sheehan, J.P., Jane, J.A., Jr., & Laws, E.R., Jr. Benign brain tumors: Sellar/ parasellar tumors. *Neurologic Clinics*, **2007**, *25*(4), 1231–1249. Available from https://doi.org/10.1016/j.ncl.2007. 07.003, xi.

[26] Louis, D.N., Perry, A., Reifenberger, G., von Deimling, A., Figarella Branger, D., Cavenee, W.K., ... Ellison, D.W. The 2016 World Health Organization Classification of Tumors of the Central Nervous System: A summary. *Acta Neuropathology*, **2016**, *131*(6), 803–820. Available from https://doi.org/10.1007/s00401-016-1545-1

[27] Sievert, A.J., & Fisher, M.J. Pediatric low-grade gliomas. *Journal of Child Neurology*, **2009**, *24*(11), 1397–1408. Available from https://doi.org/10.1177/0883073809342005.

[28] Wesseling, P., van den Bent, M., & Perry, A. Oligodendroglioma: Pathology, molecular mechanisms, and markers. *Acta Neuropathologica*, **2015**, *129*(6), 809–827. Available from https://doi.org/10.1007/s00401-015-1424-1.

[29] Van den Bent, M.J., Reni, M., Gatta, G., & Vecht, C. Oligodendroglioma. *Critical Reviews in Oncology/ Hematology*, **2008**, *66*(3), 262–272. Available from https://doi.org/10.1016/j.critrevonc.2007.11.007.

[30] Penel, N., Amela, E.Y., Decanter, G., Robin, Y.M., & Marec-Berard, P. Solitary fibrous tumors and so-called hemangiopericytoma. *Sarcoma*, **2012**, 690251. Available from https://doi.org/10.1155/201

[31] Gerstner, E.R., & Batchelor, T.T. Primary central nervous system lymphoma. *Archives of Neurology*, **2010**, *67*(3), 291–297. Available from https://doi.org/10.1001/archneurol.2010.3.

[32] McTyre, E., Scott, J., & Chinnaiyan, P. Whole brain radiotherapy for brain metastasis. *Surgical Neurology International*, **2013**, *4*(4), S236–S244. Available from https://doi.org/10.4103/2152-7806.111301

[33] Soliman, H., Das, S., Larson, D.A., & Sahgal, A. Stereotactic radiosurgery (SRS) in the modern management of patients with brain metastases. *Oncotarget*, **2016**, *7*(11), 12318–12330. Available from https://doi.org/ 10.18632/oncotarget.7131.

[34] Mrugala, M.M., Adair, J., & Kiem, H.P. Temozolomide: Expanding its role in brain cancer. *Drugs Today (Barc)*, **2010**, *46*(11), 833–846. Available from https://doi.org/10.1358/dot.2010.46.11.1549024.

[35] Hart, M.G., Garside, R., Rogers, G., Stein, K., & Grant, R. Temozolomide for high grade glioma. *Cochrane Database System Review*, **2013**, *4*, Cd007415. Available from https://doi.org/10.1002/14651858.CD007415.pub2

[36] Zhu, W., Zhou, L., Qian, J.-Q., Qiu, T.-Z., Shu, Y.-Q., & Liu, P. Temozolomide for treatment of brain metastases: A review of 21 clinical trials. *World Journal of Clinical Oncology*, **2014**, *5*(1), 19–27. Available from https://doi. org/10.5306/wjco.v5.i1.19.

[37] Gil-Gil, M.J., Mesia, C., Rey, M., & Bruna, J. Bevacizumab for the treatment of glioblastoma. Clinical Medicine Insights. *Oncology*, **2013**, *7*, 123–135. Available from https://doi.org/10.4137/CMO.S8503.

[38] Narita, Y. Bevacizumab for glioblastoma. *Therapeutics and Clinical Risk Management*, **2015**, *11*, 1759–1765. Available from https://doi. org/10.2147/TCRM.S58289

[39] Madaan, K., Kaushik, D., & Verma, T. Hydroxyurea: A key player in cancer chemotherapy. *Expert Review of Anticancer Therapy*, **2012**, *12*(1), 19–29. Available from https://doi.org/10.1586/era.11.175.

[40] Schrell, U.M., Rittig, M.G., Anders, M., Koch, U.H., Marschalek, R., Kiesewetter, F., & Fahlbusch, R. Hydroxyurea for treatment of unresectable and recurrent meningiomas. II. Decrease in the size of meningiomas in patients treated with hydroxyurea. *Journal of Neurosurgery*, **1997**, *86*(5), 840–844. Available from https://doi. org/10.3171/ jns.1997.86.5.0840.

[41] Weston, G.J., Martin, A.J., Mufti, G.J., Strong, A.J., & Gleeson, M.J. Hydroxyurea treatment of meningiomas: A pilot study. *Skull Base*, **2006**, *16*(3), 157–160. Available from https://doi.org/10.1055/s-2006-949518.

[42] Vokes, E.E., Panje, W.R., Schilsky, R.L., Mick, R., Awan, A.M., Moran, W.J., ... Weichselbaum, R.R. Hydroxyurea, fluorouracil, and

concomitant radiotherapy in poor-prognosis head and neck cancer: A phase I-II study. *Journal of Clinical Oncology*, **1989**, *7*(6), 761–768. Available from https://doi.org/10.1200/jco.1989.7.6.761.

[43] Mittal, S., Klinger, N.V., Michelhaugh, S.K., Barger, G.R., Pannullo, S.C., & Juhasz, C. Alternating electric tumor treating fields for the treatment of glioblastoma: Rationale, preclinical, and clinical studies. *Journal of Neurosurgery*, **2017**, 1–8. Available from https://doi.org/10.3171/2016.9.jns16452.

[44] Mehta, M., Wen, P., Nishikawa, R., Reardon, D., & Peters, K. Critical review of the addition of tumor treating fields (TTFields) to the existing standard of care for newly diagnosed glioblastoma patients. *Critical Reviews in Oncology/Hematology*, **2017**, *111*, 60–65. Available from https://doi.org/10.1016/j.critrevonc.2017.01.005.

[45] Kesari, S., & Ram, Z. Tumor-treating fields plus chemotherapy versus chemotherapy alone for glioblastoma at first recurrence: A post hoc analysis of the EF-14 trial. *CNS Oncology*, **2017**. Available from https://doi.org/ 10.2217/cns-2016-0049

[46] Stupp, R., Taillibert, S., Kanner, A.A., Kesari, S., Steinberg, D.M., Toms, S.A., ... Ram, Z. Maintenance therapy with tumor-treating fields plus temozolomide vs temozolomide alone for glioblastoma: A randomized clinical trial. *JAMA*, **2015**, *314*(23), 2535–2543. Available from https://doi.org/10.1001/jama.2015.16669

[47] Giladi, M., Schneiderman, R.S., Voloshin, T., Porat, Y., Munster, M., Blat, R., ... Palti, Y. mitotic spindle disruption by alternating electric fields leads to improper chromosome segregation and mitotic catastrophe in cancer cells. *Scientific Reports*, **2015**, *5*, 18046. Available from https://doi.org/10.1038/srep18046.

2

The Role of Angiogenesis in Neuronal Tumors

Abstract

Endothelial cells that line the inside of vessels migrate, expand, and differentiate during angiogenesis, which leads to the growth of new blood vessels. The tightly controlled process of angiogenesis is governed by a variety of proteins referred to as angiogenic activators and inhibitors. Angiogenesis has been linked to hypoxia, infarctions, infections, and cancer inside the brain. Human glioblastoma, a malignant brain tumor, is highly dependent on angiogenesis for life, growth, and aggressiveness. VEGF, BFGF, thrombin growth factor, ANGPT2, and hepatopoietin A are only a few of the many angiogenic factors that are important in glioblastoma angiogenesis. Novel medicines may now be developed with a focus on brain tumors based on crucial angiogenic mediators and signaling networks. This chapter provides a review of angiogenesis, its role in gliomas, and the potential of angiogenesis-targeting treatment.

2.1 Introduction

Blood is the most significant biological fluid in an individual, which transports nutrients and removes waste from the cells of the body. Vascularization serves as an essential channel for the transportation of nutrients and the elimination of waste, ensuring cellular equilibrium. Tumor cells depend on the circulatory system for the delivery of nutrition, lymphocytes, oxygen, and the removal of toxins, just like normal cells do. To satisfy their metabolic demands, tumors need a larger vascular supply as their cell count rises. Angiogenesis is a physiological process that causes the body's existing blood vessels to grow new ones, which happens to help with this [1]. Angiogenesis is necessary for the development of cancers and their spread to new locations, known as metastatic spread, which relies on angiogenesis and lymphangiogenesis [2]. As cancer progresses, angiogenesis becomes increasingly important, and tumors that lack adequate blood supply eventually undergo necrosis or apoptosis [3, 4]. Anticancer therapies that target angiogenesis-related proteins and signaling pathways show tremendous potential as angiogenesis is essential for the growth and dissemination of solid malignancies [5, 6]. In this discussion, the authors will focus on angiogenesis in the neurological system, particularly in gliomas, and investigate the most recent therapies for brain tumors that target angiogenesis.

2.2 The Central Nervous System and Angiogenesis

Understanding the neurological system is essential to comprehending the relationship between angiogenesis and brain tumors. This system cannot function without neurons, the specialist cells that make up the nervous system [7]. The human neurological system consists of two main components: the CNS and the PNS. The CNS comprises the brain and spinal columns, which regulate sensory integration and responses. It is made up of both white and gray matters, with the latter including axons that link various areas of the gray matter. This area is distinguished from gray matter by the myelin coating on its axons, which gives it a white appearance [7]. Approximately 100 billion neurons make up the CNS and PNS of a human being [8]. These excitatory neurons convey and process information. A neuron's chemical and electrical synapses allow it to communicate with other neurons in the nervous system. At synapse junctions, neurotransmitters diffuse across a small space between nerve cells, facilitating the exchange of impulses or signals [9]. The CNS is protected by the skull and spinal column. The spinal cord serves as a conduit for brain signals to go to various internal organs. Basic musculoskeletal reactions are controlled by the spinal cord and its nerves without the need for brain input. On the other hand, the brain orchestrates and regulates a variety of unconscious as well as conscious activities, playing a crucial role in integrating these activities. The brain's capabilities range from fundamental functions such as sensation and thinking to complex tasks like homeostasis control, with each function being confined to certain regions of the brain. The three primary cell types that make up the blood vessels in the typical brain are astrocytes (A), pericytes (P), and endothelial cells (EC). The BBB, which shields the CNS, is made up of these specialized cells. When primary tumors or metastases form inside the brain parenchyma and grow to a diameter of 1–2 mm in the neoplastic stage, the BBB may become physically or functionally impaired [10–14]. Angiogenesis-dependent pathways are required for various processes, including pregnancy, wound healing, ocular neovascularization, and tumor formation [10–15].

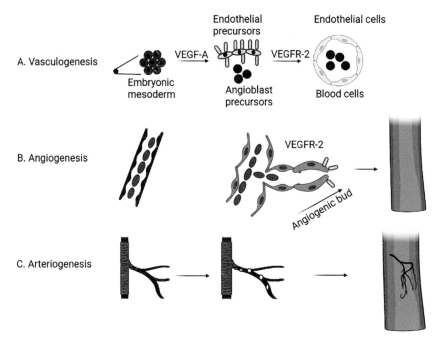

Figure 2.1 The creation of vessels and the interactions between biological mediators.

Proteolytic and mitogenic activities of endothelial cells are crucial components of angiogenesis, regulated by various factors and signaling molecules. The overall mechanism involves four steps. First, local damage is inflicted on the basement membrane tissues. Subsequently, endothelial cells migrate as a result of angiogenic chemical synthesis and release. After that, the endothelial cells multiply. Enzymes that aid in this enzymatic breakdown are released as a result of proteolysis, which breaks down the EC matrix barriers. Finally, angiogenesis is still fueled by angiogenic factors [16–19]. The migration of endothelial cells inside blood arteries depends on the interaction between tumor cell integrins and vascular ECM elements (collagens, lamins, and fibronectin) [20]. The growth of blood arteries in brain tumors and its underlying elements are shown in Figure 2.1.

2.3 Brain Cancer Angiogenesis: Cellular or Molecular Mechanism of Action

Similar to healthy brain tissue, for growth and development, brain cancer needs a constant supply of nutrients and biomolecules. The metabolic requirements of tumor cells are much higher than those of normal cells because they multiply more quickly. As a result, angiogenesis is critical in brain cancers. This section discusses the cellular and molecular biology of angiogenesis in brain tumors.

A variety of proteins, genes, and the complex process of producing new blood vessels is influenced by additional elements and signaling networks. These components can be classified into two groups: angiogenic activators/ factors and inhibitors, which work together to coordinate the process of angiogenesis.

The primary and most important element in facilitating permeability and promoting pro-angiogenesis cascades is VEGF-A, a protein known as vascular endothelial growth factor A. VEGF is increased and directly involved in neurological tumors because the blood–brain barrier is harmed during the growth and spread of the tumor. The VEGF family includes homologous factors such as PGF and seven other factors [21]. Lymphangiogenesis and lymphatic vessel growth is regulated by VEGF-C and VEGF-D effects, which largely target blood vessel creation [22–24]. VEGF-A and other vascular endothelial cell mitogens are necessary for the creation of new blood vessels [25, 26]. It has been demonstrated that many cancers overexpress VEGF-A, which is essential for angiogenesis [27]. The levels of VEGF-A, VEGF-Receptor-1, and VEGF-Receptor-2 in neural tissue decrease from the early to middle stages of embryonic development; nevertheless, they are overexpressed in neural cancer tissue [28, 29]. Additionally, six molecular variants of VEGF-A with different sequences of critical amino acids have been identified as a result of VEGF mRNA alternative splicing [30–32]. In a hypoxic environment, characterized by a lack of blood supply, VEGF-A expression is also increased [13, 33]. Hypoxia and acidosis, commonly found in solid tumors [34], are known to influence the expression of VEGF [13]. Activation of VEGF impairs vascular maturation and function, resulting in blood–brain barrier leakage, weakened BBB integrity, and cerebral edema [35–37].

Extracellular fluid builds up in the brain parenchyma in vasogenic edema, the edema brought on by BBB rupture. Fluid and plasma components build up in the nearby brain areas when the BBB is damaged by tumors or due to other reasons. Limited lymphatic vessels in the brain and restricted drainage area contribute to the development of vasogenic edema in brain cancer. Consequently, VEGF-induced vascular leakage increases interstitial fluid pressure, leading to increased edema and fluid pressure in brain tumors. It is worth noting that pathogens responsible for VEGF is attracted to the development of vasogenic edema, as well as monocytes and macrophages.

Numerous signaling systems are activated during interactions between cancer cells and endothelial cells, resulting in angiogenesis. Through its receptors, the vascular endothelial growth factor (VEGF) communicates with the nucleus of endothelial cells, causing the transcription of genes necessary for the growth of new endothelial cells. When exposed to VEGF, endothelial cells release matrix metalloproteinase (MMP) proteins, which contribute to the interstitial cells' deterioration. Integrins operate as adhesion molecules for endothelial cells, enabling them to migrate and develop into a network of blood vessels [38, 39].

VEGF signaling controls the mobility, solubility, proliferation, and activation of signaling pathways including p38 MAPK, phospholipase C, and PKC, among other characteristics of endothelial cell behavior [40–42]. VEGF receptors (VEGFRs) activate the PI3K/PTEN/Akt/mTOR pathway, which is essential for endothelial cell survival, permeability, and translation [41, 43, 44]. VEGF signalling via its receptor VEGFR2 has been identified to promote angiogenesis, particularly in gliomas [45–47].

Angiopoietins, a class of circulatory growth factors, play a role in embryogenesis and postpartum neovascularization. The main regulators of microvascular permeability have been Angiopoietin 1, Angiopoietin 2, Angiopoietin 3, and Angiopoietin 4 [48]. Angiopoietins 1, 2, and basic fibroblast growth factor (BFGF) support endothelial cell migration and proliferation in conjunction with VEGF, which helps to develop vascular networks. Angiopoietin 2 aids in the breakdown of basal membrane and interstitial tissue when combined with VEGF and enzymes like proteinases [49–51].

Interleukin-8 (IL8), a pro-angiogenic chemokine, has been associated with brain tumor angiogenesis. IL8 has been detected at high levels in the plasma and intracavity fluid of human gliomas, and these concentrations are correlated with the glioblastoma's histological grade. Hypoxia has been shown to increase IL8 production in some studies [52–54]. Glial tumors, both primary and recurrent, exhibit elevated levels of IL8 and hepatocyte growth factor (HGF) [52, 55]. CXCL12 and its corresponding receptors are also known to stimulate brain neoplasms, contributing to angiogenesis [56]. Interleukin-6, NF-kB, AP-1, CCAAT/enhancer-binding protein (C/EBP), and all have active binding sites at the IL8 promoter. Activator protein-1 has been connected to the rise of IL8 brought on by hypoxia. In glioblastomas, the putative cancer inhibitor ING-4 is essential for controlling NF-kB-mediated IL8 production and angiogenesis [57].

Notch signaling has been shown to work in conjunction with VEGF signaling to regulate angiogenesis. For example, Dll4/Notch signaling inhibits the development of tip cells and specialized vascular endothelial cells that control artery sprouting and branching in mouse retinal tissue. Researchers observed that blocking Delta-like ligand 4 (Dll4) increased blood vessel sprouting in a glioma mouse model. In brain tumor angiogenesis, pro-angiogenic/VEGF signaling is adversely regulated by notch signaling. Glioblastoma patients express two notch ligands, Dll4/Notch and JAG1, in their vascular system. Glioblastomas that are positive for DLL-4 and Jag-1 show resistance to the angiogenic inhibitor bevacizumab but are susceptible to it when DLL4 is positive and Jag-1 is negative [58–61].

Secretase-mediated N-cadherin signaling is also implicated in regulating angiogenesis. In astrocytomas and glioblastomas, in addition to impairing the insulin-like growth factor 1 (IGF1) receptor and VEGF receptor 1 (VEGFR-1), the enzyme secretase, which cleaves the Notch protein to promote Notch signaling, also promotes angiogenesis in these tumors. Secretase inhibitors show potential in the fight against brain tumor angiogenesis. VEGF promotes secretase activity in endothelial cells, which results in the cleavage of Notch I. As a result of the inhibition of secretase enzyme activity, VEGF-induced endothelial cell proliferation, migration, and viability are reduced, which lowers angiogenesis.

Transmembrane and cell-matrix signals that improve endothelial cells' adhesion to the extracellular matrix (ECM) have an impact on angiogenesis in the growth of brain tumors. The integrin family of proteins mediates the migration of vascular endothelial cells (EC) during the angiogenesis of brain tumors [62]. This class of cell-matrix receptors, such as integrins v5, v3, and v5, are examples [62].

Neurotrophins are another class of proteins that promote neuronal viability, maturation, and activity. They play a role in synaptic plasticity through their receptors, mediating signaling processes. Four structurally similar proteins, including neurotrophin-3 and neurotrophin-4, make up the neurotrophin family [63]. Both nerve growth factor (NGF) and brain-derived neurotrophic factor (BDNF) are critical for the survival and expansion of endothelial cells [64, 65]. In brain tumors, BDNF promotes the production of pro-angiogenic factors and is regulated by the activation of hypoxia-inducible factors (HIF-1) [66].

The synthesis of VEGF is hypothesized to be influenced by various genetic alterations and tumor-suppressing factors, hormones, cytokines, nitric oxide, and MAPK signaling molecules, such as Ras, Src, and TP53 (p53) [49, 67]. These factors can modulate the expression and production of VEGF, making a contribution to brain tumor angiogenesis.

2.4 BBB, Hypoxia, BBB, or Brain Tumor Vessel

Hypoxia, a condition characterized by oxygen deficiency in tissues, is a well-documented characteristic of solid tumors [68]. Hypoxia is essential for several features of human brain cancer, especially glioblastoma, including tumor formation, enhanced vascular formation, tumor growth, aggressiveness, and response to chemotherapy and radiotherapy [69–71]. During tumor growth, microvessels become irregular, dilated, and leaky, causing functional blood perfusion impairment, which causes hypoxia and ischemia inside the tumor [72]. Vascular collapse causes necrotic areas to occur. This in turn triggers the synthesis of vascular endothelial growth factor A (VEGF-A) and hypoxia-inducible factors (HIFs), which initiate vascular formation [46, 73].

HIFs are membrane proteins that become active in low-oxygen environments surrounding cells [74]. Local hypoxia has been shown to cause VEGF production and neovascularization at necrotic tumor sites [47]. Studies have shown that in cultivated glioblastoma cells, hypoxia promotes the production of VEGF genes or proteins [75]. The heterodimeric protein HIF-1, which consists of alpha and beta subunits, functions in ischemia processes connected to cancer. While the beta subunit is not oxygen-dependent, the alpha subunit is controlled by oxygen levels. Among the three alpha subunit subtypes (HIF1, HIF2, and HIF3), HIF1 has primarily been associated with ischemic processes in cancer [76]. Increased levels of HIF2A-mRNA transcript have been directly associated with mesenchymal stem cell VEGF-mRNA overexpression [77].

The cerebrospinal fluid (CSF), which surrounds the central nervous system (CNS), protects it from physical damage, a colorless fluid that also provides a special chemical environment for nerve tissue. The very selective and semipermeable blood–brain barrier (BBB), a membrane barrier in the brain and spinal cord, separates cerebral interstitial fluids from the bloodstream and maintains the specific chemical environment [78]. The BBB allows for passive diffusion and active transport of various molecules, including gases (oxygen, carbon dioxide, etc.), water (H_2O), hormones, carbohydrates, proteins, and lipid substances. However, the BBB restricts the passage of neurotoxins and other lipophilic molecules [79]. It consists of tightly sealed vascular endothelial cells connected by gap junctions. Astrocytes release angiopoietin, which regulates the distribution of macromolecules from the vascular system to neural parenchyma and prevents the efflux of hydrophobic substances and has a molecular weight of at least 500 kDa. Despite having a protective role, the BBB also poses a challenge to drug delivery to the nervous system [80]. In neural tumors, the BBB undergoes structural and functional changes, leading to increased permeability of tumor vasculature. This faulty construction contributes to vasogenic brain edema, resulting in increased permeability of tumor vasculature and become a major cause of morbidity for people with brain tumors [81, 82].

2.5 Anti-angiogenic Factors

Angiogenesis can be inhibited by various naturally occurring proteins, such as angiostatin, PF4 CXCL4, signaling protein interferons (IFNs), tissue inhibitors of metalloproteinase-1, 2, and 3, endostatin, and prolactin 16-kd fragment [83]. These proteins have shown potential in blocking tumor angiogenesis, making them promising targets for antitumor treatment strategies in early-stage research [2]. Angiotensin has an impact on endothelial and cancer cells. The correct function of vascular endothelial cells and the development of new blood vessels are both inhibited by angiotensin. It has been discovered that angiotensin therapy lowers VEGF or BFGF mRNA expression in cancers [84–86].

Endostatin, another protein found in the basement membrane, also inhibits angiogenesis. It binds to the $\alpha5\beta1/\alpha v\beta3$ integrin, preventing endothelial cells from forming focal adhesions [87, 88]. These integrin subunits are the primary receptors for fibronectin in endothelial cells. In laboratory and animal investigations, endostatin has been found to reduce pro-angiogenic growth factors like VEGF-A or BFGF and to impede cellular proliferation and migration [89, 90]. One putative mode of action for endostatin is the inhibition of VEGF and other pro-angiogenic factors [87].

2.6 Angiogenic: Transition and Homeostasis

Neoplastic vascular angiogenesis involves an angiogenic switch, which occurs when the prevascular proliferative node undergoes a transformation into an advanced tumor [91]. The altering ratio of pro- and anti-angiogenic stimuli is what causes this swing. Prostachyogenic elements, such as VEGF, angiopoietin-2, BFGF, PGF, and interleukins, promote angiogenesis, while anti-angiogenic factors, including endostatin, angiostatin, thrombospondin-1, and EMAP-2, inhibit angiogenesis [92, 93]. When the ratio of pro- to anti-angiogenic factors is out of whack, the angiogenic switch is turned on. The switch opens when this equilibrium shifts. This idea is demonstrated in Figure 2.2. The angiogenic switch may occur at different stages in the growth of a tumor [94–96]. During the angiogenic transition, cells acquire the ability to perform angiogenesis and adapt to their environment, promoting development and expansion of the tumor. Recent research has emphasized the significance of mitochondrial respiration and glycolysis as crucial components in the angiogenic transition in human gliomas [97].

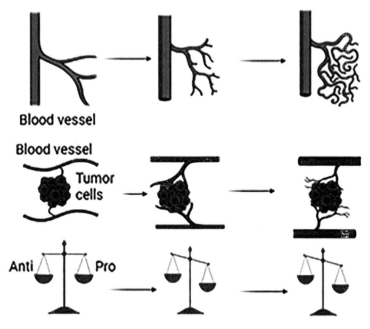

Figure 2.2   The angiogenic inducers and inhibitors are displayed by angiogenic balance.

2.7 Primary Brain Tumors and Glioblastoma Angiogenesis

For their growth, brain tumors need enough oxygen, nutrients, and meta-bolic waste disposal systems. These conditions for the growth of an invasive glioblastoma are crucially met by angiogenesis, the production of new blood vessels [98].

Low-grade gliomas, also known as astrocytomas, are tumors composed of star-shaped astrocytes and constitute the most prevalent kind of malignant tumors in the brain. These tumors often stay inside the central nervous system, growing slowly and with less distinct borders. Angiogenesis is necessary for the transformation of an astrocytoma into a heavily vascularized glioma [99].

In low-grade astrocytomas, pro-angiogenic factors such as VEGF are expressed at lower levels, whereas their expression significantly increases in glioblastomas. High-grade gliomas have more vascularity as compared to low-grade tumors and healthy brain tissues. Glioblastoma cell overexpression of VEGF promotes tumor angiogenesis and paracrinely activates endothe-lial VEGF receptors. VEGFR-1 is expressed by both low-grade and high-grade glioblastomas, while high-grade glioblastomas only express VEGFR-2 mRNA in vascular smooth muscle cells [100]. Microcirculation density and the presence of vascular endothelial growth factor protein have been linked to low-grade astrocytoma prognosis [101].

Benign brain tumors called meningiomas can develop from the meninges. As these tumors grow, they exert pressure on the surrounding brain tissue, compromising cranial nerves and blood vessels. Meningiomas account for 25% of all brain tumors. Despite being regarded as benign or low-grade tumors, they can experience periods of rapid growth. Meningiomas are highly vascularized, often deriving their profuse vascular network from the blood supply in the pia. Meningiomas express more VEGF, and peritumoral edema prevalence and severity are correlated with VEGF levels [102, 103]. The recurrence of benign meningiomas has also been linked to VEGF protein expression levels [104–106]. Capillary or capillary hemangioblastomas, which have a dense capillary network and massive, vacuolated stromal cells, are another kind of extremely vascular CNS tumor [107].

Von Hippel–Lindau disease (VHL syndrome), pancreatic cysts, and polycythemia (increased blood cell count) are all connected to hemangioblastomas. The Von Hippel–Lindau genes are involved in suppressing VEGF production, thereby limiting tumor angiogenesis. VEGF or VEGF receptor expression is constitutively present in sporadic hemangioblastomas linked with VHL [108, 109, 110, 111].

2.8 Angiogenesis in Glioblastoma

A particularly dangerous form of brain cancer is glioma, especially glioblastoma. 40% of all cases and 70% of invasive glioblastomas are glioblastomas, the most prevalent primary brain tumor [112–114]. Significant angiogenesis, or the formation of new blood vessels, is seen in some cancers. Glioblastoma is known for its extensive vascular proliferation and endothelial cell hypertrophy. Unfortunately, glioblastoma is highly vascularized and has a poor prognosis. Five years after diagnosis, 5% of patients are still alive [115].

Glioblastoma multiforme's (GBM) pathophysiology is heavily reliant on microvascular proliferation. Due to their vascular nature, GBM tumors contain mechanisms that promote the growth of many, sturdy blood vessels. Angiogenesis is aided by endothelial proliferation that is regulated by oxidative stress at the tumor site. Hypoxia-inducible factor, which encourages vascular endothelial growth factor (VEGF) transcription, is suspected to have an impact on GBM. Gliomas' metabolic needs are initially satisfied by the CNS microvasculature, but as the tumor enlarges, the available blood vessels become inadequate, which triggers the growth of additional blood vessels. Pro-angiogenic substances such as MMPs 2, VEGF-A, angiopoietin-1,

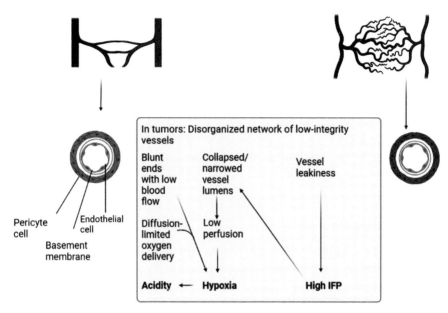

Figure 2.3 Illustration of brain tumor anticancer drugs that target the angiogenic process (bottom panel) and molecular targets utilized to decrease tumor angiogenesis (upper panel).

erythropoietin, and PGK are produced in response to hypoxia [116]. Histological grade, intra-tumoral VEGF levels, VEGF receptor expression, and level of angiogenesis in glioblastoma are related to poor prognosis [55, 117, 118–120]. Glioblastoma blood vessels' endothelial walls, basement membrane, and pericyte covering have been found to be abnormal [14, 121]. The abnormal microvasculature in glioblastoma exhibits mitotically activated endothelial and circumvascular cells forming "glomerular tufts" with multiple cell layers [107]. Angiogenesis in the brain tumor is represented as Figure 2.3.

Furthermore, genetic factors contribute to glioblastoma angiogenesis. Somatic changes in the loss of tumor suppressor P14ARF function in glioblastoma are caused by the tumor suppressor gene INK4A/ARF locus, which affects angiogenesis. The long non-coding RNA H-19 is also expressed in glioblastoma and promotes angiogenesis and metastasis [122, 123].

Research has shown a significant connection between oxygen gradients within glioblastoma and the growth of cancer stem cells called glioblastoma stem cells. These cells contribute to the recurrence of tumors and invasion and can be found in abnormal blood vessels [124, 125].

The HIF-1/VEGF axis is crucial for promoting angiogenesis and is activated by glioma stem cells [126]. Glioma stem cells have gained significant attention in angiogenesis research and are being researched as possible anti-angiogenic therapy targets. Several markers, including CD-133/Promonin-1, Nestin, Musashi-1, MAP 2, Sox-2, Neuron-tubulin, Neurofilament O4 (NFs), Noggin, GFAP, and CD-15, have aided in the characterization and identification of neuroepithelial stem cells, allowing researchers to examine their role in angiogenesis [127].

In human glioblastomas, a poor prognosis is associated with stem cell expression of CD133 [128]. Knowing how stem cells may change into tumor and endothelial cells is crucial in comprehending their involvement in the development of microvasculature [129].

2.9 Conclusion

For their growth and dissemination, new blood vessel growth is the main mechanism through which brain tumors function. The outcome is that focusing on the angiogenic route in brain tumors has tremendous promise as a cancer prevention method. Clinical studies are now testing a variety of biological and pharmaceutical treatments to stop tumor angiogenesis by inhibiting extracellular matrix proteins, transcription factors, angiogenesis-promoting factors, and enzymes. The fundamental objective of these therapies is to reduce vascular endothelial growth factor (VEGF) signaling, and tyrosine kinase inhibitors (TKIs) and monoclonal antibodies are utilized to do this. Drugs like bevacizumab, which have demonstrated the capacity to inhibit tumor development and lengthen survival in glioma patients when paired with other angiogenic therapies, have showed promising outcomes. To develop more effective anticancer therapies, gaining a thorough grasp of the mechanisms behind brain tumor angiogenesis, including elements such as brain stem cells, blood–brain barrier integrity, communication pathways, genomic instability, and epigenetic modulation, is crucial. By advancing our knowledge in these areas, researchers can pave the way for improved treatments targeting tumor angiogenesis in the brain.

References

[1] Folkman, J. What is the evidence that tumors are angiogenesis dependent? *Journal of the National Cancer Institute*, **1990**, *82*(1), 4–6.

[2] Folkman, J. Tumor angiogenesis: Therapeutic implications. *New England Journal of Medicine*, **1971**, *285*(21), 1182–1186. Available from https://doi.org/10.1056/nejm197111182852108

[3] Holmgren, L., O'Reilly, M.S., & Folkman, J. Dormancy of micrometastases: Balanced proliferation and apoptosis in the presence of angiogenesis suppression. *Nature Medicine (New York, NY, United States)*, **1995**, *1*(2), 149–153

[4] Parangi, S., O'Reilly, M., Christofori, G., Holmgren, L., Grosfeld, J., Folkman, J., & Hanahan, D. Antiangiogenic therapy of transgenic mice impairs de novo tumor growth. *Proceedings of the National Academy of Sciences of the United States of America*, **1996**, *93*(5), 2002–2007.

[5] Folkman, J. Angiogenesis in cancer, vascular, rheumatoid and another disease. *Nature Medicine (New York, NY, United States)*, **1995a**, *1*(1), 27–30.

[6] Folkman, J. Seminars in Medicine of the Beth Israel Hospital, Boston. Clinical applications of research on angiogenesis. *New England Journal of Medicine*, **1995b**, *333*(26), 1757–1763. Available from https://doi. org/10.1056/ nejm199512283332608.

[7] Garner, R. The brain and nervous system: A summary and a review. *Journal of Anatomy and Physiology*, **1881**, *15* (Pt 4), 536–579.

[8] Herculano-Houzel, S. The human brain in numbers: A linearly scaled-up primate brain. *Frontiers in Human Neuroscience*, **2009**, *3*, 31. Available from https://doi.org/10.3389/neuro.09.031.2009

[9] Vaughn, J. E. Fine structure of synaptogenesis in the vertebrate central nervous system. *Synapses*, **1989**, *3*(3), 255–285. Available from https://doi.org/10.1002/syn.890030312

[10] Bullitt, E., Zeng, D., Gerig, G., Aylward, S., Joshi, S., Smith, J.K., ... Ewend, M.G. Vessel tortuosity and brain tumor malignancy: A blinded study. *Academic Radiology*, **2005**, *12*(10), 1232–1240. Available from https://doi. org/10.1016/j.acra.2005.05.027.

[11] Deeken, J.F., & Loscher, W. The blood-brain barrier and cancer: Transporters, treatment, and Trojan horses. *Clinical Cancer Research*, **2007**, *13*(6), 1663–1674. Available from https://doi.org/10.1158/1078-0432.ccr-06- 2854.

[12] Fidler, I.J., Yano, S., Zhang, R.D., Fujimaki, T., & Bucana, C.D. The seed and soil hypothesis: Vascularisation and brain metastases. *Lancet Oncology*, **2002**, *3*(1), 53–57

[13] Fukumura, D., Xu, L., Chen, Y., Gohongi, T., Seed, B., & Jain, R.K. Hypoxia and acidosis independently up-regulate vascular endothelial growth factor transcription in brain tumors *in vivo*. *Cancer Research*, **2001**, *61*(16), 6020–6024.

[14] Yuan, F., Salehi, H.A., Boucher, Y., Vasthare, U.S., Tuma, R.F., & Jain, R.K. Vascular permeability and microcirculation of gliomas and

mammary carcinomas transplanted in rat and mouse cranial windows. *Cancer Research*, **1994**, *54*(17), 4564–4568

[15] Diaz-Flores, L., Gutierrez, R., & Varela, H. Angiogenesis: An update. *Histology and Histopathology*, **1994**, *9*(4), 807–843

[16] Auerbach, W., & Auerbach, R. Angiogenesis inhibition: A review. *Pharmacology & Therapeutics*, **1994**, *63*(3), 265–311.

[17] Ausprunk, D.H., & Folkman, J. Migration and proliferation of endothelial cells in preformed and newly formed blood vessels during tumor angiogenesis. *Microvascular Research*, **1977**, *14*(1), 53–65.

[18] Baillie, C.T., Winslet, M.C., & Bradley, N.J. Tumor vasculature a potential therapeutic target. *British Journal of Cancer*, **1995**, *72*(2), 257–267

[19] Senger, D.R. Molecular framework for angiogenesis: A complex web of interactions between extravasated plasma proteins and endothelial cell proteins induced by angiogenic cytokines. *The American Journal of Pathology*, **1996**, *149*(1), 1–7

[20] Friedlander, D.R., Zagzag, D., Shiff, B., Cohen, H., Allen, J.C., Kelly, P.J., & Grumet, M. Migration of brain tumor cells on extracellular matrix proteins *in vitro* correlates with tumor type and grade and involves alpha V and beta1 integrins. *Cancer Research*, **1996**, *56*(8), 1939–1947.

[21] Ferrara, N. Vascular endothelial growth factor: Basic science and clinical progress. *Endocrine Reviews*, **2004**, *25*(4), 581–611. Available from https://doi.org/10.1210/er.2003-0027

[22] Mandriota, S.J., Jussila, L., Jeltsch, M., Compagni, A., Baetens, D., Prevo, R., ... Pepper, M.S. Vascular endothelial growth factor-C-mediated lymphangiogenesis promotes Tumor metastasis. *EMBO Journal*, **2001**, *20*(4), 672–682. Available from https://doi.org/10.1093/emboj/20.4.672.

[23] Neufeld, G., Cohen, T., Gengrinovitch, S., & Poltorak, Z. Vascular endothelial growth factor (VEGF) and its receptors. *FASEB Journal*, **1999**, *13*(1), 9–22

[24] Rafii, S., & Skobe, M. Splitting vessels: Keeping lymph apart from blood. *Nature Medicine (New York, NY, United States)*, **2003**, *9*(2), 166–168.

[25] Conn, G., Bayne, M.L., Soderman, D.D., Kwok, P.W., Sullivan, K.A., Palisi, T.M., ... Thomas, K.A. Amino acid and cDNA sequences of a vascular endothelial cell mitogen that is homologous to platelet-derived growth factor. *Proceedings of the National Academy of Sciences of the United States of America*, **1990**, *87*(7), 2628–2632

[26] Leung, D.W., Cachianes, G., Kuang, W.J., Goeddel, D.V., & Ferrara, N. Vascular endothelial growth factor is a secreted angiogenic mitogen. *Science*, **1989**, *246*(4935), 1306–1309.

[27] Dvorak, H.F. Vascular permeability factor/vascular endothelial growth factor: A critical cytokine in tumor angiogenesis and a potential target for diagnosis and therapy. *Journal of Clinical Oncology*, **2002**, *20*(21), 4368–4380. Available from https://doi.org/10.1200/jco.2002.10.088.

[28] Kargiotis, O., Rao, J.S., & Kyritsis, A.P. Mechanisms of angiogenesis in gliomas. *Journal of Neuro-Oncology*, **2006**, *78*(3), 281–293. Available from https://doi.org/10.1007/s11060-005-9097-6.

[29] Plate, K.H., Breier, G., Weich, H.A., Mennel, H.D., & Risau, W. Vascular endothelial growth factor, and glioma angiogenesis: Coordinate induction of VEGF receptors, distribution of VEGF protein and possible *in vivo* regulatory mechanisms. *International Journal of Cancer*, **1994**, *59*(4), 520–529.

[30] Ferrara, N. Vascular endothelial growth factor. *European Journal of Cancer*, **1996**, *32a* (14), 2413–2422

[31] Ferrara, N., Houck, K., Jakeman, L., & Leung, D. W. Molecular and biological properties of the vascular endothelial growth factor family of proteins. *Endocrine Reviews*, **1992**, *13*(1), 18–32. Available from https://doi.org/ 10.1210/edrv-13-1-18.

[32] Stalmans, I., Ng, Y. S., Rohan, R., Fruttiger, M., Bouche, A., Yuce, A., ... D'Amore, P. A. Arteriolar and venular patterning in retinas of mice selectively expressing VEGF isoforms. *Journal of Clinical Investigation*, **2002**, *109* (3), 327–336. Available from https://doi.org/10.1172/jci14362.

[33] Kaur, B., Khwaja, F. W., Severson, E. A., Matheny, S. L., Brat, D. J., & Van Meir, E. G. Hypoxia and the hypoxia-inducible-factor pathway in glioma growth and angiogenesis. *Neuro-Oncology*, **2005**, *7*(2), 134–153. Available from https://doi.org/10.1215/s1152851704001115.

[34] Helmlinger, G., Yuan, F., Dellian, M., & Jain, R. K. Interstitial pH and pO2 gradients in solid tumors *in vivo*: High-resolution measurements reveal a lack of correlation. *Nature Medicine (New York, NY, United States)*, **1997**, *3*(2), 177–182.

[35] Ferrara, N. The role of VEGF in the regulation of physiological and pathological angiogenesis. *Exs*, **2005**, *94*, 209–231.

[36] Jain, R. K. Molecular regulation of vessel maturation. *Nature Medicine (New York, NY, United States)*, **2003**, *9*(6), 685–693. Available from https://doi.org/10.1038/nm0603-685

[37] Lafuente, J. V., Bulnes, S., Mitre, B., & Riese, H. H. Role of VEGF in an experimental model of cortical micronecrosis. *Amino Acids*, **2002**, *23*(1), 241–245. Available from https://doi.org/10.1007/s00726-001-0135-1.

[38] Mizejewski, G. J. Role of integrins in cancer: Survey of expression patterns. *Proceedings of the Society for Experimental Biology and Medicine*, **1999**, *222*(2), 124–138.

[39] Nelson, A. R., Fingleton, B., Rothenberg, M. L., & Matrisian, L. M. Matrix metalloproteinases: Biologic activity and clinical implications. *Journal of Clinical Oncology*, **2000**, *18*(5), 1135–1149. Available from https://doi. org/10.1200/jco.2000.18.5.1135.

[40] Jones, M. K., Itani, R. M., Wang, H., Tomikawa, M., Sarfeh, I. J., Szabo, S., & Tarnawski, A. S. Activation of VEGF and Ras genes in gastric mucosa during angiogenic response to ethanol injury. *American Journal of Physiology*, **1999**, *276*(6 Pt 1), G1345-G1355.

[41] Lal, B. K., Varma, S., Pappas, P. J., Hobson, R. W., 2nd, & Duran, W. N. VEGF increases permeability of the endothelial cell monolayer by activation of PKB/akt, endothelial nitric-oxide synthase, and MAP kinase pathways. *Microvascular Research*, **2001**, *62*(3), 252–262. Available from https://doi.org/10.1006/mvre.2001.2338.

[42] Takahashi, T., Ueno, H., & Shibuya, M. VEGF activates protein kinase C-dependent, but Ras-independent Raf-MEK-MAP kinase pathway for DNA synthesis in primary endothelial cells. *Oncogene*, **1999**, *18*(13), 2221–2230. Available from https://doi.org/10.1038/sj.onc.1202527

[43] Six, I., Kureishi, Y., Luo, Z., & Walsh, K. Akt signaling mediates VEGF/VPF vascular permeability *in vivo*. *FEBS Letters*, **2002**, *532*(12), 67–69.

[44] Takahashi, M., Matsui, A., Inao, M., Mochida, S., & Fujiwara, K. ERK/MAPK-dependent PI3K/Akt phosphorylation through VEGFR-1 after VEGF stimulation in activated hepatic stellate cells. *Hepatology Research*, **2003**, *26* (3), 232–236.

[45] Fischer, I., Gagner, J. P., Law, M., Newcomb, E. W., & Zagzag, D. Angiogenesis in gliomas: Biology and molecular pathophysiology. *Brain Pathology*, **2005**, *15*(4), 297–310.

[46] Holash, J., Maisonpierre, P. C., Compton, D., Boland, P., Alexander, C. R., Zagzag, D., ... Wiegand, S. J. Vessel cooption, regression, and growth in tumors mediated by angiopoietins and VEGF. *Science*, **1999**, *284*(5422), 1994–1998

[47] Plate, K. H., Breier, G., Weich, H. A., & Risau, W. Vascular endothelial growth factor is a potential Tumor angiogenesis factor in human gliomas *in vivo*. *Nature*, **1992**, *359*(6398), 845–848. Available from https:// doi.org/ 10.1038/359845a0.

[48] Valenzuela, D. M., Griffiths, J. A., Rojas, J., Aldrich, T. H., Jones, P. F., Zhou, H., ... Yancopoulos, G. D. Angiopoietins 3 and 4: Diverging gene counterparts in mice and humans. *Proceedings of the National Academy of Sciences of the United States of America*, **1999**, *96*(5), 1904–1909.

[49] Carmeliet, P., & Jain, R. K. Angiogenesis in cancer and other diseases. *Nature*, **2000**, *407*(6801), 249–257. Available from https://doi. org/10.1038/35025220.

[50] Reiss, Y., Machein, M. R., & Plate, K. H. The role of angiopoietins during angiogenesis in gliomas. *Brain Pathology*, **2005**, *15*(4), 311–317

[51] Yancopoulos, G. D., Davis, S., Gale, N. W., Rudge, J. S., Wiegand, S. J., & Holash, J. Vascular-specific growth factors and blood vessel formation. *Nature*, **2000**, *407*(6801), 242–248. Available from https://doi.org/10.1038/35025215.

[52] Salmaggi, A., Eoli, M., Frigerio, S., Silvani, A., Gelati, M., Corsini, E., ... Boiardi, A. Intracavitary VEGF, BFGF, IL-8, IL-12 levels in primary and recurrent malignant glioma. *Journal of Neuro-Oncology*, **2003**, *62*(3), 297–303

[53] Melder, R. J., Koenig, G. C., Witwer, B. P., Safabakhsh, N., Munn, L. L., & Jain, R. K. During angiogenesis, vascular endothelial growth factor and basic fibroblast growth factor regulate natural killer cell adhesion to tumor endothelium. *Nature Medicine (New York, NY, United States)*, **1996**, *2*(9), 992–997.

[54] Shweiki, D., Itin, A., Soffer, D., & Keshet, E. Vascular endothelial growth factor induced by hypoxia may mediate hypoxia-initiated angiogenesis. *Nature*, **1992**, *359*(6398), 843–845. Available from https://doi.org/10.1038/ 359843a0.

[55] Schmidt, N. O., Westphal, M., Hagel, C., Ergun, S., Stavrou, D., Rosen, E. M., & Lamszus, K. Levels of vascular endothelial growth factor, hepatocyte growth factor/scatter factor and basic fibroblast growth factor in human gliomas and their relation to angiogenesis. *International Journal of Cancer*, **1999**, *84*(1), 10–18.

[56] Li, M., & Ransohoff, R. M. The roles of chemokine CXCL12 in embryonic and brain tumor angiogenesis. *Seminars in Cancer Biolog*, **2009**, *19*(2), 111–115. Available from https://doi.org/10.1016/j.semcancer.2008.11.001.

[57] Garkavtsev, I., Kozin, S. V., Chernova, O., Xu, L., Winkler, F., Brown, E., ... Jain, R. K. The candidate Tumor suppressor protein ING4 regulates brain Tumor growth and angiogenesis. *Nature*, **2004**, *428*(6980), 328–332. Available from https://doi.org/10.1038/ nature02329

[58] Hellstrom, M., Phng, L. K., Hofmann, J. J., Wallgard, E., Coultas, L., Lindblom, P., ... Betsholtz, C. Dll4 signalling through Notch1 regulates formation of tip cells during angiogenesis. *Nature*, **2007**, *445*(7129), 776–780. Available from https://doi.org/10.1038/nature05571.

[59] Ridgway, J., Zhang, G., Wu, Y., Stawicki, S., Liang, W. C., Chanthery, Y., ... Yan, M. Inhibition of Dll4 signalling inhibits Tumor growth by deregulating angiogenesis. *Nature*, **2006**, *444*(7122), 1083–1087. Available from https://doi.org/10.1038/nature05313.

[60] Noguera-Troise, I., Daly, C., Papadopoulos, N. J., Coetzee, S., Boland, P., Gale, N. W., ... Thurston, G. Blockade of Dll4 inhibits Tumor growth by promoting non-productive angiogenesis. *Nature*, **2006**, *444*(7122), 1032–1037. Available from https://doi.org/10.1038/nature05355.

[61] Jubb,A.M.,Browning,L.,Campo,L.,Turley,H.,Steers,G.,Thurston,G.,... Ansorge, O. Expression of vascular Notch ligands Delta-like 4 and Jagged-1 in glioblastoma. *Histopathology*, **2012**, *60*(5), 740–747. Available from https://doi.org/10.1111/j.1365-2559.2011.04138.x.

[62] Hood, J. D., & Cheresh, D. A. Role of integrins in cell invasion and migration. *Nature Reviews Cancer*, **2002**, *2*(2), 91–100. Available from https://doi.org/10.1038/nrc727.

[63] Hallbook, F., Wilson, K., Thorndyke, M., & Olinski, R. P. Formation and evolution of the chordate neurotrophin and Trk receptor genes. *Brain, Behavior and Evolution*, **2006**, *68*(3), 133–144. Available from https://doi.org/ 10.1159/000094083.

[64] Kraemer, R., & Hempstead, B. L. Neurotrophins: Novel mediators of angiogenesis. *Frontiers in Bioscience*, **2003**, *8*, s1181–s1186.

[65] Nico, B., Mangieri, D., Benagiano, V., Crivellato, E., & Ribatti, D. Nerve growth factor as an angiogenic factor. *Microvascular Research*, **2008**, *75*(2), 135–141. Available from https://doi.org/10.1016/j. mvr.2007.07.00

[66] Nakamura, K., Martin, K. C., Jackson, J. K., Beppu, K., Woo, C. W., & Thiele, C. J. Brain-derived neurotrophic factor activation of TrkB induces vascular endothelial growth factor expression via hypoxia-inducible factor-1alpha in neuroblastoma cells. *Cancer Research*, **2006**, *66*(8), 4249–4255. Available from https://doi.org/ 10.1158/0008-5472.can-05-2789.

[67] Fukumura, D., Kashiwagi, S., & Jain, R. K. The role of nitric oxide in Tumor progression. *Nature Reviews Cancer*, **2006**, *6*(7), 521–534. Available from https://doi.org/10.1038/nrc1910.

[68] Brown, J. M. Tumor hypoxia in cancer therapy. *Methods in Enzymology*, **2007**, *435*, 295–321.

[69] Blouw, B., Song, H., Tihan, T., Bosze, J., Ferrara, N., Gerber, H.-P., ... Bergers, G. The hypoxic response of tumors is dependent on their microenvironment. *Cancer Cell*, **2003**, *4*(2), 133–146. Available from https://doi.org/ 10.1016/S1535-6108(03)00194-6.

[70] Méndez, O., Zavadil, J., Esencay, M., Lukyanov, Y., Santovasi, D., Wang, S.-C., ... Zagzag, D. Knock down of HIF-1α in glioma cells reduces migration *in vitro* and invasion *in vivo* and impairs their ability to form tumor spheres. *Molecular Cancer*, **2010**, *9*. Available from https://doi.org/10.1186/1476-4598-9-133, 133-133.

[71] Sullivan, R., & Graham, C. H. Hypoxia-driven selection of the metastatic phenotype. *Cancer and Metastasis Reviews*, **2007**, *26*(2), 319–331. Available from https://doi.org/10.1007/s10555-007-9062-2.

[72] Hashizume, H., Baluk, P., Morikawa, S., McLean, J. W., Thurston, G., Roberge, S., ... McDonald, D. M. Openings between defective endothelial cells explain tumor vessel leakiness. *American Journal of Pathology*, **2000**, *156*(4), 1363–1380. Available from https://doi.org/10.1016/s0002-9440(10)65006-7.

[73] Zagzag, D., Zhong, H., Scalzitti, J. M., Laughner, E., Simons, J. W., & Semenza, G. L. Expression of hypoxia-inducible factor 1alpha in brain tumors: Association with angiogenesis, invasion, and progression. *Cancer*, **2000**, *88*(11), 2606–2618

[74] Smith, T. G., Robbins, P. A., & Ratcliffe, P. J. The human side of hypoxia-inducible factor. *British Journal of Haematology*, **2008**, *141*(3), 325–334. Available from https://doi.org/10.1111/j.1365-2141.2008.07029.x.

[75] Ikeda, E., Achen, M. G., Breier, G., & Risau, W. Hypoxia-induced transcriptional activation and increased mRNA stability of vascular endothelial growth factor in C6 glioma cells. *Journal of Biological Chemistry*, **1995**, *270*(34), 19761–19766.

[76] Wiesener, M. S., Jurgensen, J. S., Rosenberger, C., Scholze, C. K., Horstrup, J. H., Warnecke, C., ... Eckardt, K. U. Widespread hypoxia-inducible expression of HIF-2alpha in distinct cell populations of different organs. *FASEB Journal*, **2003**, *17*(2), 271–273. Available from https://doi.org/10.1096/fj.02-0445fje.

[77] Flamme, I., Krieg, M., & Plate, K. H. Up-regulation of vascular endothelial growth factor in stromal cells of hemangioblastomas is correlated with up-regulation of the transcription factor HRF/HIF-2α. *The American Journal of Pathology*, **1998**, *153*(1), 25–29.

[78] Engelhardt, B., & Sorokin, L. The blood-brain and the blood-cerebrospinal fluid barriers: Function and dysfunction. *Seminars in Immunopathology*, **2009**, *31*(4), 497–511. Available from https://doi.org/10.1007/s00281-009- 0177-0.

[79] Ballabh, P., Braun, A., & Nedergaard, M. The blood-brain barrier: An overview: Structure, regulation, and clinical implications. *Neurobiology of Disease*, **2004**, *16*(1), 1–13. Available from https://doi.org/10.1016/j.nbd.2003.12.016.

[80] Lee, S. W., Kim, W. J., Choi, Y. K., Song, H. S., Son, M. J., Gelman, I. H., ... Kim, K. W. SSeCKS regulates angiogenesis and tight junction formation in blood-brain barrier. *Nature Medicine (New York, NY, United*

States), **2003**, *9*(7), 900–906. Available from https://doi.org/10.1038/nm889.

[81] Jain, R. K., di Tomaso, E., Duda, D. G., Loeffler, J. S., Sorensen, A. G., & Batchelor, T. T. Angiogenesis in brain Tumors. *Nature Reviews Neuroscience*, **2007**, *8*(8), 610–622. Available from https://doi.org/10.1038/nrn2175.

[82] Jain, R. K., Tong, R. T., & Munn, L. L. Effect of vascular normalization by antiangiogenic therapy on interstitial hypertension, peritumor edema, and lymphatic metastasis: Insights from a mathematical model. *Cancer Research*, **2007**, *67*(6), 2729–2735. Available from https://doi.org/10.1158/0008-5472.can-06-4102.

[83] Nishida, N., Yano, H., Nishida, T., Kamura, T., & Kojiro, M. Angiogenesis in Cancer. *Vascular Health and Risk Management*, **2006**, *2*(3), 213–219.

[84] Claesson-Welsh, L., Welsh, M., Ito, N., Anand-Apte, B., Soker, S., Zetter, B., ... Folkman, J. Angiostatin induces endothelial cell apoptosis and activation of focal adhesion kinase independently of the integrin binding motif RGD. *Proceedings of the National Academy of Sciences of the United States of America*, **1998**, *95*(10), 5579–5583.

[85] Lucas, R., Holmgren, L., Garcia, I., Jimenez, B., Mandriota, S. J., Borlat, F., ... Pepper, M. S. Multiple forms of angiostatin induce apoptosis in endothelial cells. *Blood*, **1998**, *92*(12), 4730–4741.

[86] Kirsch, M., Strasser, J., Allende, R., Bello, L., Zhang, J., & Black, P. M. Angiostatin suppresses malignant glioma growth *in vivo*. *Cancer Research*, **1998**, *58*(20), 4654–4659.

[87] Folkman, J. Antiangiogenesis in cancer therapy endostatin and its mechanisms of action. *Experimental Cell Research*, **2006b**, *312*(5), 594–607. Available from https://doi.org/10.1016/j.yexcr.2005.11.015.

[88] Rehn, M., Veikkola, T., Kukk-Valdre, E., Nakamura, H., Ilmonen, M., Lombardo, C., ... Vuori, K. Interaction of endostatin with integrins implicated in angiogenesis. *Proceedings of the National Academy of Sciences of the United States of America*, **2001**, *98*(3), 1024–1029. Available from https://doi.org/10.1073/ pnas.031564998.

[89] O'Reilly, M. S., Boehm, T., Shing, Y., Fukai, N., Vasios, G., Lane, W. S., ... Folkman, J. Endostatin: An endogenous inhibitor of angiogenesis and tumor growth. *Cell*, **1997**, *88*(2), 277–285.

[90] Olsson, A. K., Johansson, I., Akerud, H., Einarsson, B., Christofferson, R., Sasaki, T., ... Claesson-Welsh, L. The minimal active domain of endostatin is a heparin-binding motif that mediates inhibition of tumor vascularization. *Cancer Research*, **2004**, *64*(24), 9012–9017. Available from https://doi.org/10.1158/0008-5472.can-04-2172.

[91] Sirois, M. G., & Edelman, E. R. VEGF effect on vascular permeability is mediated by synthesis of plateletactivating factor. *American Journal of Physiology*, **1997**, *272*(6 Pt 2), H2746–H2756.

[92] Dameron, K. M., Volpert, O. V., Tainsky, M. A., & Bouck, N. Control of angiogenesis in fibroblasts by p53 regulation of thrombospondin-1. *Science*, **1994**, *265*(5178), 1582–1584.

[93] Good, D. J., Polverini, P. J., Rastinejad, F., Le Beau, M. M., Lemons, R. S., Frazier, W. A., & Bouck, N. P. A tumor suppressor-dependent inhibitor of angiogenesis is immunologically and functionally indistinguishable from a fragment of thrombospondin *Proceedings of the National Academy of Sciences of the United States of America*, **1990**, *87*(17), 6624–6628.

[94] Bergers, G., & Benjamin, L. E. Tumorigenesis and the angiogenic switch. *Nature Reviews Cancer*, **2003**, *3*(6), 401–410. Available from https://doi.org/10.1038/nrc1093

[95] Carmeliet, P. Angiogenesis in health and disease. *Nature Medicine (New York, NY, United States)*, **2003**, *9*(6), 653–660. Available from https://doi.org/10.1038/nm0603-653.

[96] Fidler, I. J., & Ellis, L. M. Neoplastic angiogenesisnot all blood vessels are created equal. *New England Journal of Medicine*, **2004**, *351*(3), 215–216. Available from https://doi.org/10.1056/NEJMp048080.

[97] Talasila, K.M., Rosland, G.V., Hagland, H.R., Eskilsson, E., Flones, I.H., Fritah, S., ... Miletic, H. The angiogenic switch leads to a metabolic shift in human glioblastoma. *Neuro-Oncology*, **2017**, *19*(3), 383–393. Available from https://doi.org/10.1093/neuonc/now175.

[98] Folkman, J. Angiogenesis. *Annual Review of Medicine*, **2006a**, *57*, 1–18. Available from https://doi.org/10.1146/ annurev.med.57.121304.131306.

[99] Machein, M. R., & Plate, K. H. VEGF in brain tumors. *Journal of Neuro-Oncology*, **2000**, *50*(12), 109–120.

[100] Hatva, E., Kaipainen, A., Mentula, P., Ja¨a¨skela¨inen, J., Paetau, A., Haltia, M., & Alitalo, K. Expression of endothelial cell-specific receptor tyrosine kinases and growth factors in human brain tumors. *The American Journal of Pathology*, **1995**, *146*(2), 368–378.

[101] Abdulrauf, S. I., Edvardsen, K., Ho, K. L., Yang, X. Y., Rock, J. P., & Rosenblum, M. L. Vascular endothelial growth factor expression and vascular density as prognostic markers of survival in patients with low-grade astrocytoma. *Journal of Neurosurgery*, **1998**, *88*(3), 513–520. Available from https://doi.org/10.3171/ jns.1998.88.3.0513.

[102] Berkman, R. A., Merrill, M. J., Reinhold, W.C., Monacci, W.T., Saxena, A., Clark, W.C., ... Oldfield, E.H. Expression of the vascular

permeability factor/vascular endothelial growth factor gene in central nervous system neoplasms. *Journal of Clinical Investigation*, **1993**, *91*(1), 153–159. Available from https://doi.org/10.1172/ jci116165.

[103] Christov, C., Lechapt-Zalcman, E., Adle-Biassette, H., Nachev, S., & Gherardi, R. K. Vascular permeability factor/vascular endothelial growth factor (VPF/VEGF) and its receptor flt-1 in microcystic meningiomas. *Acta Neuropathologica*, **1999**, *98*(4), 414–420.

[104] Goldman, C.K., Bharara, S., Palmer, C.A., Vitek, J., Tsai, J.C., Weiss, H.L., & Gillespie, G.Y. Brain edema in meningiomas is associated with increased vascular endothelial growth factor expression. *Neurosurgery*, **1997**, *40*(6), 1269–1277.

[105] Yoshioka, H., Hama, S., Taniguchi, E., Sugiyama, K., Arita, K., & Kurisu, K. Peritumoral brain edema associated with meningioma: Influence of vascular endothelial growth factor expression and vascular blood supply. *Cancer*,**1999**, *85*(4), 936–944

[106] Yamasaki, F., Yoshioka, H., Hama, S., Sugiyama, K., Arita, K., & Kurisu, K. Recurrence of meningiomas. *Cancer*, **2000**, *89*(5), 1102–1110.

[107] Kleihues, P., Cavenee, W. K., & International Agency for Research on Cancer. Pathology and genetics of Tumors of the nervous system. *Lyon: IARC Press*, **2000**.

[108] Levy, A.P., Levy, N.S., Iliopoulos, O., Jiang, C., Kaplin, W.G., Jr., & Goldberg, M.A. Regulation of vascular endothelial growth factor by hypoxia and its modulation by the von Hippel-Lindau tumor suppressor gene. *Kidney International*, **1997**, *51*(2), 575–578.

[109] Wang, G.L., Jiang, B.H., Rue, E.A., & Semenza, G.L. Hypoxia-inducible factor 1 is a basic-helix-loophelix-PAS heterodimer regulated by cellular O2 tension. *Proceedings of the National Academy of Sciences of the United States of America*, **1995**, *92*(12), 5510–5514.

[110] Morii, K., Tanaka, R., Washiyama, K., Kumanishi, T., & Kuwano, R. Expression of vascular endothelial growth factor in capillary hemangioblastoma. *Biochemical and Biophysical Research Communications*, **1993**, *194*(2), 749–755. Available from https://doi.org/10.1006/ bbrc.1993.1885.

[111] Wizigmann-Voos, S., Breier, G., Risau, W., & Plate, K.H. Up-regulation of vascular endothelial growth factor and its receptors in von Hippel-Lindau disease-associated and sporadic hemangioblastomas. *Cancer Research*, **1995**, *55*(6), 1358–1364.

[112] Furnari, F.B., Fenton, T., Bachoo, R.M., Mukasa, A., Stommel, J.M., Stegh, A., ... Cavenee, W.K. Malignant astrocytic glioma: Genetics,

biology, and paths to treatment. *Genes & Development*, **2007**, *21*(21), 2683–2710. Available from https://doi.org/10.1101/gad.1596707.

[113] Louis, D.N., Ohgaki, H., Wiestler, O.D., Cavenee, W.K., Burger, P.C., Jouvet, A., ... Kleihues, P. The 2007 WHO classification of Tumors of the central nervous system. *Acta Neuropathologica*, **2007**, *114*(2), 97–109. Available from https://doi.org/10.1007/s00401-007-0243-4.

[114] Meyer, M. A. Malignant gliomas in adults. *New England Journal of Medicine*, **2008**, *359*(17), 18–50. Available from https://doi.org/10.1056/NEJMc086380, author reply1850

[115] Behin, A., Hoang-Xuan, K., Carpentier, A.F., & Delattre, J.Y. Primary brain Tumors in adults. *Lancet*, **2003**, *361* (9354), 323–331. Available from https://doi.org/10.1016/s0140-6736(03)12328-8.

[116] Fong, G. H. Mechanisms of adaptive angiogenesis to tissue hypoxia. *Angiogenesis*, **2008**, *11*(2), 121–140. Available from https://doi.org/10.1007/s10456-008-9107-3.

[117] Samoto, K., Ikezaki, K., Ono, M., Shono, T., Kohno, K., Kuwano, M., & Fukui, M. Expression of vascular endothelial growth factor and its possible relation with neovascularization in human brain tumors. *Cancer Research*, **1995**, *55*(5), 1189–1193.

[118] Ke, L.D., Shi, Y. X., Im, S.A., Chen, X., & Yung, W.K. The relevance of cell proliferation, vascular endothelial growth factor, and basic fibroblast growth factor production to angiogenesis and tumorigenicity in human glioma cell lines. *Clinical Cancer Research*, **2000**, *6*(6), 2562–2572.

[119] Lafuente, J.V., Adan, B., Alkiza, K., Garibi, J.M., Rossi, M., & Cruz-Sanchez, F. F. Expression of vascular endothelial growth factor (VEGF) and platelet-derived growth factor receptor-beta (PDGFR-beta) in human gliomas. *Journal of Molecular Neuroscience*, **1999**, *13*(12), 177–185. Available from https://doi.org/10.1385/jmn:13:1–2:177.

[120] Plate, K. H. Mechanisms of angiogenesis in the brain. *Journal of Neuropathology & Experimental Neurology*, **1999**, *58*(4), 313–320.

[121] Plate, K.H., & Mennel, H. D. Vascular morphology and angiogenesis in glial tumors. *Experimental and Toxicologic Pathology*, **1995**, *47*(23), 89–94. Available from https://doi.org/10.1016/s0940-2993(11)80292-7.

[122] Zerrouqi, A., Pyrzynska, B., Febbraio, M., Brat, D.J., & Van Meir, E.G. P14ARF inhibits human glioblastoma-induced angiogenesis by upregulating the expression of TIMP3. *Journal of Clinical Investigation*, **2012**, *122*(4), 1283–1295. Available from https://doi.org/10.1172/jci38596.

[123] Jiang, X., Yan, Y., Hu, M., Chen, X., Wang, Y., Dai, Y., ... Xia, H. Increased level of H19 long noncoding RNA promotes invasion, angiogenesis, and stemness of glioblastoma cells. *Journal of Neurosurgery*, **2016**, *124*(1), 129–136. Available from https://doi.org/10.3171/2014.12.jns1426

[124] Pistollato, F., Abbadi, S., Rampazzo, E., Persano, L., Della Puppa, A., Frasson, C., ... Basso, G. Intratumoral hypoxic gradient drives stem cells distribution and MGMT expression in glioblastoma. *Stem Cells*, **2010**, *28*(5), 851–862. Available from https://doi.org/10.1002/stem.415.

[125] Gilbertson, R. J., & Rich, J. N. Making a Tumor's bed: Glioblastoma stem cells and the vascular niche. *Nature Reviews Cancer*, **2007**, *7*(10), 733–736. Available from https://doi.org/10.1038/nrc2246

[126] Folkins, C., Shaked, Y., Man, S., Tang, T., Lee, C.R., Zhu, Z., ... Kerbel, R. S. Glioma tumor stem-like cells promote tumor angiogenesis and vasculogenesis via vascular endothelial growth factor and stromalderived factor 1. *Cancer Research*, **2009**, *69*(18), 7243–7251. Available from https://doi.org/10.1158/0008-5472. CAN-09-0167.

[127] Dell'Albani, P. Stem cell markers in gliomas. *Neurochemical Research*, **2008**, *33*(12), 2407–2415. Available from https://doi.org/10.1007/s11064-008-9723-8.

[128] Germano, I., Swiss, V., & Casaccia, P. Primary brain tumors, neural stem cell, and brain tumor cancer cells: Where is the link? *Neuropharmacology*, **2010**, *58*(6), 903–910. Available from https://doi.org/10.1016/j. neuropharm.2009.12.019.

[129] Scully, S., Francescone, R., Faibish, M., Bentley, B., Taylor, S.L., Oh, D., ... Shao, R. Transdifferentiation of glioblastoma stem-like cells into mural cells drives vasculogenic mimicry in glioblastomas. *Journal of Neuroscience*, **2012**, *32*(37), 12950–12960. Available from https://doi.org/10.1523/jneurosci.2017-12.2012.

3

Methods of Transduction and the Physiology of the Blood–Brain Barrier

Abstract

The blood–brain barrier (BBB) complicates the treatment of neurological and cancer conditions, which hinders medications from reaching their intended sites in high enough concentrations. Some differences between BBB capillaries and capillaries in other organs include enhanced mitochondrial concentration, a scarcity of fenestration, and little fluid endocytotic activity. Additionally, the BBB capillaries include tight connections. The ECs, or endothelial cells, are surrounded by Rouget cells or astroglia foot processes, establishing consistent morphological enzymatic hindrance. Understanding the physiological changes of the blood–brain barrier and the process of absorption through this barrier is crucial to overcoming these barriers to innovation and finding effective and safe treatments for the growing population of people suffering from neurological disorders and cancer.

3.1 Introduction

More than 1.5 billion individuals worldwide suffer from neurological conditions including cancer, neurodegenerative diseases, infections, pain, or psychological issues, and if appropriate therapies are not developed, this number is anticipated to rise [1]. The blood–brain barrier (BBB) hinders therapeutic drugs from reaching the nervous system, which extends the time needed for drug development and increases the likelihood of clinical study failure [2, 3].

Paul Ehrlich made the first experimental discovery of the BBB when he saw that peripheral tissues discolored after receiving an intravenous injection of a water-soluble dye, but the central nervous system (CNS) was unaffected [4]. Trypan blue injection into the cerebrospinal fluid (CSF) induced strong brain cell coloring without staining neighboring organs, demonstrating the existence of the BBB [5]. The idea put out by Lina Stern in 1921

51

that cerebral capillaries act as the structural foundation for a physiological barrier to shield the brain from poisons or infectious agents in the blood is still relevant today [6]. The limitation of solute movement between the brain and circulation is further aided by endothelial tight junction complexes [7].

A layer of highly specialized endothelial cells (ECs), a blood–CSF barrier created by the choroid plexus epithelium, and a layer of arachnoid epithelium that separates the blood from the subarachnoid cerebrospinal fluid make up the three layers that constitutes the blood–brain barrier (BBB). The layer of ECs, which divides human blood from the brain interstitial fluid (BIF), makes up the majority of the BBB [8].

In contrast to other tissues, the central nervous system's blood capillaries have a unique design. The abluminal membrane and the luminal membrane of the nervous system capillary endothelium, which are separated by around 0.3 m of endothelial ground plan, make up the two parallel cell membranes that make up the BBB [1, 3]. Small, big polar, or lipid-insoluble molecules cannot pass through the capillary walls to enter the brain because of a continuous lipid bilayer, with the exception of gas exchange. BBB cells differ from peripheral cells by having a larger concentration of mitochondria, a lack of fenestrations [9], a restricted amount of pinocytotic activity [10], and the presence of tight junctions (TJs) [11, 12]. The endothelial cells are surrounded by an architectural and enzymatic barrier made up of pericytes and astrocyte foot processes. In the area between ECs and the brain tissue surrounding penetrating arteries in the central nervous system (CNS), perivascular macrophages carry out immunological tasks. In the neurovascular unit (NVU), interactions and communication occur due to the close proximity of neurons to astrocytes, microglia, pericytes, and blood vessels (Figure 3.1). The neurovascular unit's innermost luminal component is made up of ECs that border the brain's capillaries and have a greater number or volume of mitochondria. A 30–40 nm thick basement membrane made up of laminin, HSPG, fibronectin, other extracellular matrix proteins, and collagen IV surrounds the cerebral blood vessels. A number of transmembrane protein molecules that poke through or block the intercellular pathway form tight junctions called zonula occludens, which increase the BBB's impermeability [13–15]. To successfully block the entry of polar compounds from bodily fluids into the interstitial fluid through paracellular aqueous pathways, claudin and occludin interact intimately with other tight junctional proteins [12]. The carboxyl and amino termini of occludin, as well as two transmembrane domains, are directed toward the cytoplasm, which increases the electrical resistance in tissues with tight junctions [16, 17]. The initial adhesion of adjacent plasma membranes is thought to be facilitated by homophilic contacts

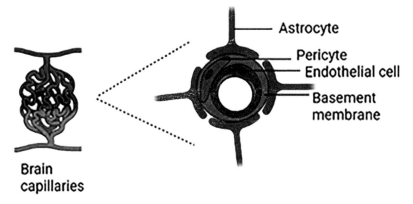

Figure 3.1 Schematic representations of cerebral capillaries or the link between the neurovascular component depict the blood–brain barrier.

between adhesion molecules, such as JAMs or ESAMs, members of the immunoglobulin superfamily [15, 18].

Intracellular proteins bind to first-order extracellular proteins, such as ZO and Ca^{2+}-dependent serine protein kinases (CASK). Cingulin or JACOP serves as the key second-order extender molecule [15, 18]. The cell uses regulatory and signaling proteins such as multi-PDZ-protein 1, ZONAB, PAR 3/6, afadin/AF6, RGS5, and MAGI-13. Different adaptors or regulatory/signaling proteins control how the cytoskeleton and membrane interact [15, 18]. Between tight and adhesive junctions, epithelial and endothelial cells make a clear differentiation. Vascular endothelial cadherin is the most crucial molecule in endothelial cell-to-cell adhesion junctions. PECAM also plays a role in homophilic adhesion. Catenins, including desmoplakin and p120 catenin (p120ctn), are the primary linker molecules that connect adherent junctions to the cytoskeleton [12]. The endothelium exhibits a higher trans-epithelial direct current inductance of 1500–2000 Ωcm^2 [19].

The basement membrane, which surrounds the cerebral blood vessels and is in close proximity to the end foot cell membranes of neuroglia, encompasses Rouget cells (granular or filamentous) and ECs [15]. The pericytes to EC ratio is 1:3 [20]. At some stage during the development of the BBB, Rouget cells appear to be essential in regulating tissue survival or managing cerebral blood flow through the adventitial cell body's actin fibers [21, 22].

In order to keep the BBB working properly and the concentration of transmitters outside of cells, water, metabolic products, astroglia, water, and ions are essential. Astrocyte-neuron cell interactions influence synaptic propagation, plasticity, chemical transmitter clearance, and blood circulation [23].

Due to their high cholesterol content, noncerebral capillaries cannot passively diffuse through the plasma bilayer, leading to denser packing of membrane components [24]. In other words, the BBB limits ions' passage in both directions by free diffusion and stops them from entering the brain from the blood, confining the movement of ions to transcellular transport only.

3.2 BBB's Advancement

Throughout fetal development, neural cells establish communication with the embryonic endothelium to form the BBB, which reaches full development by birth [25–27]. A CNS-specific vascular system and the specialization of the BBB in the vascular endothelium are induced by neuroepithelial signaling via the Wnt/-catenin pathway [22, 28, 29]. In humans and a 14-week-old fetus, claudin-5 may be seen near the cell margins, indicating an early BBB feature [30]. Evidence of a trypan-blue barrier during the 12th week of pregnancy has been found from postmortem studies of perinatal deaths and stillborn children [31]. Astrocytes are essential for preserving the BBB's tightness [32].

Circumventricular organs (CVOs) are parts of the CNS that lack the BBB and have open capillaries that let solutes to readily move between bodily fluids and peripheral tissues. CVOs include the neurohypophysis, choroid plexus, pineal glands, median eminence, OVLT, subcommissural organ, postrema region, and subfornical organ. However, the tight blood vessels of the BBB have a contact area of roughly 1:5000 compared to the porous and fenestrated blood vessels in CVOs, rendering these areas useless for changing the extracellular fluid of the brain's bulk composition and impracticable for drug administration [33].

The cells that make up the avascular arachnoid membrane, which covers the whole central nervous system (CNS), have tight connections [34].

3.3 The BBB's Physiology

Obstacles like the BBB, transport, metabolism, and immune response are supported by the plica choroidea epithelium, and arachnoid matter epithelium, respectively. These barriers are permeable to gases that are inhalable anesthetics, including helium, xenon, nitrogen, and other gases [35]. With a distance of approximately 650 kilometers or an area of 12 square meters, the BBB effectively protects the brain from polar chemicals [36]. Lipid-soluble compounds can diffuse through the BBB, but polar metabolites like glucose and amino acids require ECs to express significant levels of transport proteins to cross [37].

The BBB poses both a physical and enzymatic challenge, making drug delivery increasingly difficult. Biologically active compounds must contend with metabolic enzymes such as alkaline phosphatase, -glutamyl transpeptidase, dipeptidyl(amino)-peptidase IV, aromatic acid decarboxylase, or aminopeptidase A and N, which are oriented toward metabolizing nervous system stimulants or other entities associated with the barrier but unable to cross it [12].

On their luminal membrane, the ECs of the BBB also include efflux transporters [38]. P-glycoprotein (ABCB1) and breast cancer resistance protein (ABCG2) are two ABC transporters that are essential for the efflux of medicines from the nervous system, whereas ABCC1 is critical for the efflux of medications from CSF to the circulation [39–41]. The P-glycoprotein efflux pump at the BBB is upregulated during disease states like epilepsy, strengthening the barrier. Alterations in the BBB, particularly in the way ABC transporters function, have also been linked to the etiology of neurological disorders like presenile dementia and primary Parkinsonism [42–46].

The BBB is impenetrable, although there are a number of highly controlled routes that pass across it (Figure 3.1). The movement of polar substances paracellularly is significantly constrained by the existence of tight junctions. However, leukocytes and ions are able to cross the BBB via altering or evading the tight junctions. Integrins such as VLA-4 tether and roll leukocytes, while adhesive substances like VCAM-1, PECAM-1, and ICAM-1 assist certain subsets of leukocytes in adhering to or migrating through the cytokine-stimulated brain endothelium [47, 48]. Because of their lipid solubility, lipophilic or amphiphilic solutes may readily pass across the large surface area of the lipid cell membrane. Through passive or secondarily active carrier-mediated influx, critical polar molecules such as monocarboxylates, amino acids, and short peptides, as well as other polar chemicals, are delivered into the nervous system. Proteins and peptides can penetrate the intracranial endothelium through a process known as receptor-mediated transcytosis (RMT). When positively charged biomolecules, such as cationized albumin, are taken up by the BBB, a process known as adsorption-mediated transcytosis (AMT) takes place. These four channels are essential for drug distribution via the cerebral endothelium, with passive transport accounting for the majority of CNS-active drug entry into the brain.

3.3.1 Transcellular diffusion

Barbiturates and benzodiazepines are examples of lipophilic compounds that may passively travel through the endothelial cell membrane and readily breach the blood–brain barrier. Its lipid solubility determines how quickly an ionized or neutral solute enters the central nervous system [49, 50]. If lipophilic chemicals are not substrates for ABC efflux transporters, they will build up in the brain [38]. Another important chemical characteristic for passive transport across the BBB is the polar surface area (PSA). PSAs below 60–70 A are typical for drugs that can penetrate the BBB via passive transport, according to the linear correlation found in the PSA data of 45 different medicines [51]. Ligands with low rotational freedom (preferably eight ligands) and low hydrogen-bonding capacity (six hydrogen bonds) are advantageous for BBB penetration [52]. The capacity to traverse the BBB is correlated with the molecule shape (spherical or rod-shaped) [53]. The higher net free energy required for transitioning from water to the plasma membrane bilayer impedes the transcellular transport of blood into brain endothelial cells from the bloodstream [49]. Zwitterions and neutral chemicals often have lower CNS permeability than basic substances, which are followed by basic compounds and then zwitterions [54]. In this situation, the ionization state is crucial. Since biological bases are positively charged at neutral pH, they can interact with the phospholipid head groups of the plasma membrane or the pericellular matrix, which are negatively charged, to make it easier for them to enter the cell membrane. The pKa range of 4–10 is therefore thought to be crucial for BBB penetration [55]. A study found that substances with tertiary amines and pH 7–8 are likely to promote BBB permeability [56]. Strong acids and bases, such as carboxylic acids, have difficulty in crossing the BBB [53].

Additionally, a therapeutic medication can only be transported through the BBB in its unbound form. Consequently, the BBB's ability to transport plasma proteins, especially albumin, is compromised. Lipophilicity and molecular weight contribute to the binding of plasma proteins. Molecular weights between 500 and 700 Da indicate that the majority of medicines with large molecular weights are very protein-bound (98.2%) [54]. The ionization state can affect the levels of unbound drugs since acids, neutral substances, zwitterions, and bases have varying degrees of attachment to plasma proteins. Increased lipophilicity, however, can increase the binding of zwitterions and basic substances to proteins, which can hinder their overall transport [54]. The brain-free unbound fraction is the only portion of the drug that can elicit a pharmacological response, but it has received less attention compared to systemic protein binding. To ensure effective delivery to the CNS, both the extent of cerebral penetration and the degree of binding to neural tissue need to be considered. The metabolic stability of the therapeutic agent is crucial since a higher metabolic activity can quickly eliminate the drug from the bloodstream without allowing sufficient time for BBB permeation. Certain drug types, such as proteins and peptides, may not maintain 80% of the dosage after 1 hour, as seen with extensively distributed drugs [54].

3.3.1.1 ATP-binding cassette transporters and efflux transporters

When a drug becomes lipidized or acquires molecular weight, the probability that it will act as a substrate for P-glycoprotein rises [39]. P-glycoprotein is thought to play a part in preventing the buildup of lipophilic medications including paclitaxel, loperamide, vinblastine, and cyclosporine since it is extensively expressed in the luminal layer of brain micro-vessel endothelial cells [12, 57, 58]. ABC efflux transporters have been circumvented through co-administration of an efflux carrier blocker and the creation of drug analogues that are not substrates for efflux carriers. For instance, co-administration of valspodar with paclitaxel has been demonstrated to boost the anticancer drug's brain penetration and decrease tumor volume in mice [59].

3.3.2 Ion transportation

In order to maintain the ideal conditions for synaptic and neuronal function, the blood–brain barrier (BBB) needs to be controlled in terms of ion content and water flow. Cerebrospinal fluid (CSF) and brain interstitial fluid potassium levels are comparable to plasma levels, around 2.5–2.9 mM, although they can fluctuate due to factors such as activity, diet, and pathological conditions like epilepsy [60–62]. Normally, divalent ions like calcium ($Ca2+$) and magnesium ($Mg2+$) do not pass through the BBB. When neurons are active, the BBB is essential for buffering electrolytes, and it tightly controls the pH of the brain. These processes are interconnected with the regulation of extracellular potassium and neurotransmitter levels. Neuronal glucose metabolism during activity also generates water, which needs to be appropriately managed [63–65].

Ion and water homeostasis in the brain are significantly maintained by astrocytes. They can recycle neurotransmitters directly or through their interactions with neurons, distribute potassium ions, and remove excess water from the brain. The BBB and the astrocytes' perivascular endfeet are in close proximity to one other and have a specific function in the homeostatic processes that regulate the extracellular environment during ongoing neural activity [66]. Through gap junctions, astrocytic endfeet and their neighboring cells receive accumulated potassium ions from neural activity, utilizing the electrochemical gradient within the astrocyte. By depositing potassium ions in the perivascular region, astrocytic endfeet with high levels of inward recti-fying potassium channels (Kir4.1) are well-suited for spatial buffering, help-ing to maintain ion balance [66, 67]. Similarly, the increased expression of aquaporin-4 (AQP-4) water channels in astrocytic endfeet surrounding blood vessels allows for the redistribution of water, aiding in the regulation of brain fluid volume.

Cerebrospinal fluid (CSF) plays a role in removing metabolic waste from the extracellular space of the brain. Similar to how excitatory amino acid transporters (EAAT-1 or EAAT-2) are used by astrocytes to move glutamate out of the body, CSF is absorbed by astrocytes via a sodium-dependent mech-anism. This process is followed by the overall absorption of ions and fluid, which are equally cleared at the BBB and the Virchow–Robin space [66].

3.3.3 Carrier-mediated transportation

Targeting one of the several carrier systems that the blood–brain barrier (BBB) has will make it easier to transport drugs or drug-loaded nanoparticles (NPs) to the brain. Polar substances that cannot directly cross the plasma membrane, such as glucose, nucleosides, or amino acids, must instead enter the central nervous system (CNS) via carrier-mediated transport. Strategies to improve the delivery of medicinal drugs can be devised by using the BBB carrier systems that already exist.

Levodopa, a prescription used to treat Parkinson's disease, is an exam-ple of a drug that uses carrier-mediated transport to cross the BBB. The large neutral amino acid transporter crosses the BBB carrying levodopa, the precur-sor to dopamine. Levodopa contains the necessary functional groups (−COO and −NH2) for recognition and transport by this carrier system [68]. Similar approaches can be employed by chemically modifying pharmacologically active compounds to make them suitable substrates for endogenous carrier systems. For instance, biphalin, a dimeric encephalin analog, transports BBB via the neutral amino acid carrier [69]. The transport recognizes the −COOH or −NH2 group as a covalent link to a similar carbon, allowing the compound to be transported.

A glucose transporter protein known as GLUT1 is expressed by astro-cytes, the choroid plexus, and the endothelial cells of brain micro-vessels. It is essential for the movement of glucose into the brain. GLUT1 is highly selective in its substrate requirements and can transport substances that closely mimic D-glucose [70]. While hyperglycemia does not seem to affect GLUT1 concentrations, hypoglycemia does. Various glucose transporters, such as GLUT-4, are also present at the BBB [71–73].

Glycopeptides and opioid peptides offer long-lasting analgesia and are more stable and bioavailable than other opioid peptides. The chemical glycosylation of opioids or proteins can enhance analgesic effects by increasing BBB transport and slowing down clearance rates [74, 75]. The transport of glycopeptides across the BBB is not solely attributed to passive diffusion, but it also involves stimulation of negative membrane curvature, leading to increased endocytosis and transport [76, 77].

Transporters associated with glutathione (GSH), such as the glutathione transporter-1, have been utilized for the delivery of particles with GSH functionalities. For example, pegylated liposomes containing GSH tags and doxorubicin showed increased brain–blood ratio compared to non-GSH-tagged liposomes [78]. Similarly, pegylated liposomes functionalized with GSH has been utilized to carry antiviral drugs to the brain, and paclitaxel nanoparticles coated with GSH have been studied for the treatment of brain tumors.

Hexose and big neutral amino acid carriers are among the prominent choices for delivering substrates to the brain due to their carrying capacity. However, successful strategies for BBB transport require a comprehensive understanding of both the drug and the transporter involved [12].

3.3.4 Receptor-mediated transcytosis

The composition of cerebrospinal fluid (CSF) differs from that of plasma, particularly in terms of protein content. Due to their hydrophilic nature, size, or chemical-bonding ability, most plasma proteins cannot reach the brain [79]. However, peptides, proteins, macromolecules, and particulates, such as drug conjugates, antibodies, fusion proteins, or bifunctional nanoparticles, may transcytose (RMT) via receptors and enter the brain.

RMT entails the alteration of cell surface receptors for cellular membranes by ligands, leading to membrane invagination that may or may not be covered by clathrin. Endocytotic vesicles are formed and may fuse with endosomes, which are pre-lysosomal compartments with an acidic pH. This fusion releases the receptor from the ligand, allowing it to return to the cell surface. Various receptor proteins can be utilized for transportation. For example, the transferrin receptor, widely distributed on the cell surface, moves to vesicles after binding to its ligand. Coated pits can also be observed on the membrane surface, even without a ligand coupling, allowing for the transport of substances through LDL receptors [80]. Another receptor, LRP1, enables bidirectional transport, either exocytosing substances to cross the BBB or fusing with lysosomes for degradation [81]. An example of lysosomal degradation is the transport of iron from intracellular ferritin to transferrin [82]. Endosomes carrying intact receptor–ligand complexes may be transported to the innermost small sac of the Golgi complex, where they can be degraded by enzymes and released in vesicles that ultimately undergo lysosomal degradation [83].

The BBB's rejection of the lysosomal route may be a unique characteristic in comparison to several other cells and tissues, potentially to maintain homeostasis and cytogenesis of various biomolecules. Several macromolecules, including insulin, transferrin, cytokines, and leptin, have been demonstrated to cross the BBB *in vivo* using RMT. Important chemicals can be sent to the brain through this procedure.

3.3.4.1 Utilizing transcytosis-mediated by receptors

The utilization of NPs or biomacromolecule-NP conjugation has recently advanced, making it one of the most efficient ways to deliver treatments to the central nervous system (CNS). The effectiveness of this strategy has been established by innovative pre-clinical investigations, such as the positive phase 2 trial of ANG-1005, a peptide-ligand for LRP1 (Angiopep2) combined with paclitaxel, which showed promising results in patients with breast tumors and LRP1 deficiency.

The goal of earlier research was to deliver medications to the brain by using receptors that carry large endogenous substances like transferrin and human insulin. Current research suggests that a signaling receptor like NAC could be utilized for drug transport to brain cells. For an approach to be effective, it should have a strong affinity for the receptors and be able to release its payload in the neural parenchyma.

To avoid conflicts between the delivery vectors and endogenous ligands for binding site occupancy within the blood–brain barrier (BBB), it is important to maintain low levels of endogenous ligands. Despite extensive research on transferrin, no clinical products have been developed from this study. The receptor affinity of the vector conjugate can be influenced by the linker or spacer utilized, and plasma concentrations of transferrin are substantially greater than Kd values. Adequate brain uptake of the vector conjugate is crucial to provide a therapeutic dosage; around 2% of the prescribed dosage per gram of brain serves as a good goal for drug delivery in mice. It is significant to highlight that insulin and other vectors having pharmacological effects might not be ideal for the best outcomes. To guarantee targeted delivery to certain brain regions while minimizing side effects in other body parts, it is ideal for receptors to be expressed in the endothelium of blood vessels in the brain. Brain receptor exclusivity is uncommon, though [84].

3.3.4.1.1 *Transferrin and insulin receptors*

Molecular Trojan horses are created by coupling medicinal chemicals to specific transferrin or insulin ligand antibodies and their corresponding endogenous receptors [85–87]. The absorption of iron coupled to transferrin is mediated by the transferrin receptor (TfR). However, because it is present throughout the body, brain-targeting TfR lacks selectivity and specificity, including the liver, spleen, and lungs. When used as a brain delivery route, the Tf conjugate faces competition from high concentrations of endogenous transferrin [88].

To achieve gene expression specifically in the brain, the use of TfR-targeted receptors and CNS-specific gene regulators is required. In research utilizing immunoliposomes containing glial-derived neurotrophic factor and an anti-TfR monoclonal antibody (OX26) shown beneficial effect in Parkinson's disease. In rats, full recovery from Parkinson's disease brought on by neurotoxicity was seen [89]. In contrast to the post-capillary compartment, brain endothelial cells were shown to have a higher concentration of OX26 antibody coupling, indicating that the strong binding affinity of these antibodies for TfR may make dissociation from the receptor challenging in the post-capillary compartment [90]. Therefore, low-affinity antibodies should be considered for effective dissociation. Advances in anti-TfR antibody design have led to the development of single-chain therapeutic antibodies coupled with TfR-specific monoclonal antibodies, resulting in higher brain concentrations (3.5% of the administered dosage/gram of brain) for the treatment of senile dementia [91, 92]. Using bi-specific low-affinity anti-TfR antibodies coupled with an anti-BACE-1 antibody, which has low affinity for TfR, showed promising results in slowing down the progression of dementia and a ten-fold increase in levels [93]. This method allows the delivery of therapeutic antibodies with high specificity to patients with various CNS diseases.

In addition to the TfR, human insulin receptor (HIR) and other BBB receptor-specific antibodies have been used singly or in combination. Intravenous administration of chimeric HIRmAbs coupled with a tumor necrotic attribute decoy receptor resulted in a 30% increase in cerebral levels in Rhesus monkeys, equivalent to 3% of the administered dosage (also 4.5% in the liver) [94]. Liposomal drugs delivered by HIRmAbs have also shown success in crossing the BBB. Using HIRmAbs coupled to pegylated-liposomes through a 2000 Da PEG linker, siRNA directed against tyrosine hydroxylase was transported across the blood–brain barrier in a mouse animal model of Parkinson's disease [95]. More advanced delivery methods using HIRmAbs can be developed, such as unique tri-functional fusion antibodies consisting of a HIRmAb for brain entry, a neuritic beta for disrupting neuritic plaques, or newborn Fc-receptors for brain-to-blood efflux [96].

3.3.4.1.2 LDL-receptor or related proteins 1 and 2

Lipoprotein particles containing apolipoprotein E and B100 (ApoB100) bind to the LDL receptor and undergo internalization through endocytosis [97]. The lipoprotein receptor-related protein (LRP), which interacts with a variety of receptors including APOE, TPA, APP, and lactoferrin, among others, mediates this process. LRP is expressed in a variety of organs, including the brain and tumors [98]. Overexpression of LRP has been observed in malignant astrocytomas, glioblastomas, as well as in the cerebellum, neurons, and astrocytes [99].

The transport of melanotransferrin across the blood–brain barrier has been linked to the LRP1 receptor [100]. LRP1 offers greater capacity for BBB delivery compared to TfR, making it a potential target. In an animal model of intracranial tumors, doxorubicin conjugates were transported to melanotransferrin via LRP1, leading to improved survival rates. Lactoferrin, naturally present in low quantities in the body, can be utilized as a vector for targeting LRP1. By attaching lactoferrin to polyamidoamine dendrimers using a PEG spacer, neuroprotective benefits were achieved in rats with induced Parkinson's disease [101].

Additionally, in ongoing clinical studies (Phase II completed), peptides generated from ligands are being utilized in the creation of medications for the treatment of early-stage or malignant brain tumors [102]. Based on the aprotinin structure, Angiochem has created peptides dubbed Angiopeps that are BBB-permeable. These peptides exhibit high rates of LRP1 or LRP2 ligand transcytosis. In tests employing in situ cerebral perfusion, a 19-amino acid peptide generated from the "Kunitz domain" of bovine pancreatic trypsin inhibitor demonstrated enhanced drug delivery to the brain. This coupling of peptides to drug vectors resulted in enhanced survival in animal models of intracranial tumors [103].

3.3.4.1.3 Leptin receptors

In order to access the cerebral parenchyma, leptin interacts with the leptin receptor, which might be seen on the endothelial cells of brain capillaries or within the choroid plexus [104].

Leptin 61-90 conjugated to a pegylated poly-(lysine) dendrimer complexed with DNA, according to studies in rats, boosted gene expression in the brain in a manner comparable to the effects seen with natural leptin 61-90 [105].

3.3.4.1.4 NAchR or the nicotinic acetylcholine receptor

The transport of RGV29 molecules across the blood–brain barrier (BBB) has been discovered to be made possible by the ligand RVG29. Peptide complexes of RGV29 and D-arginine-9vbmer with siRNA were shown to cross the BBB through this ligand, possibly explaining their absorption into the brain. The complexes were connected by a triglycine spacer [106].

It was observed that bunarotoxin, a ligand for the nicotine acetylcholine receptor, reduced the uptake of these complexes, indicating that RVG-29 reaches the brain through these ligands, specifically the α-7 subunit of the receptor [106]. By attaching RVG-29 to ionic liposomal small interfering RNA (siRNA) compounds, gene silencing of the cellular prion protein gene was achieved [107]. Although it is impossible to disregard the GABAB receptor's role in the absorption, absorption of the RVG-29 coupled polyamidoamine dendrimer gene sequences cannot be prevented by nicotinic agonists and antagonists [108, 109].

3.3.4.1.5 Diptheria toxin receptor

Mutants of the diphtheria toxin that are not poisonous have been investigated as possible therapeutic delivery systems for the brain [110]. In studies, these mutants have been used as brain delivery vectors in human immunization. Additionally, when paired with the receptor-specific protein vector CRM 197 or functionalizing liposomes containing horseradish peroxidase, it has been demonstrated that horseradish peroxidase may traverse the blood–brain barrier (BBB) in a guinea pig model [12]. However, it is important to note that this method may not be suitable for repeated injections due to potential concerns regarding immunogenicity.

3.3.5 Transcytosis via adsorptive means

Transcytosis through adsorptive means allows large-molecular-weight biopharmaceuticals to enter the brain. This process requires endocytosis and transcytosis of acidic conjugated proteins, as the molecule needs to possess an increased positive charge at neutral pH to electrostatically interact with anionic on the cell's exterior [111, 112]. In terms of the processes required, endocytosis in the context of AMT is comparable to receptor-mediated endocytosis. Various compounds, such as histone [113], avidin [112], cationized polyclonal bovine IgG [114], E2078, and other cell-penetrating peptides [115] like the TAT protein [116], have been shown to enter the brain through AMT [117].

Originally recognized for its intracellular function in viral gene expression, the TAT peptide is a non-amphipathic, arginine-rich cell-penetrating peptide generated from the TAT protein of HIV-1 [79]. The exact mechanism by which exogenous TAT reaches cells is still not fully understood, although it has been shown that TAT protein binds to LDLR family members and heparin-sulfate proteoglycans [79]. Strong cell attachment and translocation are facilitated by the highly cationic cluster in TAT, which is made up of six arginine or two lysine motifs (RKKKRRQRRR), regardless of cell ligands or temperature [118]. It has also been discovered that other arginine-rich peptides, such as SynB5 (RGGRLAYLRRRWAVLGR) and pAnt(4358) (RQIKIWFQNRRMKWKK), improve brain penetration by AMT [119, 120].

However, the use of cationic drugs for brain delivery is limited due to their higher absorption in the liver or excretion through the kidneys, resulting in low amounts reaching the brain (typically below 0.1% of the intravenously administered dose). Immunological complex formation and nonspecific permeability in the brain and peripheral vessels are additional challenges associated with cationized proteins that may restrict their therapeutic use for brain delivery. The usage of myristoylated polyarginine vectors is one method that has been investigated to get around the problems caused by excessive cationic charges [121].

3.4 Conclusion

By strictly controlling the entry of chemicals into the brain, the blood–brain barrier (BBB) serves a critical function in preserving brain homeostasis. This specialized barrier allows only less than a tenth of the intravenous dosage of medication to be absorbed, posing challenges for CNS disease treatment. However, there are highly regulated transport mechanisms that can be harnessed to deliver medications and nanotheranostics across the BBB. When developing drugs, pharmacokinetic factors and physicochemical characteristics that aid passive diffusion should be taken into account. Among, various transport modalities, only endocytotic mechanisms, such as receptor-mediated endocytosis, have demonstrated success in delivering therapeutics, including antibodies and biomolecules, to the CNS. Utilizing carrier-mediated and receptor-mediated endocytosis through nanoparticulate devices has showed potential, with higher-capacity transporters being particularly effective. Clinical research is now being done to improve these methods of improving medication delivery to the brain.

References

[1] Lalatsa, A., & Barbu, E. Carbohydrate Nanoparticles for Brain Delivery. *International Review of Neurobiology*, **2016**, *130*, 115–153. Available from https://doi.org/10.1016/bs.irn.2016.05.004.

[2] Kola, I., & Landis, J. Can the pharmaceutical industry reduce attrition rates? *Nature Reviews Drug Discovery*, **2004**, *3*(8), 711–715. Available from https://doi.org/10.1038/nrd1470.

[3] Pardridge, W.M. The blood-brain barrier and neurotherapeutics. *NeuroRx*, **2005**, *2*(1), 1–2. Available from https://doi.org/10.1602/neurorx.2.1.1.

[4] Ehrlich, P. Das Sauerstoff-Bedürfniss des Organismus:eine farbenanalytische Studie. Berlin: Hirschwald, **1885**.

[5] Goldmann, E. (1913). Vitalfarbung am zentralnervensystem. *Abhandl Konigl preuss Akad Wiss.*, **1913**, *1*, 1–60.

[6] Bradbury, M.W.B. The concept of the blood-brain barrier. *Chichester: Wiley*, **1979**

[7] Reese, T.S., & Karnovsky, M.J. Fine structural localization of a blood-brain barrier to exogenous peroxidase. *Journal of Cell Biology*, **1967**, *34*(1), 207–217.

[8] Abbott, N.J. Ronnback, L., & Hansson, E. Astrocyte-endothelial interactions at the blood-brain barrier. *Nature Reviews Neuroscience*, **2006**, *7*(1), 41–53. Available from https://doi.org/10.1038/nrn1824.

[9] Fenstermacher, J., Gross, P., Sposito, N., Acuff, V., Pettersen, S., & Gruber, K. Structural and functional variations in capillary systems within the brain. *Annals of the New York Academy of Sciences*, **1988**, *529*, 21–30

[10] Sedlakova, R., Shivers, R.R., & Del Maestro, R.F. Ultrastructure of the blood-brain barrier in the rabbit. *Journal of Submicroscopic Cytology and Pathology*, **1999**, *31*(1), 149–161.

[11] Kniesel, U., & Wolburg, H. Tight junctions of the blood-brain barrier. *Cellular and Molecular Neurobiology*, **2000**, *20*(1), 57–76.

[12] Lalatsa, A., Schatzlein, A., & Uchegbu, I. Nanostructures overcoming the blood-brain barrier: Physiological considerations and mechanistic issues. In M. J. Alonso, & N. S. Csaba (Eds.), *Nanostructured Biomaterials for Overcoming Biological Barriers*, **2012**, 329–363

[13] Oldendorf, W.H. The blood-brain barrier. *Experimental Eye Research*, **1977**, *25*, Suppl, 177–190.

[14] Oldendorf, W.H., Cornford, M.E., & Brown, W.J. The large apparent work capability of the blood-brain barrier: A study of the mitochondrial

content of capillary endothelial cells in the brain and other tissues of the rat. *Annals of Neurology*, **1977**, *1*(5), 409–417. Available from https://doi.org/10.1002/ana.410010502.

[15] Hawkins, B.T., & Davis, T.P. The blood-brain barrier/neurovascular unit in health and disease. *Pharmacological Reviews*, **2005**, *57*(2), 173–185. Available from https://doi.org/10.1124/pr.57.2.4.

[16] Furuse, M., Hirase, T., Itoh, M., Nagafuchi, A., Yonemura, S., Tsukita, S., & Tsukita, S. Occludin: A novel integral membrane protein localizing at tight junctions. *Journal of Cell Biology*, **1993**, *123*(6 Pt 2), 1777–1788.

[17] Wong, V., & Gumbiner, B.M. A synthetic peptide corresponding to the extracellular domain of occludin perturbs the tight junction permeability barrier. *Journal of Cell Biology*, **1997**, *136*(2), 399–409

[18] Wolburg, H., Wolburg-Buchholz, K., Liebner, S., & Engelhardt, B. Claudin-1, claudin-2 and claudin-11 are present in tight junctions of choroid plexus epithelium of the mouse. *Neuroscience Letters*, **2001**, *307*(2), 77–80

[19] Butt, A.M., Jones, H.C., & Abbott, N.J. (1990). Electrical resistance across the blood-brain barrier in anaesthetized rats: A developmental study. *Journal of Physiology (Cambridge, United Kingdom)*, **1990**.

[20] Shepro, D., & Morel, N.M. Pericyte physiology. *FASEB Journal*, **1993**, *7*(11), 1031–1038

[21] Daneman, R., Zhou, L., Kebede, A.A., & Barres, B.A. Pericytes are required for blood-brain barrier integrity during embryogenesis. *Nature*, **2010**, *468*(7323), 562–566. Available from https://doi.org/10.1038/nature09

[22] Hamilton, N.B., Attwell, D., & Hall, C. N. Pericyte-mediated regulation of capillary diameter: A component of neurovascular coupling in health and disease. *Front Neuroenergetics*, **2010**, 2. Available from https://doi.org/ 10.3389/fnene.2010.00005.

[23] Wong, A.D., Ye, M., Levy, A.F., Rothstein, J.D., Bergles, D.E., & Searson, P.C. The blood-brain barrier: An engineering perspective. *Frontiers in Neuroengineering*, **2013**, *6*, 7. Available from https://doi.org/10.3389/ fneng.2013.00007.

[24] Schirmacher, A., Winters, S., Fischer, S., Goeke, J., Galla, H.J., Kullnick, U., ... Stogbauer, F. Electromagnetic fields (1.8 GHz) increase the permeability to sucrose of the blood-brain barrier *in vitro*. *Bioelectromagnetics*, **2000**, *21*(5), 338–345.

[25] Keep, R.F., Ennis, S.R., Beer, M.E., & Betz, A.L. Developmental changes in blood-brain barrier potassium permeability in the rat:

Relation to brain growth. *Journal of Physiology (Cambridge, United Kingdom)*, **1995**, *488*(Pt 2), 439–448.

[26] Olsson, Y., Klatzo, I., Sourander, P., & Steinwall, O. Blood-brain barrier to albumin in embryonic new born and adult rats. *Acta Neuropathologica*, **1968**, *10*(2), 117–122.

[27] Saunders, N.R., Knott, G.W., & Dziegielewska, K.M. Barriers in the immature brain. *Cellular and Molecular Neurobiology*, **2000**, *20*(1), 29–40.

[28] Liebner, S., & Plate, K.H. Differentiation of the brain vasculature: The answer came blowing by the Wnt. *Journal of Angiogenesis Research*, **2010**, *2*, 1. Available from https://doi.org/10.1186/2040-2384-2-1.

[29] Stenman, J.M., Rajagopal, J., Carroll, T.J., Ishibashi, M., McMahon, J., & McMahon, A.P. Canonical Wnt signaling regulates organ-specific assembly and differentiation of CNS vasculature. *Science*, **2008**, *322*(5905), 1247–1250. Available from https://doi.org/10.1126/science.1164594.

[30] Virgintino, D., Errede, M., Robertson, D., Capobianco, C., Girolamo, F., Vimercati, A., ... Roncali, L. Immunolocalization of tight junction proteins in the adult and developing human brain. *Histochemistry and Cell Biology*, **2004**, *122*(1), 51–59. Available from https://doi.org/10.1007/s00418-004-0665-1.

[31] Grontoft, O. Intracranial haemorrhage and blood-brain barrier problems in the new-born, a pathologicoanatomical and experimental investigation. *Acta Pathologica et Microbiologica Scandinavica, Supplementum*, **1954**, *100*, 8–10

[32] Hartmann, C., Zozulya, A., Wegener, J., & Galla, H.J. The impact of glia-derived extracellular matrices on the barrier function of cerebral endothelial cells: An *in vitro* study. *Experimental Cell Research*, **2007**, *313*(7), 1318–1325. Available from https://doi.org/10.1016/j.yexcr.2007.01.024

[33] Begley, D.J. The blood-brain barrier: Principles for targeting peptides and drugs to the central nervous system. *Journal of Pharmacy and Pharmacology*, **1996**, *48*(2), 136–146.

[34] Begley, D.J. Delivery of therapeutic agents to the central nervous system: The problems and the possibilities. *Pharmacology & Therapeutics*, **2004b**, *104*(1), 29–45. Available from https://doi.org/10.1016/j.pharmthera.2004.08.001

[35] Bradbury, M.W. Transport of iron in the blood-brain-cerebrospinal fluid system. *Journal of Neurochemistry*, **1997**, *69*(2), 443–454.

[36] Misra, A., Ganesh, S., Shahiwala, A., & Shah, S. P. Drug delivery to the central nervous system: A review. *Journal of Pharmacy & Pharmaceutical Sciences*, **2003**, *6*(2), 252–273.

[37] Begley, D.J., & Brightmann, M.W. (2003). Peptide transport and delivery into the central nervous system. In L. P.-T. Prokai (Ed.), *Progress in Drug Research*, **2003**, 39.

[38] Begley, D.J. ABC transporters and the blood-brain barrier. *Current Pharmaceutical Design*, **2004a**, *10*(12), 1295–1312.

[39] Terasaki, T., & Hosoya, K. The blood-brain barrier efflux transporters as a detoxifying system for the brain. *Advanced Drug Delivery Reviews*, **1999**, *36*(2-3), 195–209.

[40] Shen, S., & Zhang, W. ABC transporters and drug efflux at the blood-brain barrier. *Reviews of Neuroscience*, **2010**, *21*(1), 29–53.

[41] Shen, S., Callaghan, D., Juzwik, C., Xiong, H., Huang, P., & Zhang, W. ABCG2 reduces ROS-mediated toxicity and inflammation: A potential role in Alzheimer's disease. *Journal of Neurochemistry*, **2010**, *114*(6), 1590–1604. Available from https://doi.org/10.1111/j.1471-4159.2010.06887.x.

[42] Loscher, W., & Potschka, H. Blood-brain barrier active efflux transporters: ATP-binding cassette gene family. *NeuroRx*, **2005a**, *2*(1), 86–98. Available from https://doi.org/10.1602/neurorx.2.1.86.

[43] Loscher, W., & Potschka, H. Drug resistance in brain diseases and the role of drug efflux transporters. *Nature Reviews Neuroscience*, **2005b**, *6*(8), 591–602. Available from https://doi.org/10.1038/nrn1728.

[44] Loscher, W., & Potschka, H. Role of drug efflux transporters in the brain for drug disposition and treatment of brain diseases. *Progress in Neurobiology*, **2005c**, *76*(1), 22–76. Available from https://doi.org/10.1016/j. pneurobio.2005.04.006.

[45] Volk, H., Potschka, H., & Loscher, W. Immunohistochemical localization of P-glycoprotein in rat brain and detection of its increased expression by seizures are sensitive to fixation and staining variables. *Journal of Histochemistry and Cytochemistry*, **2005**, *53*(4), 517–531. Available from https://doi.org/10.1369/jhc.4A6451.2005.

[46] ElAli, A., & Hermann, D.M. ATP-binding cassette transporters and their roles in protecting the brain. *Neuroscientist*, **2011**, *17*(4), 423–436. Available from https://doi.org/10.1177/1073858410391270.

[47] Laschinger, M., & Engelhardt, B. Interaction of alpha4-integrin with VCAM-1 is involved in adhesion of encephalitogenic T cell blasts to brain endothelium but not in their transendothelial migration *in vitro*. *Journal of Neuroimmunology*, **2000**, *102*(1), 32–43.

[48] Greenwood, J., Amos, C.L., Walters, C.E., Couraud, P.O., Lyck, R., Engelhardt, B., & Adamson, P. Intracellular domain of brain endothelial

intercellular adhesion molecule-1 is essential for T lymphocyte-mediated signaling and migration. *Journal of Immunology*, **2003**, *171*(4), 20

[49] Clark, D.E. In silico prediction of blood-brain barrier permeation. *Drug Discovery Today*, **2003**, *8*(20), 927–933

[50] Kramer, S.D. Absorption prediction from physicochemical parameters. *Pharmaceutical Science & Technology Today*, **1999**, *2*(9), 373–380.

[51] Kelder, J., Grootenhuis, P.D., Bayada, D.M., Delbressine, L.P., & Ploemen, J.P. Polar molecular surface as a dominating determinant for oral absorption and brain penetration of drugs. *Pharmaceutical Research*, **1999**, *16*(10), 1514–1519.

[52] Abbott, N.J., Patabendige, A.A., Dolman, D.E., Yusof, S.R., & Begley, D.J. Structure and function of the blood-brain barrier. *Neurobiology of Disease*, **2010**, *37*(1), 13–25. Available from https://doi.org/10.1016/j.nbd.2009.07.030.

[53] Fong, C.W. Permeability of the blood-brain barrier: Molecular mechanism of transport of drugs and physiologically important compounds. *Journal of Membrane Biology*, **2015**, *248*(4), 651–669. Available from https://doi. org/10.1007/s00232-015-9778-9.

[54] Gleeson, M.P. Generation of a set of simple, interpretable ADMET rules of thumb. *Journal of Medicinal Chemistry*, **2008**, *51*(4), 817–834. Available from https://doi.org/10.1021/jm701122q.

[55] Fischer, H., Gottschlich, R., & Seelig, A. Blood-brain barrier permeation: Molecular parameters governing passive diffusion. *Journal of Membrane Biology*, **1998**, *165*(3), 201–211

[56] Goodwin, J.T., & Clark, D.E. In silico predictions of blood-brain barrier penetration: Considerations to "keep in mind". *Journal of Pharmacology and Experimental Therapeutics*, **2005**, *315*(2), 477–483. Available from https:// doi.org/10.1124/jpet.104.075705.

[57] Drion, N., Lemaire, M., Lefauconnier, J.M., & Scherrmann, J.M. Role of P-glycoprotein in the blood-brain transport of colchicine and vinblastine. *Journal of Neurochemistry*, **1996**, *67*(4), 1688–1693.

[58] Kemper, E.M., van Zandbergen, A.E., Cleypool, C., Mos, H.A., Boogerd, W., Beijnen, J. H., & van Tellingen, O. Increased penetration of paclitaxel into the brain by inhibition of P-Glycoprotein. *Clinical Cancer Research*, **2003**, *9*(7), 2849–2855.

[59] Fellner, S., Bauer, B., Miller, D.S., Schaffrik, M., Fankhanel, M., Spruss, T., ... Fricker, G. Transport of paclitaxel (Taxol) across the blood-brain barrier *in vitro* and *in vivo*. *Journal of Clinical Investigation*, **2002**, *110*(9), 1309–1318. Available from https://doi.org/10.1172/JCI15451.

[60] Medbo, J.I., & Sejersted, O. M. Plasma pwotassium changes with high intensity exercise. *Journal of Physiology (Cambridge, United Kingdom)*, **1990**, *421*, 105–122.

[61] Bradbury, M.W., Stubbs, J., Hughes, I.E., & Parker, P. The Distribution of Potassium, Sodium, Chloride and Urea between Lumbar Cerebrospinal Fluid and Blood Serum in Human Subjects. *Clinical Science*, **1963**, *25*, 97–105.

[62] Hansen, A. J. Effect of anoxia on ion distribution in the brain. *Physiological Reviews*, **1985**, *65*(1), 101–148.

[63] Jeong, S.M., Hahm, K.D., Shin, J.W., Leem, J.G., Lee, C., & Han, S.M. Changes in magnesium concentration in the serum and cerebrospinal fluid of neuropathic rats. *Acta Anaesthesiologica Scandinavica*, **2006**, *50*(2), 211–216. Available from https://doi.org/10.1111/j.1399-6576.2006.00925.x.

[64] Michalke, B., & Nischwitz, V. Review on metal speciation analysis in cerebrospinal fluid-current methods and results: A review. *Analytica Chimica Acta*, **2010**, *682*(1-2), 23–36. Available from https://doi.org/10.1016/j. aca.2010.09.054

[65] Rapoport, S. Blood-brain barrier in physiology and Medicine. *New York, USA: Raven,* **1976.**

[66] Simard, M., & Nedergaard, M. The neurobiology of glia in the context of water and ion homeostasis. *Neuroscience*, **2004**, *129*(4), 877–896. Available from https://doi.org/10.1016/j.neuroscience.2004.09.053.

[67] Brasko, C., Hawkins, V., De La Rocha, I.C., & Butt, A.M. Expression of Kir4.1 and Kir5.1 inwardly rectifying potassium channels in oligodendrocytes, the myelinating cells of the CNS. *Brain Structure & Function*, **2017**, *222* (1), 41–59. Available from https://doi.org/10.1007/s00429-016-1199-8.

[68] Wade, L.A., & Katzman, R. Synthetic amino acids and the nature of L-DOPA transport at the blood-brain barrier. *Journal of Neurochemistry*, **1975**, *25*(6), 837–842

[69] Thomas, S.A., Abbruscato, T.J., Hruby, V.J., & Davis, T.P. The entry of [D-penicillamine2,5] enkephalin into the central nervous system: Saturation kinetics and specificity. *Journal of Pharmacology and Experimental Therapeutics*, **1997**, *280*(3), 1235–1240.

[70] Carruthers, A., DeZutter, J., Ganguly, A., & Devaskar, S.U. Will the original glucose transporter isoform please stand up!. *American Journal of Physiology: Endocrinology and Metabolism*, **2009**, *297*(4), E836–848. Available from https://doi.org/10.1152/ajpendo.00496.2009.

[71] Devaskar, S., Zahm, D.S., Holtzclaw, L., Chundu, K., & Wadzinski, B.E. Developmental regulation of the distribution of rat brain insulin-insensitive

(Glut 1) glucose transporter. *Endocrinology*, **1991**, *129*(3), 1530–1540. Available from https://doi.org/10.1210/endo-129-3-1530.

[72] Simpson,I.A.,Appel,N.M.,Hokari,M.,Oki,J.,Holman,G.D.,Maher,F.,… Smith, Q. R. Blood-brain barrier glucose transporter: Effects of hypo- and hyperglycemia revisited. *Journal of Neurochemistry*, **1999**, *72*(1), 238–247

[73] Simpson, I.A., Vannucci, S.J., DeJoseph, M.R., & Hawkins, R.A. Glucose transporter asymmetries in the bovine blood-brain barrier. *Journal of Biological Chemistry*, **2001**, *276*(16), 12725–12729. Available from https://doi. org/10.1074/jbc.M010897200.

[74] Egleton, R.D., Mitchell, S.A., Huber, J.D., Janders, J., Stropova, D., Polt, R., … Davis, T. P. Improved bioavailability to the brain of glyco-sylated Met-enkephalin analogs. *Brain Research*, **2000**, *881*(1), 37–46

[75] Polt, R., Porreca, F., Szabo, L.Z., Bilsky, E.J., Davis, P., Abbruscato, T.J., … Hruby, V.J. Glycopeptide enkephalin analogues produce analgesia in mice: Evidence for penetration of the blood-brain barrier. *Proceedings of the National Academy of Sciences of the United States of America*, **1994**, *91*(15), 7114–7118.

[76] Dhanasekaran, M., Palian, M.M., Alves, I., Yeomans, L., Keyari, C.M., Davis, P., … Polt, R. Glycopeptides related to beta-endorphin adopt helical amphipathic conformations in the presence of lipid bilayers. *Journal of the American Chemical Society*, **2005**, *127*(15), 5435–5448. Available from https://doi.org/10.1021/ja0432158.

[77] Egleton, R.D., Bilsky, E.J., Tollin, G., Dhanasekaran, M., Lowery, J., Alves, I., … Porreca, F. Biousian glycopeptides penetrate the blood-brain barrier. *Tetrahedron: Asymmetry*, **2005**, *16*(10), 65–75.

[78] Birngruber, T., Raml, R., Gladdines, W., Gatschelhofer, C., Gander, E., Ghosh, A., … Sinner, F. Enhanced doxorubicin delivery to the brain administered through glutathione PEGylated liposomal doxorubicin (2B3- 101) as compared with generic Caelyx,((R))/Doxil((R))-a cerebral open flow microperfusion pilot study. *Journal of Pharmaceutical Sciences*, **2014**, *103*(7), 1945–1948. Available from https://doi. org/10.1002/jps.23994.

[79] Lalatsa, A., Schatzlein, A.G., & Uchegbu, I.F. Strategies to deliver peptide drugs to the brain. *Molecular Pharmaceutics*, **2014**, *11*(4), 1081–1093. Available from https://doi.org/10.1021/mp400680d.

[80] Bickel, U., Yoshikawa, T., & Pardridge, W.M. Delivery of peptides and proteins through the blood-brain barrier. *Advanced Drug Delivery Reviews*, **2001**, *46*(1-3), 247–279.

[81] Herz, J., & Marschang, P. Coaxing the LDL receptor family into the fold. *Cell*, **2003**, *112*(3), 289–292.

[82] Broadwell, R.D., Balin, B.J., & Salcman, M. Transcytotic pathway for blood-borne protein through the blood-brain barrier. *Proceedings of the National Academy of Sciences of the United States of America*, **1988**, *85*(2), 632–636.

[83] Willingham, M.C., Hanover, J.A., Dickson, R.B., & Pastan, I. Morphologic characterization of the pathway of transferrin endocytosis and recycling in human KB cells. *Proceedings of the National Academy of Sciences of the United States of America*, **1984**, *81*(1), 175–179.

[84] Pardridge, W.M. Biopharmaceutical drug targeting to the brain. *Journal of Drug Targeting*, **2010**, *18*(3), 157–167. Available from https://doi.org/10.3109/10611860903548354.

[85] Boado, R.J., & Pardridge, W.M. Brain and organ uptake in the rhesus monkey *in vivo* of recombinant iduronidase compared to an insulin receptor antibody-iduronidase fusion protein. *Molecular Pharmaceutics*, **2017**, *14* (4), 1271–1277. Available from https://doi.org/10.1021/acs.molpharmaceut.6b01166

[86] Chang, R., Knox, J., Chang, J., Derbedrossian, A., Vasilevko, V., Cribbs, D., ... Sumbria, R.K. Blood-brain barrier penetrating biologic TNF-alpha inhibitor for Alzheimer's disease. *Molecular Pharmaceutics*, **2017**, *14*(7), 2340–2349. Available from https://doi.org/10.1021/acs.molpharmaceut.7b00200.

[87] Pardridge, W.M. Brain drug development and brain drug targeting. *Pharmaceutical Research*, **2007a**, *24*(9), 1729–1732. Available from https://doi.org/10.1007/s11095-007-9387-0.

[88] Shi, N., Zhang, Y., Zhu, C., Boado, R.J., & Pardridge, W.M. Brain-specific expression of an exogenous gene after i.v. administration. *Proceedings of the National Academy of Sciences of the United States of America*, **2001**, 98 (22), 12754–12759. Available from https://doi.org/10.1073/pnas.221450098.

[89] Zhang, Y., & Pardridge, W.M. Near complete rescue of experimental Parkinson's disease with intravenous, non-viral GDNF gene therapy. *Pharmaceutical Research*, **2009**, *26*(5), 1059–1063. Available from https://doi. org/10.1007/s11095-008-9815-9.

[90] Moos, T., & Morgan, E.H. Restricted transport of anti-transferrin receptor antibody (OX26) through the blood-brain barrier in the rat. *Journal of Neurochemistry*, **2001**, *79*(1), 119–129.

[91] Boado, R.J., Zhou, Q.H., Lu, J.Z., Hui, E.K., & Pardridge, W.M. Pharmacokinetics and brain uptake of a genetically engineered bifunctional fusion antibody targeting the mouse transferrin receptor. *Molecular Pharmaceutics*, **2010**, *7*(1), 237-244. Available from https://doi.org/10.1021/mp900235k.

[92] Zhou, Q.H., Fu, A., Boado, R.J., Hui, E.K., Lu, J.Z., & Pardridge, W.M. Receptor-mediated abeta amyloid antibody targeting to Alzheimer's disease mouse brain. *Molecular Pharmaceutics*, **2011**, *8*(1), 280–285. Available from https://doi.org/10.1021/mp1003515

[93] Yu, Y.J., Zhang, Y., Kenrick, M., Hoyte, K., Luk, W., Lu, Y., ... Dennis, M.S. Boosting brain uptake of a therapeutic antibody by reducing its affinity for a transcytosis target. *Science Translational Medicine*, **2011**, *3*(84), 84ra44. Available from https://doi.org/10.1126/scitranslmed.3002230.

[94] Boado, R.J., Hui, E.K., Lu, J.Z., Zhou, Q.H., & Pardridge, W.M. Selective targeting of a TNFR decoy receptor pharmaceutical to the primate brain as a receptor-specific IgG fusion protein. *Journal of Biotechnology*, **2010**, *146*(1-2), 84–91. Available from https://doi.org/10.1016/j.jbiotec.2010.01.011.

[95] Pardridge, W.M. shRNA and siRNA delivery to the brain. *Advanced Drug Delivery Reviews*, **2007b**, *59*(2-3), 141–152. Available from https://doi.org/10.1016/j.addr.2007.03.008.

[96] Boado, R.J., Zhang, Y., Zhang, Y., Xia, C.F., & Pardridge, W.M. Fusion antibody for Alzheimer's disease with bidirectional transport across the blood-brain barrier and abeta fibril disaggregation. *Bioconjugate Chemistry*, **2007**, *18*(2), 447–455. Available from https://doi.org/10.1021/bc060349x

[97] Spencer, B.J., & Verma, I.M. Targeted delivery of proteins across the blood-brain barrier. *Proceedings of the National Academy of Sciences of the United States of America*, **2007**, *104*(18), 7594–7599. Available from https://doi.org/ 10.1073/pnas.0702170104.

[98] Rebeck, G.W., Reiter, J.S., Strickland, D.K., & Hyman, B.T. Apolipoprotein E in sporadic Alzheimer's disease: Allelic variation and receptor interactions. *Neuron*, **1993**, *11*(4), 575–580.

[99] Yamamoto, M., Ikeda, K., Ohshima, K., Tsugu, H., Kimura, H., & Tomonaga, M. Increased expression of low density lipoprotein receptor-related protein/alpha2-macroglobulin receptor in human malignant astrocytomas. *Cancer Research*, **1997**, *57*(13), 2799–2805.

[100] Karkan, D., Pfeifer, C., Vitalis, T.Z., Arthur, G., Ujiie, M., Chen, Q., ... Jefferies, W.A. A unique carrier for delivery of therapeutic compounds beyond the blood-brain barrier. *PLoS One*, **2008**, *3*(6), e2469. Available from https://doi.org/10.1371/journal.pone.0002469.

[101] Huang, R., Ke, W., Han, L., Liu, Y., Shao, K., Jiang, C., & Pei, Y. Lactoferrin-modified nanoparticles could mediate efficient gene delivery to the brain *in vivo*. *Brain Research Bulletin*, **2010**, *81*(6), 600–604. Available from https://doi.org/10.1016/j.brainresbull.2009.12.008.

[102] O'Sullivan, C.C., Lindenberg, M., Bryla, C., Patronas, N., Peer, C.J., Amiri-Kordestani, L., ... Bates, S.E. ANG1005 for breast cancer brain metastases: Correlation between 18F-FLT-PET after first cycle and MRI in response assessment. *Breast Cancer Research and Treatment*, **2016**, *160*(1), 51–59. Available from https://doi.org/ 10.1007/ s10549-016-3972-z.

[103] Demeule,M.,Currie,J.C.,Bertrand,Y.,Che,C.,Nguyen,T.,Regina,A.,... Beliveau, R. Involvement of the low-density lipoprotein receptor-related protein in the transcytosis of the brain delivery vector angio-pep-2. *Journal of Neurochemistry*, **2008**, *106*(4), 1534–1544. Available from https://doi.org/10.1111/j.1471-4159.2008.05492.x.

[104] Banks, W.A., Kastin, A.J., Huang, W., Jaspan, J.B., & Maness, L.M. Leptin enters the brain by a saturable system independent of insulin. *Peptides*, **1996**, *17*(2), 305–311.

[105] Barrett, G.L., Trieu, J., & Naim, T. The identification of leptin-derived peptides that are taken up by the brain. *Regulatory Peptides*, **2009**, *155*(1-3), 55–61. Available from https://doi.org/10.1016/j. regpep.2009.02.008

[106] Kumar,P.,Wu,H.,McBride,J.L.,Jung,K.E.,Kim,M.H.,Davidson,B.L.,... Manjunath, N. Transvascular delivery of small interfering RNA to the central nervous system. *Nature*, **2007**, *448*(7149), 39–43. Available from https://doi.org/10.1038/nature05901.

[107] Pulford, B., Reim, N., Bell, A., Veatch, J., Forster, G., Bender, H., ... Zabel, M. D. Liposome-siRNA-peptide complexes cross the blood-brain barrier and significantly decrease PrP on neuronal cells and PrP in infected cell cultures. *PLoS One*, **2010**, *5*(6), e11085. Available from https://doi.org/10.1371/journal.pone.0011085

[108] Wilkins, M.E., Li, X., & Smart, T. Tracking cell surface GABAB receptors using an alpha-bungarotoxin tag. *Journal of Biological Chemistry*, **2008**, *283*(50), 34745–34752. Available from https://doi. org/10.1074/jbc. M803197200.

[109] Vorbrodt, A.W. Ultracytochemical characterization of anionic sites in the wall of brain capillaries. *Journal of Neurocytology*, **1989**, *18*(3), 359–368.

[110] Sauer, I., Dunay, I.R., Weisgraber, K., Bienert, M., & Dathe, M. An apo-lipoprotein E-derived peptide mediates uptake of sterically stabilized liposomes into brain capillary endothelial cells. *Biochemistry*, **2005**, *44*(6), 2021–2029. Available from https://doi.org/10.1021/bi048080x.

[111] Sauer, J.M., Ring, B.J., & Witcher, J.W. Clinical pharmacokinetics of atomoxetine. *Clinical Pharmacokinetics*, **2005**, *44*(6), 571–590. Available from https://doi.org/10.2165/00003088-200544060-00002

[112] Pardridge, W.M. Peptide drug delivery to the brain. *New York: Raven Press Ltd*, **1991**.

[113] Pardridge, W.M., Triguero, D., & Buciak, J. Transport of histone through the blood-brain barrier. *Journal of Pharmacology and Experimental Therapeutics*, **1989**, *251*(3), 821–826.

[114] Triguero, D., Buciak, J.B., Yang, J., & Pardridge, W.M. Blood-brain barrier transport of cationized immunoglobulin G: Enhanced delivery compared to native protein. *Proceedings of the National Academy of Sciences of the United States of America*, **1989**, *86*(12), 4761–4765

[115] Terasaki, T., Deguchi, Y., Sato, H., Hirai, K., & Tsuji, A. *In vivo* transport of a dynorphin-like analgesic peptide, E-2078, through the blood-brain barrier: An application of brain microdialysis. *Pharmaceutical Research*, **1991**, *8*(7), 815–820.

[116] Frankel, A.D., & Pabo, C.O. Cellular uptake of the tat protein from human immunodeficiency virus. *Cell*, **1988**, *55*(6), 1189–1193.

[117] Kumagai, A.K., Eisenberg, J.B., & Pardridge, W.M. Absorptive-mediated endocytosis of cationized albumin and a beta-endorphin-cationized albumin chimeric peptide by isolated brain capillaries. Model system of blood-brain barrier transport. *Journal of Biological Chemistry*, **1987**, *262*(31), 15214–15219.

[118] Subrizi, A., Tuominen, E., Bunker, A., Rog, T., Antopolsky, M., & Urtti, A. Tat(48-60) peptide amino acid sequence is not unique in its cell penetrating properties and cell-surface glycosaminoglycans inhibit its cellular uptake. *Journal of Controlled Release*, **2012**, *158*(2), 277–285. Available from https://doi.org/10.1016/j. jconrel.2011.11.007.

[119] Mitchell, D.J., Kim, D.T., Steinman, L., Fathman, C.G., & Rothbard, J.B. Polyarginine enters cells more efficiently than other polycationic homopolymers. *Journal of Peptide Research*, **2000**, *56*(5), 318–325.

[120] Drin, G., Cottin, S., Blanc, E., Rees, A.R., & Temsamani, J. Studies on the internalization mechanism of cationic cell-penetrating peptides. *Journal of Biological Chemistry*, **2003**, *278*(33), 31192–31201. Available from https:// doi.org/10.1074/jbc.M303938200.

[121] Pham, W., Zhao, B.Q., Lo, E.H., Medarova, Z., Rosen, B., & Moore, A. Crossing the blood-brain barrier: A potential application of myristoylated polyarginine for *in vivo* neuroimaging. *NeuroImage*, **2005**, *28*(1), 287–292. Available from https://doi.org/10.1016/j. neuroimage.2005.06.007.

4

Specific Brain Tumor Treatments Supplied using Active Nanotechnology Delivery Systems

Abstract

Brain tumors, which originate within the brain and swiftly infiltrate the surrounding tissue, stand as one of the most perilous manifestations of cancer globally, thereby presenting a considerable public health issue. The discovery of adaptive nanocarriers that can pass the blood–brain barrier (BBB) and advances in nanotechnology are revolutionizing the treatment of brain tumors. The utilization of ligand-conjugated nanoparticle systems for treating brain tumors represents a novel and effective approach. Various ligands, including peptides, aptamers, antibodies, transferrin, and folic acid, are conjugated to brain tumor markers and employed in drug/gene delivery systems and imaging agents that specifically target brain tumors. When a specific marker is targeted toward a tumor tissue, the BBB endothelial cells facilitate transcytosis and allow the carrier to penetrate the malignant tissue. Recent research has utilized various ligand-conjugated nanoparticles to transport and image brain tumors, which will be discussed in detail in this chapter.

4.1 Introduction

The most extensively employed treatments for brain tumors are combined modality therapies, encompassing chemotherapy, surgery, and radiation [1]. However, surgeons and tumor researchers may unintentionally damage the healthy brain tissue surrounding the tumor [2]. Despite standard treatment options, the infiltrative development of gliomas is linked to a poor prognosis and quick recurrence. Consequently, completely removing glioma-infiltrated tissues without causing harm to a healthy brain tissue poses a significant challenge for oncologists [3]. Additionally, a high proportion of treatment failures in glioma patients is caused by the toxicity of standard chemotherapy and the adverse effects of radiation [4].

Unfortunately, because brain tumors are elusive and can spread across the brain parenchyma, local therapy is frequently futile [5]. The blood–brain barrier (BBB), which prevents the transport of chemotherapy drugs to the brain after systemic therapy, is another component.

According to a study, the aggressiveness and molecular heterogeneity of malignant brain tumors, as well as the high rates of treatment resistance observed in high-grade gliomas, are all primary causes of chemotherapy failure in brain tumors [6]. Malignant brain tumors may be defeated and patient survival rates increased by creating innovative therapy platforms with molecularly targeted mechanisms. For instance, customized nanoparticulate devices allow for both active and passive targeted drug delivery to brain tumors [7]. Scientists have been working on this problem for quite some time in order to minimize the amount of medication that needs to pass through healthy brain and peripheral tissues to reach the tumor.

Encapsulated drugs for the treatment of brain tumors are now distributed more effectively, thanks to the use of active targeted drug delivery systems [8]. Transcending the blood–brain barrier in the treatment of brain tumors, understanding the tumor microenvironment, and taking into consideration the physiology of tumor cells are only a few of the things that need to be done. Brain tumors possess unique characteristics and behaviors that distinguish them from other types of cancer. The use of new nanoscale vehicles in the treatment of many illnesses has shown promising outcomes. This chapter examines several ligands for the delivery of drugs that are particular to brain tumors, as summarized in Table 4.1.

4.2   Transcending the Blood–Brain Barriers via Transcytosis Mediated by Receptors

The convergence point of blood arteries and brain tissue is commonly referred to as the blood–brain barrier (BBB). It acts as a protective barrier, allowing only specific structures of molecules to pass through, thus safeguarding the brain from harmful substances [31]. Figure 4.1 provides a conceptual illustration of the complex transportation network within the BBB. Targeted medication delivery, which utilizes receptor-mediated transcytosis, plays a crucial role in achieving high selectivity, affinity, and specificity when combating brain tumors [32].

Table 4.1 Nanoscale therapeutic or imaging agents for brain tumors can be produced by conjugating a variety of ligands, including peptides, aptamers, folic acid antibodies, transferrin, and lactoferrin.

Ligand class	The receptor's name	Carrier class	Type of cell	Strategies	Important point	Ref.
Transferrin	TfR1	Liposome	Cellular types C6 and C6/ADR	Tetrandrine liposomes combined with tweaked TF vincristine were developed	Tetrandrine liposomes and vincristine modified by Tf have the potential to significantly prolong the period of circulation, clearly accumulating in the brain site of the tumor.	9
	TfR1	Carbon dots	SJGBM2 cells	The covalent compound of carbon dots and transferrin doxorubicin (CDots–Trans–Dox) was created	C-Dots–Trans- Dox at 10 nM dramatically reduced viability by 14%–45% across numerous paediatric brain tumour cell lines and was significantly more cytotoxic than Dox alone.	10
	TfR1	Cationic-pegylated liposome	GBM, LN229, U87 MG, and U373	Targeted cationic liposome with pegylation for transferrin	Results from mice who had received U373MG xenografts showed that the targeted NPs had a strong anticancer effect but that free zoledronic acid did not affect the tumors.	11
	TfR1	PAMAM dendrimer	C6 cells	Polyamidoamine dendrimer (PAMAM) modified with transferrin (Tf) and TRAIL-encoding plasmid in condensed form	According to the Tf-modified NPs, the TUNEL test could significantly increase tumor apoptosis. Rats treated with PAMAM-PEG-Tf/TRAIL compared to other groups possessed a greater median survival time (28.5 days).	12

(Continued)

Table 4.1 *Continued.*

Ligand class	The receptor's name	Carrier class	Type of cell	Strategies	Important point	Ref.
	TfR1	Micelle	C6 cells	Polyethylene glycol 1000 succinate that has been loaded with docetaxel (DTX) of D-alpha tocopheryl attached to transferrin (vitamin E-TPGS or TPGS) micelles	Transferrin-targeted TPGS micelles may be a suitable carrier for brain targeting, according to *in vivo* data.	13
Lactoferrin	LfR	Solid lipid nanoparticle (SLN)	Microvascular endothelial cells from the human brain (HBMECs)	SLNs loaded with changed BCNU's Lf and TX (TX-Lf-BCNU-SLN)	The permeability coefficient of the BBB through the BCNU rose by almost five times, thanks to TX-Lf-BCNU-SLNs.	14
	LfR	Iron oxide nanoparticles	C6 glioma cells	Having a median center, monodisperse nanoparticles of iron oxide, surfaces between 14 and 26 nm in size were created and joined to lactoferrin	C6 cells were shown to preferentially take up lactoferrin-conjugated iron oxide nanoparticles (Lf-IONPs), which displayed a high degree of cytotoxicity fivefold increase in MPS signal when compared to IONPs without lactoferrin.	15
	LfR	Micelles made of polycaprolactone and polyethylene glycol	C6 glioma cells	The preparation of PG-PCL micelles involved encapsulating iron oxide nanoparticles that are superparamagnetic and hydrophobic (SPIONs) using the solvent-evaporation technique inside the core of micelles	According to the *in vivo* experiments, the Lf-containing nanoparticles efficiently collected in glioma cells and extended the duration of frequent fainting at the tumour site by 48 hours.	16
	LfR	Pro-cationic liposome	BCECs and C6 cells	Pro-cationic liposome modified with lactoferrin and loaded with	It can prevent C6 from growing more.	

	LfR	Prodrug of hyaluronic acid	C6 cells	doxorubicin (DOX-Lf-PCL) has been created	Effectively *in vitro* compared to other DOX formulations.	17
				Combining doxorubicin through hyaluronic acid and an acid-labile hydrazone bond (HA-DOX)	The greatest median survival time was seen in glioma-bearing mice treated with Lf-HA-DOX, which was twice as long as that of the saline group.	18
Folic acid	FR	Superparamagnetic iron oxide nanoparticles coated with BSA	U251 cells	Folic acid (FA) was added after iron oxide nanoparticles were combined with bovine serum albumin (BSA)	Effective cellular uptake and motion-dependent MRI imaging.	19
	FR	PAMAM G5 dendrimer	HBMEC and C6 cells	PAMAM G5 dendrimers modified with borneol and folic acid and full with doxorubicin	According to an *in vivo* investigation, using the developed formulation boosted DOX accumulation in brain tumors and lengthened the half-life and area under the curve.	20
	FR	Hybrid polymer-lipid nanoparticles	T98G cells	Paclitaxel is encapsulated in folic acid hybrid nanoparticle-enhanced polymer lipids that have undergone cyclo-[Arg-Gly-Asp-D-Phe-Lys] modification of the sequence (cRGDfK)	Clearly, in a living organism, anticancer tests demonstrated that the developed formulation significantly extended Balb/C mice's median survival time.	21
	FR	Polymeric micelles of Pluronic P105	C6 cells	DOX-filled polymeric micelles of Pluronic P105 that are coupled to the folic acid receptor and the glucose transporter	Following intravenous administration of the created tailored formulation, a high suppression ratio of tumor development was seen.	22
	FR	Nanocrystalline cellulose	DBTRG05MG, H4, and C6 cells	Cellulose nanocrystals conjugated to folic acid for the administration of chemotherapy drugs	High absorption by cells via clathrin-mediated endocytosis.	23

(Continued)

Table 4.1 *Continued.*

Ligand class	The receptor's name	Carrier class	Type of cell	Strategies	Important point	Ref.
Antibodies	Melanotransferrin AB	Solid nanoparticles of lipid	HBMECs U87MG	Specialized medication delivery	–	24
	GLUT1 scfv	Polymeric micelles based on PEG-PE	U87MG 2D and 3D models	Specialized medication delivery	Reduced steric hindrance was caused by the much GLUT-1 scFv molecules are smaller than GLUT-1 IgG molecules.	25
	CD133 AB	Liposome	Glioblastoma stem cells, U87 segregated	Specialized medication delivery	An agent that specifically targets glioblastoma stem cells.	26
Aptamer	AS1411	PEG-PLGA	Glioma cells C6 Rat with C6 intracranial bearings, mice harboring C6 xenografts	Specialized medication delivery	–	27
	AS1411	PGG	U87 MG mice with xenografts of U87 MG-PMT48-Luc	Specialized medication delivery	–	28
Peptide	RGD	mPEG-b-PDPA	Glioma cells U87MG	Specialized medication delivery	Metastasis into the tumor mass deeply.	29
	cRGD	PEG-SS-PCL	Glioma cells U87MG	Specialized medication delivery	Had fewer downsides and better inhibition of tumor growth in comparison to PEG-SS-PCL that is non-targeting, and its cRGD20/ PEG-PCL equivalents are reduction-insensitive.	30

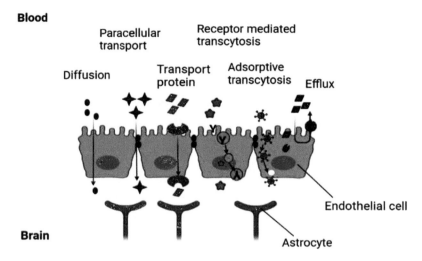

Figure 4.1 Blood–brain barrier transportation.

4.3 Based on Transferrin Targeting

Transferrin, an 80-kilodalton glycoprotein, consists of two identical mono-mers and forms a transmembrane homodimer. Disulfide bonds are formed between each monomer at Cys89 and Cys98, creating a ring structure [33, 34]. The affinity and selectivity of transferrin receptor 1 (TfR1) for binding two molecules of transferrin can reach 105–1010 M21 [35]. Variations in the structural characteristics of cell receptors can have a major impact on the affinity of these receptors for transferrin molecules [36].

To precisely treat mouse gliomas, Zhang created paclitaxel-loaded transferrin-modified polyphosphoester hybrid micelles (TPM). In mice with intracranial U87 MG gliomas, TPM demonstrated improved anti-glioma potency and prolonged life. Due to its highly expressed surface on BBB endothelial cells, transferrin is an attractive option for targeted drug delivery systems to brain tumors [37].

However, transferrin's suitability in designing future brain-specific drug delivery systems is limited due to competition with natural ligands [38]. To overcome the limitations of standard glioblastoma treatments, vincristine/tetrandrine liposomes with Tf modification were created by Song et al. and had anti-inflammatory and anticancer properties [9]. Conjugated transferrin improved BBB transport, cellular uptake, decreased multidrug resistance (MDR), prevented cancer cell invasion, and blocked microvascular channels *in vitro* (VM channels) considerably. Tetrandrine and vincristine liposomes were used in *in vivo* investigations that indicated the anticancer medications' longer half-lives at the location of brain tumors and their high anticancer activity in mice with brain tumors [9].

To increase the bioavailability of bioactive compounds across the BBB, Jain et al. created PLGA nanoparticles (NPs) coated with polysorbate 80 and loaded with methotrexate and transferrin. After being intravenously injected into glioma-bearing albino rats, the nanoparticles demonstrated good penetration and biodistribution, demonstrating better BBB permeability and faster migration to the tumor site. The interaction between polysorbate 80 coating, glioma cells' surface transferrin receptor 1 (TfR1), and transferrin-conjugated nanoparticles contributed to the success of this cancer therapy intervention. These nanoparticles demonstrated good compatibility with various vehicles, low organ toxicity, prolonged release, and ease of adaptability [39].

Drug administration with dual targets can improve the therapeutic index of anticancer medications for brain tumors. Targeting C6 cells and tumors, Qin et al. created liposomes containing paclitaxel with RGD peptide and transferrin (Tf) conjugation. The dual-targeting approach using RGD/TF-liposomes showed promising results for glioma detection and treatment [40].

Resveratrol, a natural chemical with several beneficial properties against tumors, including anti-tumor efficacy, reversal of multidrug resistance (MDR), synergistic activity with conventional anticancer drugs, and low damage to normal tissues, was investigated by Guo et al. Studies using Tf-PEG-PLA-RSV showed that RSV-polymer conjugates reduced tumor volume and increased survival time in C6 glioma-bearing rats, compared to free resveratrol [41]. This method could offer a unique and effective approach for targeted treatment of gliomas using resveratrol as an anti-glioma drug.

Malignant brain gliomas are difficult to treat with chemotherapy because of a number of factors, including poor BBB transport and blood–tumor barrier (BTB) penetration. These restrictions were overcome by Cui, Xu, Chow, Wang, and Wang by creating MNP-MSN-PLGA-Tf nanoparticles that were co-loaded with paclitaxel and DOX that had been modified with transferrin. Magnetic induction of these nanoparticles showed potent anti-glioma action in brain xenografts in BALB/c nude mice. The co-delivery of DOX and paclitaxel in these magnetic nanoparticles under magnetic fields could be a potential strategy for enhancing the therapeutic index of systemic therapy [42].

Transferrin ligands can be utilized for targeting gliomas due to the understanding of the interaction between transferrin and its receptor, as well as the fate of transferrin once it leaves the body. Exploiting nanoscale carriers, anticancer medications may be directed to brain tumors by exploiting transferrin receptor overexpression on malignant cells. Due to the long history of transferrin usage in cancer biology research, this may have therapeutic applications [43].

4.4 Targeting Relying on Lactoferrin

Lactoferrin (Lf), an 80-kDa globular glycoprotein with two lobes, belongs to the family of transferrin glycoproteins [43]. Iron is transported across these cells through the lactoferrin receptor (LfR), which is abundantly expressed on microvascular endothelial cells in the brain and gliomas [44]. Conjugating Lf with a receptor molecule facilitates Lf transcytosis across the blood–brain barrier (BBB) and subsequent endocytic absorption by glioma cells. The expression of cyclin D1 and D4 is likewise inhibited by Lf, which prevents the proliferation of malignant U87MG cells [44]. Lf can therefore act as a glioma therapy as well as an anticancer ligand.

To improve the stability and BBB transport of carmustine (BCNU) for the treatment of glioblastoma multiforme (GBM), Kuo and Cheng created a novel formulation employing solid lipid nanoparticles (SLNs) loaded with tamoxifen (TX) and conjugated with Lf [14]. The penetration of BCNU through the BBB was dramatically increased by almost 10 times when lipids were included in the formulation. Through the use of endocytosis-based drug delivery, *in vitro* experiments also showed higher cellular absorption of the manufactured SLNs.

A pH-responsive prodrug system made up of doxorubicin (DOX), hyaluronic acid (HA), and Lf (Lf-HA-DOX) was created by Yin et al. [18]. The HA-DOX conjugate was made to encourage Lf transport across the BBB. BALB/C mice C6 glioma tumors displayed increased Lf-HA-DOX accumulation in real-time fluorescence imaging. Treatment with Lf-HA-DOX has shown its effectiveness in increasing the delivery of anti-glioma chemotherapy to the location of the brain tumor by dramatically extending survival when compared to the control group.

In a research by Fang et al., lactoferrin (Lf) was utilized as a tether to create dual-modal nanocapsules with complex magnetism [45]. The magnetic nanostructure consisted of hydrophilic core and hydrophobic shell regions encapsulating doxorubicin (Dox) and curcumin (Cur), respectively (Lf-MDCs). The cellular absorption of Lf-receptor overexpressed RG2 glioma cells was enhanced by the application of an external magnetic field and Lf modification. In tumor-bearing mice, intravenous administration of the Lf-MDCs led to considerable accumulation at the tumor site and maximum tumor growth inhibition.

Although liposomes have been considered as a possible anti-cancer medication delivery method, they have shown limited efficacy in brain cancer treatment due to poor BBB penetration. Chen et al. developed doxorubicin-conjugated pro-cationic liposomes (DOX-Lf-PCL) to enhance the therapeutic effectiveness against gliomas [17]. In brain capillary endothelial cells and C6 glioma cells, pro-cationic liposomes and lactoferrin-conjugated pro-cationic liposomes showed enhanced cell uptake. When compared to other therapies, *in vivo* investigations on rats receiving DOX-Lf-PCLs revealed longer longevity, highlighting the potential of this liposomal platform for glioma treatment.

Multidrug resistance (MDR) is a significant challenge in glioma treatment [46]. To solve this problem, Pang et al. created lactoferrin-conjugated polymersomes that included doxorubicin and tetrandrine, a bis-benzylisoquinoline alkaloid that has the ability to reverse MDR [47]. The developed system inhibited MDR with encapsulated tetrandrine while simultaneously targeting the BBB and glioma with the lactoferrin moiety. This strategy demonstrated increased absorption by C6 glioma cells and significant tumor growth suppression in a glioma-bearing rat model.

Lf, when conjugated with nanoparticles or liposomes, can enhance drug delivery to gliomas by utilizing its brain-targeting properties and interaction with glioma cells. Lf has been shown to possess BBB transcytosis and targeting abilities, making it a promising ligand for glioma treatment. Conjugation of Lf to drug delivery vehicles can improve their specificity and enhance medication delivery to glioma cells, potentially enhancing therapeutic effects.

4.5 Based on Folic Acid Targeting

Cascade targeting is a strategic approach that entails the coupling of two ligands to nanocarriers, thereby enhancing the targeting of brain tumors. This method enables more precise localization of brain metastases or the blood–brain barrier (BBB), leading to enhanced drug delivery at the site of the tumor [48–51]. For example, Kuo and Chen developed etoposide-coated PLGA nanoparticles conjugated with lactoferrin (Lf) and folic acid (FA) for enhanced transport through human brain microvascular endothelial cells (HBMECs) and subsequent suppression of U87MG cell proliferation [52]. The study demonstrated an approximately twofold increase in the BBB penetration coefficient of the Lf/FA/PLGA nanoparticles, suggesting improved delivery of etoposide to gliomas. This dual-targeted drug delivery system shows promise as a safe and biodegradable approach for potential clinical trials.

To improve medication accumulation and retention at the tumor site, Niu et al. modified Pluronic P105 polymeric micelles encapsulating doxorubicin (GF-DOX) with a glucose transporter and folic acid [22]. According to the study, GF-DOX is delivered to brain tumors more effectively than in the control group due to enhanced transport across a BBB model. Active targeting of cancer cells was made possible by the nanoparticles' surface coating of the folic acid ligand. An efficient and secure method of chemotherapy for brain tumors involved combining folic acid receptor-mediated endocytosis for active cancer cell targeting with glucose transporter-mediated endocytosis for brain targeting.

Chen et al. created polymersomal GFP-D to improve doxorubicin BBB transit and precisely target glioma cells [53]. The GFP-D formulation was shown to successfully cross the BBB and specifically target cancer cells, highlighting its promise as a means of treating brain tumors.

Using two ligands in conjunction on nanocarriers, cascade targeting, holds promise for overcoming the barriers posed by the BBB and the glioma tumor barrier. By employing this strategy, drugs can be more efficiently delivered to brain tumors, improving treatment options for gliomas and other brain malignancies.

4.6 Targeting using Antibodies

4.6.1 Delivery of drugs

Drug transport via the BBB may be improved by targeting specific delivery mechanisms to the brain's vasculature. Antibodies (AB) are often employed to enhance receptor-mediated transcytosis (RMT), which is crucial when treating brain tumors with therapeutic medicines.

4.6.1.1 Antibody against melanotransferrin

Melanotransferrin on these cells can be precisely targeted with a monoclonal melanotransferrin antibody (MA) on HBMECs [24]. The blood–brain barrier (BBB) may be crossed by MA-TX-ETP-SLNs, which are SLNs with tamoxifen grafted on them and etoposide trapped within. By enabling better contact between SLNs and HBMECs, MA enhances the permeability coefficient of the BBB, encouraging endocytosis activity as a result. This is ascribed to the BBB structure collapsing briefly as a result of surface-attached MA. The flow through the "back door" (MA-TX-ETP-SLN) is increased by the same HBMEC-lipid NP fusion that makes MA possible. It was established that the two factors most significantly affecting the feasibility of HBMEC are control and SLNs. The combination of etoposide (ETP), tamoxifen (TX), and solid lipid nanoparticles (SLNs) is referred to by the abbreviation MA-TX-ETP-SLNs. Due to the enhanced absorption made possible by MA in HBMECs, ETP is more cytotoxic than other ETP-SLNs, but TX slows down the efflux of ETP from cancer cells and shortens ETP's residence time in cells [24].

4.6.1.2 Glucose transporter-1 antibody

Brain tumors were treated with a combination therapy, which included the use of antibodies. This strategy combines two anticancer medications to enhance effectiveness. To effectively treat the GB 3D multicellular model [25], a polymeric micelle-based system was developed using PEG-PE. The system incorporated the anti-glucose transporter-1 (GLUT1) antibody along with doxorubicin (DOX) and curcumin (CUR). GB, a form of cancer, is known for overexpressing a membrane protein called GLUT1. Drugs can reach GBs by focusing on GLUT1, which is located in the plasma membrane of the blood–brain barrier (BBB). The micelles' interaction with GB cells was improved by the inclusion of GLUT1-scFv, a single-chain variable fragment, in a concentration- and time-dependent manner. Steric hindrance was overcome by the presence of more than 0.5% GLUT1-scFv by reducing the cell-associated micelles. Glioblastoma cell nuclei absorbed micelles carrying DOX-GLUT1-scFv similarly to non-targeted micelles. Targeting GLUT-1 has an important impact on lowering the formulation's off-site toxicity.

Moreover, when rhodamine-labeled micelles were tracked, targeted DOXCUR micelles demonstrated superior penetration and distribution as contrasted with untargeted micelles. Models of spheroid, which mimic the 3D architecture of *in vivo* malignancies, were recommended for studying these effects. Non-targeted micelles were hindered in peripheral cells and had limited penetration into deeper layers of the body. In contrast, GLUT-1-targeted micelles easily entered 3D spheroids, overcoming physical barriers and enhancing cell contact. The micelle surface was coated with GLUT-1 scFv, which boosted intracellular drug transport and had a synergistic effect on therapeutic efficacy. The CUR IC50 was considerably lowered by targeting GLUT-1, down from 14.8 to 6.5 M at 0.025 M DOX [54]. In addition, GLUT-1 receptor blockage caused glucose starvation in cancer cells, which resulted in cell death. These findings suggest a novel pathway where glucose uptake in U87MG cells could be hindered. Using scFv instead of total IgG antibodies offers several advantages. The smaller size of GLUT-1 scFv reduces steric hindrance during conjugation with nanoparticles (NPs), resulting in an 81% conjugation yield, higher than the 65%–70% obtained with whole IgG antibodies [25].

4.6.1.3 Prominin-1 antibody

Another antibody, anti-CD133 (antiprominin-1), was employed in combination treatment for GBM. CD133 is a glycoprotein that may protect the cell membrane topology. It is overexpressed on glioblastoma stem cells' (GSCs) outside, which are seen in brain tumors. Anti-CD133 was used in liposomes containing gemcitabine and bevacizumab (GEM-BV-L) to target GSCs using this protein [55]. It was determined that each liposome contained 15 anti-CD133 antibodies. An anti-CD133 coupled to a non-targeted GEM-L dramatically suppressed GSC formation, according to *in vitro* experiments. Anti-CD133-GEM-L formulation also reduced endogenous neovascularization in host mouse. After intravenous injection of GSC tumor xenografts into BALB/c nude mice, tumor volume was evaluated to assess the anticancer efficacy of the anti-CD133-GEM-BV-L therapy. After 55 days of treatment, non-targeted GEM-BV-L tumor sizes were over 1000 mm^3, but those treated with anti-CD133-GEM-BV-L had tumor volumes of approximately 250 mm^3. Anti-CD133 antibodies that were conjugated to GEM-encapsulated liposomes dramatically increased the ability of GSCs to inhibit cell proliferation. Furthermore, targeting GSCs with anti-CD133-GEM-L led to a reduction in the dosage of bevacizumab required to achieve the same antiangiogenesis effect compared to non-targeted GEM-L [55].

4.6.1.4 Interleukin-13 receptor

Interleukin-13 (IL-13) has two types of receptors, IL-13/4R and IL-13Ra2, one of which is present in healthy cells and the other in high-grade astrocytomas, often known as GBM. The IL-13Ra2 receptor is overexpressed in many GBs, according to recent studies [56, 57]. The IL-13Ra2 receptor can be used to deliver anticancer drugs to a variety of brain cancers as a result of its upregulation. The absence of detectable IL-13Ra2 in normal cells, which do not overexpress the IL-13 receptor, is consistent with the lack of uptake shown when healthy cells were exposed to IL-13-targeted DOX-encapsulated liposomes for the same exposure duration. On the other hand, when IL-13-targeted liposomes were exposed to U251 glioma cells, the intrinsic fluorescence of DOX demonstrates that it was substantially more accumulated and retained inside cells as compared to cells exposed to free DOX or non-targeted DOX-liposomes. The greater cytotoxicity shown with IL-13-targeted liposomes may be explained by the better doxorubicin absorption and retention in glioma cells. Furthermore, when comparing IL-13-targeted liposomes to non-targeted DOX-liposomes, *in vivo* experiments showed a 500% reduction in tumor volume [56]. Targeting the IL-13 receptor with DOX-liposomes significantly reduced the number of brain tumors in nude

U87 xenograft mice [58]. Therefore, IL-13 receptor-targeted nanovesicles could be utilized for specific drug delivery to GB.

4.6.2 Tumor imaging

Histology is currently the only technique available for accurately diagnosing glioblastoma in patients, which can be divided into mesenchymal, proneural, neural, and classical kinds. However, each of these subtypes has distinct molecular markers and weaknesses that are relevant to treatment approaches [59].

In the treatment of glioblastoma, patients typically undergo surgery as the initial treatment, followed by radiation therapy and chemotherapy. Molecular imaging using nanotechnology and biomarkers holds promise in addressing the current therapeutic challenges. This approach enables the identification of specific glioma subtypes, allowing for the development of customized treatment strategies tailored to individual patients. To facilitate this technique, an effective contrast agent and a suitable targeting molecule are necessary. In this article, researchers discuss the successful application of antibodies (ABs) linked to targeted imaging compounds for glioblastoma [60].

4.6.2.1 Heat shock protein 70 antibody

Antibodies such as cmHsp70.1 have been utilized to visualize gliomas by binding to the 72-kDa heat shock protein Hsp70. This protein is expressed in high-grade gliomas, distinguishing them from healthy cells of the same type [61]. Membrane Hsp70 (mHsp70) is a viable candidate for brain targeting because of its quick internalization into tumor cells. Superparamagnetic iron oxide nanoparticles (SPIONs) were coupled with cmHsp70.1, resulting in SPION-cmHsp70.1, to enable magnetic resonance imaging (MRI).

Studies have demonstrated that SPION-cmHsp70.1 exhibits dose-dependent selectivity for both benign and malignant cells. In glioma-bearing mice, tumors absorbed more SPION-cmHsp70.1 than a healthy brain tissue, according to biodistribution studies. Additionally, SPION-cmHsp70.1 accumulation was improved after gliomas that expressed Hsp70 received a single dose of ionizing radiation (10 Gy) to test if they would respond. However, because SPION-cmHsp70.1 was only taken up by living cells and the necrotic alterations brought on by the increased radiation dosage were restricted to the nucleus, increasing the radiation dose to 20 Gy had no additional impact on absorption. Since brain tumors are radiosensitive, combining radiation with Hsp70-targeted medications works better since it encourages the magnetic complex's quick growth. Moreover, the development of cmHsp70.1

conjugates has facilitated the quantification of Hsp70 in biological fluids using a highly sensitive NMR technique, detecting concentrations as low as 5 pg/mL. The ability of SPION-cmHsp70.1 to detect gliomas may open doors to innovative therapeutic approaches [61].

4.6.2.2 IgG type I receptor for epidermal growth factor

Glioblastoma (GBM) and other malignancies, notably those with overexpression and activation of the epidermal growth factor receptor (EGFR), have been related. This association provides enhanced surgical contrast for tumor identification because it is possible to distinguish clearly between the margins of tumors and the surrounding normal tissue when using EGFR-targeted near-infrared (NIR) fluorescent dyes. Effective imaging agents such as AntiEGFRcany, when combined with fluorescent and radio-labeled nanomaterials, have proven productive for imaging purposes [62].

Anti-EGFR antibodies may be used to target GB cells using polymeric nanoscale imaging agents (NIAs) based on poly(L-malic acid). These anti-EGFR antibody-containing NIAs can cross the blood–brain barrier (BBB) and target cancer cells in particular, enabling more precise imaging of malignancies [63]. Utilizing anti-EGFR on NIAs, it may be possible to differentiate between brain metastases and other separate lesions, such as primary brain tumors, on MRI. EGFR-targeting NIAs demonstrate longer-lasting and more gradual side effects compared to non-targeted NIAs. According to biodistribution studies, tumor cells encircled by blood vessels exhibit a large buildup of the contrast agent, whereas blood arteries only exhibit a trace quantity of non-targeted NIA [63].

For targeted imaging of glioblastoma, the utilization of an anti-EGFR antibody-like AbB (panitumumab) in association with nanoparticles (NPs) such as AuNPs has been explored, taking advantage of the NPs' surface-enhanced Raman scattering (SERS) characteristics. SERS-NPs offer greater photostability than fluorescent dyes, making them ideal for applications requiring permanent surgical procedures. Panitumumab, a potent GB-targeting medication, has been found to identify overlapping epitopes in the human EGFR's EC3 region. Through MRI-guided transcranial focused ultrasound (TcMRgFUS) and SERS imaging, the blood–brain barrier may be crossed by 50 nm AuNPs coated with polyethylene glycol (PEG), allowing them to enter the healthy brain parenchyma. TcMRgFUS may rupture the BBB, which allows anti-EGFR AB in combination with AuNPs to target the tumor location (anti-EGFR-SERS-NPs). Studies on cells showed that anti-EGFR-SERS-NPs were distributed intracellularly in a perinuclear manner, primarily in multivesicular structures. Anti-EGFR-SERS-NPs showed preferential absorption by GB cells in the brain parenchyma as compared to PEG-SERS NPs. Anti-EGFR-SERS-NPs were specifically localized in the brain parenchyma around the tumor, according to *in vivo* distribution studies [64]. Notably, compared to earlier research using non-targeted SERS-NPs to scan tumors in mouse brains, this novel approach needed around 20 times less NPs (per gram of body weight) [65].

Another type of NP that can be utilized for anti-EGFR imaging of GB is superparamagnetic iron oxide nanoparticles (SPIONs) [66]. Conjugates of anti-EGFR-SPIONs were found to exhibit superior BBB transport and tumor retention compared to non-targeted SPIONs in rats when administered intravenously. The anti-EGFR-SPIONs were visible in MRIs 24 hours after injection, with increasing signal intensity at 48 hours. Importantly, anti-EG-FR-SPIONs were specifically observed in the cytoplasm of tumor cells and not in a healthy tissue [66]. Magnetic targeting techniques demonstrated a significant increase in NP accumulation within tumors, owing to the highly magnetically sensitive iron oxide core of SPIONs [67].

Conjugated iron oxide nanoparticles (IONPs) coated with domain-1 recombinant epidermal growth factor (EGF1) generated from human coagulation factor VII have also proved successful in achieving targeted magnetic resonance imaging (MRI) of gliomas. EGF1-EGFP-IONPs showed high specificity and enhanced MR contrast in U87MG glioma tissue with positive tissue factor expression. Understanding the subtypes of gliomas can lead to improved treatment strategies for patients with brain tumors, encompassing molecular imaging, targeted therapy, and therapeutic monitoring [62]. However, the presence of EGFRvIII, a mutant variant of the protein, poses considerable challenges during MRI. Biopsy confirmation and molecular data are often required due to the association of EGFRvIII, a constitutively active mutation, with increased invasiveness and resistance. Labeling components such as near-infrared quantum dots (Qd800) can be used with a monoclonal antibody against EGFRvIII (EGFRvIIIsd) to enhance Qd800 internalization in U87MG-EGFRvIII cells. Studies conducted in both the lab and on animals have demonstrated that EGFRvIIIsd-Qd800 is superior to EGFRhFc-Qd800. Furthermore, it is hypothesized that the use of near-infrared Qdots as contrast agents will increase the effectiveness of EGFRvIIIsd targeting [60].

4.6.2.3 Vascular endothelial growth factor

High-grade gliomas exhibit necrosis and hypoxia, encouraging the synthesis of vascular endothelial growth factor (VEGF) and angiogenesis [68]. Increased development of tumor blood vessels is a result of VEGF buildup in the tumor [69]. Macromolecules and nanoparticles can enter the brain through the BBB, especially in tumor-containing areas [70]. VEGF-BSA-MNPs can enhance MRI angiography for the early detection of glioma microvessels, with specific accumulation in VEGF-positive cells and active neoangiogenesis [71].

4.6.3 Gene delivery

Gene therapy using antibodies is a successful method for treating malignant tumor [72]. *In vitro* studies demonstrated improved apoptosis and cell death in glioblastoma cells (U87MG and LN229) while employing human serum albumin nanoparticles that contain certain microRNA plasmids targeted at the survivin inhibitor protein and mHsp70 antibody (cmHsp70.1). Compared to control antibody and non-targeted nanoparticles, cells showed enhanced receptivity to cmHsp70.1 antibody-conjugated nanoparticles, causing an increase in caspase 3/7 activation and a reduction in the survival of clonogenic cells. These findings support the use of cmHsp70.1 antibody-targeted nanoparticles as promising gene carriers for specific targeting of cancer cells [72].

4.6.4 Radiotherapy

NPs with an AB could be utilized to treat GBs in addition to other methods, such as the delivery of genes or targeted therapy.

4.6.4.1 Epidermal growth factor receptor antibody

In cases of radioresistant glioblastomas (GBs), the use of EGFR-targeting nanoparticles (NPs) has shown promising results in increasing radiosensitivity [73]. A specific subgroup of GB patients expressing the mutant EGFR, known as EGFRvIII, can exhibit resistance to radiation and chemotherapy. Various mechanisms contribute to this resistance and include better DNA double-strand break repair after radiation treatment, increased cell proliferation, and antiapoptotic effects [73, 74].

Iron oxide nanoparticles (IONPs) can be combined with the well-known recombinant monoclonal antibody cetuximab (Erbitux, IMC-C225), which targets EGFRvIII, to deliver NPs directly to the tumor location. Studies employing EGFRvIII-expressing human glioblastoma multiforme (GBM) cells and healthy astrocytes have showed promise for cetuximab-IONPs. The astrocytes were not appreciably affected by single or fractionated radiation after the cetuximab-IONPs had been removed after 24 hours. When paired with radiation, cetuximab-IONPs enhanced EGFR internalization and disrupted EGFR cell signaling, which increased apoptosis. Cetuximab has been shown to enhance radiosensitivity in GBM due to its effects on apoptosis, cell proliferation, and radiation-induced damage repair [75]. Additionally, it has been demonstrated that increased levels of untargeted IONPs can also radiosensitize recurrent GBM [76].

Cetuximab-IONPs have demonstrated stronger tumor-fighting effectiveness than cetuximab by itself or free IONPs. The concentration of free IONPs was 100 times lower when cetuximab was conjugated to them [76]. Cetuximab-IONPs, which enhance EGFR cell uptake and inhibit the EGFR signaling pathway, have been found to be more effective than conventional treatments in inducing GBM cell death [77]. Furthermore, cetuximab-IONPs have been shown to impair DNA double-strand break repair when exposed to radiation. In investigations of GBM cells, when compared to pre-IR treatments with free IONPs or cetuximab alone, the cetuximab-IONPs therapy dramatically enhanced intracellular reactive oxygen species (ROS) generation. The cytotoxicity induced by cetuximab-IONPs was found to be mediated by protein and DNA damage [77].

In mice with aggressive, radioresistant GBM xenografts, cetuximab-IONPs have been shown to improve radiosensitivity. Compared to therapy with cetuximab alone, cetuximab-IONPs greatly increased animal survival rates and decreased tumor development [73]. These findings suggest that EGFR-targeting NPs, such as cetuximab-IONPs, hold promise as a strategy to enhance the effectiveness of radiation therapy in radioresistant GBs.

4.7 Peptide-based Targeting

A new targeted delivery strategy has been developed keeping this in mind, in an effort to boost its penetration into tumors and successfully cross the BBB. Some studies showed that peptides were more effective at penetrating the brain than ABs [78].

4.7.1 Delivery of drugs

4.7.1.1 RGD peptide

Scientists have developed a targeted drug delivery strategy using specific tumor-triggered, programmable, worm-like micelles to treat gliomas, a particular kind of brain tumor [29]. Methoxy poly(ethylene glycol) block poly(2-diisopropyl methacrylate) and bio-reducible (RGDfK) make up these micelles. Conjugated C peptides, which are pH-sensitive, can deliver cytotoxic emtansine (DM1) to the tumor site [29]. The micelles, known as RNW, exhibit pinpoint targeting, profound tumor penetration, and effective absorption of glioma cells.

Another targeting approach involves cyclic RGD (cRGD), which is a method for precise drug delivery to glioblastomas (GBs) [30, 78]. Micelles with a biodegradable intracellular shell composed of tocopherol-stabilized poly(caprolactone)-poly(ethylene glycol) (PEG-SS-PCL) and cRGD release the drug more efficiently, suppress tumor growth, and minimize adverse effects in xenograft models of GB [30]. Similar to this, it was demonstrated that docetaxel-loaded c(RGDyK)/DTX-PLA-PEG micelles accumulated in brain tumor tissues, inhibited tumor growth, and stopped the formation of tumors without causing any negative effects [79, 80].

Combining targeting peptides, such as RGD and interleukin-13 (IL-13), can enhance GB delivery efficacy. RGD-IL-13-functionalized nanoparticles exhibited improved cellular uptake and penetration of tumor spheroids, outperforming mono-modified nanoparticles in delivering their payload to GBMs [81]. Additionally, the inclusion of a "helper" peptide, such as the TH peptide, which can facilitate escape from lysosomes in endothelial cells, potentially improves the ability of cRGD-targeted nanocarriers to penetrate glioma cores and cross the BBB [82, 83].

Studies conducted *in vitro* and *in vivo* have shown that these targeted delivery methods are effective at eliminating cancer stem cells, vascular mimicry channels, and glioma cells, among other things, and improving treatment efficacy in brain gliomas [82, 83]. The medication paclitaxel (PTX) was encapsulated in cRGD-TH liposomes (cRGD-TH-Lip), which offered hope for lowering the dangers of unchecked blood–brain barrier leakage and boosting both *in vitro* and *in vivo* therapeutic effectiveness [82, 83].

These studies demonstrate the potential of peptide-based targeted drug delivery systems to increase penetration of brain tumors, increase therapeutic effectiveness, and reduce side effects.

4.8 Conclusion

Precision plays a pivotal role in various techniques used for treating individuals with brain tumors. Molecular characterization of brain cancers has significantly advanced. However, there is still a delay between discoveries and the implementation of improved targeted therapies for brain tumors, which could enhance patient outcomes. Considering that malignant brain tumors are relatively uncommon compared to other cancers, the progress of clinical trials focusing on tailored nanomedicines for targeted treatment has been hindered by a limited number of participants. Achieving targeted brain tumor treatment with tailored nanomedicine may be feasible if patients' tumor molecular profiles are prepared but only for carefully selected individuals with specific molecular routes or targets. To conduct experiments in human medicine using precise methods of administration, information on the various types of brain tumors and several biological variables is required. The creation of tailored medication delivery systems for the treatment of brain tumors can overcome these issues, which would expedite clinical trials. For successful clinical trials involving malignant brain tumors, patients and samples must be prepared for genetic and molecular analysis. Findings from other studies can be utilized to design more precise and logical trials for brain tumor treatment. While there are apparent obstacles in the path toward glioma-focused treatment, if the medical community works together to enhance patient outcomes, they are not insurmountable.

References

[1] Reygagne, E., Du Boisgueheneuc, F., & Berger, A. Brain metastases: Focal treatment (surgery and radiation therapy) and cognitive consequences. *Bulletin du Cancer*, **2017**, *104*(4), 344–355

[2] Reardon, D.A., & Mitchell, D.A. The development of dendritic cell vaccine-based immunotherapies for glioblastoma. Paper presented at the Seminars in Immunopathology, **2017**.

[3] Mehdorn, H. M., Schwartz, F., & Becker, J. (2017). Awake craniotomy for tumor resection: Further optimizing therapy of brain tumors. *Trends in Reconstructive Neurosurgery*, **2017**, 309–313

[4] Preusser, M., & Marosi, C. Neuro-oncology in 2016: Advances in brain Tumor classification and therapy. *Nature Reviews Neurology*, **2017**, *13*(2), 71–72

[5] Lee, D., Ryu, H., Won, H., & Kwon, S. Advances in epigenetic glioblastoma therapy. *Oncotarget*, **2017**, *8*(11), 18577–18589.

[6] Lin, L., Cai, J., & Jiang, C. Recent advances in targeted therapy for glioma. *Current Medicinal Chemistry*, **2016**, *24* (13), 1365–1381

[7] Polivka, J., Holubec, L., Kubikova, T., Priban, V., Hes, O., Pivovarcikova, K., & Treskova, I. Advances in experimental targeted therapy and immunotherapy for patients with glioblastoma multiforme. *Anticancer Research*, **2017**, *37*(1), 21–33.

[8] Birk, H. S., Han, S. J., & Butowski, N. A. (2017). Treatment options for recurrent high-grade gliomas. *CNS Oncology*, **2017**, *6*(1), 61–70.

[9] Song, X.-I, Liu, S., Jiang, Y., Gu, L.-y, Xiao, Y., Wang, X., ... Li, X.-t. Targeting vincristine plus tetrandrine liposomes modified with

DSPE-PEG 2000-transferrin in the treatment of brain glioma. *European Journal of Pharmaceutical Sciences*, **2017**, *96*, 129–140.

[10] Li, S., Amat, D., Peng, Z., Vanni, S., Raskin, S., De Angulo, G., ... Leblanc, R.M. (2016). Transferrin conjugated nontoxic carbon dots for doxorubicin delivery to target pediatric brain tumor cells. *Nanoscale*, **2016**, *8*(37), 16662–16669.

[11] Salzano, G., Zappavigna, S., Luce, A., D'Onofrio, N., Balestrieri, M., Grimaldi, A., ... Porru, M. Transferrin-targeted nanoparticles containing zoledronic acid as a potential tool to inhibit glioblastoma growth. *Journal of Biomedical Nanotechnology*, **2016**, *12*(4), 811–830.

[12] Gao, S., Li, J., Jiang, C., Hong, B., & Hao, B. Plasmid pORF-hTRAIL targeting to glioma using transferrinmodified polyamidoamine dendrimer. *Drug Design, Development and Therapy*, **2016**, *10*, 1.

[13] Sonali, Agrawal, P., Singh, R.P., Rajesh, C.V., Singh, S., Vijayakumar, M.R., ... Muthu, M.S. Transferrin receptor-targeted vitamin E TPGS micelles for brain cancer therapy: Preparation, characterization and brain distribution in rats. *Drug Delivery*, **2016**, *23*(5), 1788–1798.

[14] Kuo, Y.-C., & Cheng, S.-J. Brain targeted delivery of carmustine using solid lipid nanoparticles modified with tamoxifen and lactoferrin for antitumor proliferation. *International Journal of Pharmaceutics*, **2016**, *499*(1), 10–19

[15] Tomitaka, A., Arami, H., Gandhi, S., & Krishnan, K.M. Lactoferrin conjugated iron oxide nanoparticles for targeting brain glioma cells in magnetic particle imaging. *Nanoscale*, **2015**, *7*(40), 16890–16898

[16] Zhou, Q., Mu, K., Jiang, L., Xie, H., Liu, W., Li, Z., ... Zhu, Y. Glioma-targeting micelles for optical/magnetic resonance dual-mode imaging. *International Journal of Nanomedicine*, **2015**, *10*, 1805.

[17] Chen, H., Qin, Y., Zhang, Q., Jiang, W., Tang, L., Liu, J., & He, Q. Lactoferrin modified doxorubicin-loaded procationic liposomes for the treatment of gliomas. *European Journal of Pharmaceutical Sciences*, **2011**, *44*(1), 164–173.

[18] Yin, Y., Fu, C., Li, M., Li, X., Wang, M., He, L., ... Peng, Y. A pH-sensitive hyaluronic acid prodrug modified with lactoferrin for glioma dual-targeted treatment. *Materials Science and Engineering: C*, **2016**, *67*, 159–169.

[19] Wang, X., Tu, M., Tian, B., Yi, Y., Wei, Z., & Wei, F. Synthesis of tumor-targeted folate conjugated fluorescent magnetic albumin nanoparticles for enhanced intracellular dual-modal imaging into human brain tumor cells. *Analytical Biochemistry*, **2016**, *512*, 8–17

[20] Xu, X., Li, J., Han, S., Tao, C., Fang, L., Sun, Y., ... Li, F. A novel doxorubicin loaded folic acid conjugated PAMAM modified with borneol, a

nature dual-functional product of reducing PAMAM toxicity and boosting BBB penetration. *European Journal of Pharmaceutical Sciences*, **2016**, *88*, 178–190.

[21] Agrawal, U., Chashoo, G., Sharma, P. R., Kumar, A., Saxena, A.K., & Vyas, S. Tailored polymerlipid hybrid nanoparticles for the delivery of drug conjugate: Dual strategy for brain targeting. *Colloids and Surfaces B: Biointerfaces*, **2015**, *126*, 414–425.

[22] Niu, J., Wang, A., Ke, Z., & Zheng, Z. Glucose transporter and folic acid receptor-mediated Pluronic P105 polymeric micelles loaded with doxorubicin for brain tumor treating. *Journal of Drug Targeting*, **2014**, *22*(8), 712–723

[23] Dong, S., Cho, H.J., Lee, Y.W., & Roman, M. Synthesis and cellular uptake of folic acid-conjugated cellulose nanocrystals for cancer targeting. *Biomacromolecules*, **2014**, *15*(5), 1560–1567.

[24] Kuo, Y.-C., & Wang, I. H. Enhanced delivery of etoposide across the bloodbrain barrier to restrain brain tumor growth using melanotransferrin antibody- and tamoxifen-conjugated solid lipid nanoparticles. *Journal of Drug Targeting*, **2016**, *24*(7), 645–654. Available from https://doi.org/10.3109/1061186X.2015.1132223

[25] Sarisozen, C., Dhokai, S., Tsikudo, E.G., Luther, E., Rachman, I.M., & Torchilin, V.P. Nanomedicine based curcumin and doxorubicin combination treatment of glioblastoma with scFv-targeted micelles: *In vitro* evaluation on 2D and 3D tumor models. *European Journal of Pharmaceutics and Biopharmaceutics*, **2016**, *108*, 54–67. Available from https://doi.org/10.1016/j.ejpb.2016.08.013.

[26] Shin, D.H., Lee, S.-J., Kim, J.S., Ryu, J.-H., & Kim, J.-S. Synergistic effect of immunoliposomal gemcitabine and bevacizumab in glioblastoma stem cell-targeted therapy. *Journal of Biomedical Nanotechnology*, **2015**, *11*(11), 1989–2002. Available from https://doi.org/10.1166/jbn.2015.2146

[27] Guo, J., Gao, X., Su, L., Xia, H., Gu, G., Pang, Z., ... Chen, H. Aptamer-functionalized PEG-PLGA nanoparticles for enhanced anti-glioma drug delivery. *Biomaterials*, **2011**, *32*(31), 8010–8020. Available from https://doi.org/10.1016/j.biomaterials.2011.07.004.

[28] Luo, Z., Yan, Z., Jin, K., Pang, Q., Jiang, T., Lu, H., ... Jiang, X. Precise glioblastoma targeting by AS1411 aptamer-functionalized poly (l-gamma-glutamylglutamine)-paclitaxel nanoconjugates. *Journal of Colloid and Interface Science*, **2017**, *490*, 783–796. Available from https://doi.org/10.1016/j.jcis.2016.12.004.

[29] Zeng, L., Zou, L., Yu, H., He, X., Cao, H., Zhang, Z., ... Li, Y. Treatment of malignant brain tumor by tumor-triggered programmed

wormlike micelles with precise targeting and deep penetration. *Advanced Functional Materials*, **2016**, *26*(23), 4201–4212. Available from https://doi.org/10.1002/adfm.201600642

[30] Zhu, Y., Zhang, J., Meng, F., Deng, C., Cheng, R., Feijen, J., & Zhong, Z. \ cRGD-functionalized reductionsensitive shell-sheddable biodegradable micelles mediate enhanced doxorubicin delivery to human glioma xenografts *in vivo*. *Journal of Controlled Release*, **2016**, *233*, 29–38. Available from https://doi.org/10.1016/j. jconrel.2016.05.014.

[31] Reynolds, J.L., & Mahato, R.I. Nanomedicines for the Treatment of CNS Diseases. *Journal of Neuroimmune Pharmacology*, **2017**, *12*(1), 1–5.

[32] Nguyen, K., Pham, M., Vo, T., Duan, W., Tran, P., & Thao, T. Strategies of engineering nanoparticles for treating neurodegenerative disorders. *Current Drug Metabolism*, **2017**, *18*, 1–12.

[33] Wadajkar, A.S., Dancy, J.G., Hersh, D.S., Anastasiadis, P., Tran, N.L., Woodworth, G.F., ... Kim, A.J. Tumor-targeted nanotherapeutics: Overcoming treatment barriers for glioblastoma. *Wiley Interdisciplinary Reviews: Nanomedicine and Nanobiotechnology,* **2016.**

[34] Lopes, A.M., Chen, K.Y., & Kamei, D.T. A transferrin variant as the targeting ligand for polymeric nanoparticles incorporated in 3-D PLGA porous scaffolds. *Materials Science and Engineering: C*, **2017**, *73*, 373–380

[35] Sun, H., Li, H., & Sadler, P.J. Transferrin as a metal ion mediator. *Chemical Reviews*, **1999**, 99(9), 2817–2842.

[36] Cheng, Y., Zak, O., Aisen, P., Harrison, S.C., & Walz, T. Structure of the human transferrin receptortransferrin complex. *Cell*, **2004**, *116*(4), 565–576

[37] Zhang, P., Hu, L., Yin, Q., Zhang, Z., Feng, L., & Li, Y. Transferrin-conjugated polyphosphoester hybrid micelle loading paclitaxel for brain-targeting delivery: Synthesis, preparation and *in vivo* evaluation. *Journal of Controlled Release*, **2012**, *159*(3), 429–434

[38] Zhang, H., Hou, L., Jiao, X., Ji, Y., Zhu, X., & Zhang, Z. Transferrin-mediated fullerenes nanoparticles as Fe 2 1 -dependent drug vehicles for synergistic anti-tumor efficacy. *Biomaterials*, **2015**, *37*, 353–366

[39] Jain, A., Jain, A., Garg, N.K., Tyagi, R.K., Singh, B., Katare, O.P., ... Soni, V. Surface engineered polymeric nanocarriers mediate the delivery of transferrinmethotrexate conjugates for an improved understanding of brain cancer. *Acta Biomaterialia*, **2015**, *24*, 140–151

[40] Qin, L., Wang, C.Z., Fan, H.J., Zhang, C.J., Zhang, H.W., Lv, M.H., & Cui, S.D. A dual-targeting liposome conjugated with transferrin and

arginine-glycine-aspartic acid peptide for glioma-targeting therapy. *Oncology Letters*, **2014**, *8*(5), 2000–2006

[41] Guo, W., Li, A., Jia, Z., Yuan, Y., Dai, H., & Li, H. Transferrin modified PEG-PLA-resveratrol conjugates: *In vitro* and *in vivo* studies for glioma. *European Journal of Pharmacology*, **2013**, *718*(1), 41–47

[42] Cui, Y., Xu, Q., Chow, P.K.-H., Wang, D., & Wang, C.-H. Transferrin-conjugated magnetic silica PLGA nanoparticles loaded with doxorubicin and paclitaxel for brain glioma treatment. *Biomaterials*, **2013**, *34*(33), 8511–8520

[43] Roy, K., Kanwar, R.K., & Kanwar, J.R. (2015). Molecular targets in arthritis and recent trends in nanotherapy. *International Journal of Nanomedicine*, **2013**, *10*, 5407.

[44] Roy, K., Patel, Y.S., Kanwar, R.K., Rajkhowa, R., Wang, X., & Kanwar, J.R. Biodegradable Eri silk nanoparticles as a delivery vehicle for bovine lactoferrin against MDA-MB-231 and MCF-7 breast cancer cells. *International Journal of Nanomedicine*, **2016**, *11*, 25.

[45] Fang, J.H., Lai, Y.H., Chiu, T.L., Chen, Y.Y., Hu, S. H., & Chen, S.Y. Magnetic coreshell nanocapsules with dual-targeting capabilities and co-delivery of multiple drugs to treat brain gliomas. *Advanced Healthcare Materials*, **2014**, *3*(8), 1250–1260

[46] Bender, H.R., Kane, S., & Zabel, M.D. Delivery of therapeutic siRNA to the CNS using cationic and anionic liposomes. *JoVE (Journal of Visualized Experiments)*, **2016**, *113*, e54106–e54106.

[47] Pang, Z., Gao, H., Yu, Y., Guo, L., Chen, J., Pan, S., ... Jiang, X. Enhanced intracellular delivery and chemotherapy for glioma rats by transferrin-conjugated biodegradable polymersomes loaded with doxorubicin. *Bioconjug Chem*, **2011**, *22*(6), 1171–1180.

[48] Legrand, D., Pierce, A., Elass, E., Carpentier, M., Mariller, C., & Mazurier, J. Lactoferrin structure and functions. *Bioactive components of milk*, **2008**, 163–194.

[49] Yi, Y.-S. Folate receptor-targeted diagnostics and therapeutics for inflammatory diseases. *Immune Network*, **2016**, *16*(6), 337–343.

[50] Gupta, A., Kaur, C.D., Saraf, S., & Saraf, S. Targeting of herbal bioactives through folate receptors: A novel concept to enhance intracellular drug delivery in cancer therapy. *Journal of Receptors and Signal Transduction*, **2017**, 110.

[51] Xu, X., Li, J., Han, S., Tao, C., Fang, L., Sun, Y., ... Li, F. A novel doxorubicin loaded folic acid conjugated PAMAM modified with borneol, a nature dual-functional product of reducing PAMAM toxicity and boosting BBB penetration. *European Journal of Pharmaceutical Sciences*, **2016**, *88*, 178–190.

[52] Kuo, Y.-C., & Chen, Y.-C. Targeting delivery of etoposide to inhibit the growth of human glioblastoma multiforme using lactoferrin-and folic acid-grafted poly (lactide-co-glycolide) nanoparticles. *International Journal of Pharmaceutics*, **2015**, *479*(1), 138–149.

[53] Chen, Y.-C., Chiang, C.-F., Chen, L.-F., Liang, P.-C., Hsieh, W.-Y., & Lin, W.-L. Polymersomes conjugated with des-octanoyl ghrelin and folate as a BBB-penetrating cancer cell-targeting delivery system. *Biomaterials*, **2014**, *35*(13), 4066–4081

[54] Shibuya, K., Okada, M., Suzuki, S., Seino, M., Seino, S., Takeda, H., & Kitanaka, C. Targeting the facilitative glucose transporter GLUT1 inhibits the self-renewal and tumor-initiating capacity of cancer stem cells. *Oncotarget*, **2015**, *6*(2), 651–661. Available from https://doi.org/10.18632/oncotarget.2892

[55] Shin, D.H., Lee, S.-J., Kim, J.S., Ryu, J.-H., & Kim, J.-S. Synergistic effect of immunoliposomal gemcitabine and bevacizumab in glioblastoma stem cell-targeted therapy. *Journal of Biomedical Nanotechnology*, **2015**, *11*(11), 1989–2002. Available from https://doi.org/10.1166/jbn.2015.2146

[56] Madhankumar, A.B., Slagle-Webb, B., Mintz, A., Sheehan, J.M., & Connor, J.R. Interleukin-13 receptortargeted nanovesicles are a potential therapy for glioblastoma multiforme. *Molecular Cancer Therapeutics*, **2006**, *5* (12), 3162–3169. Available from https://doi.org/10.1158/1535-7163.mct-06-0480.

[57] Moretti, I.F., Silva, R., Oba-Shinjo, S.M., Carvalho, P.O.D., Cardoso, L.C., Castro, I.d, & Marie, S.K.N. The impact of interleukin-13 receptor expressions in cell migration of astrocytomas. *MedicalExpress*, **2015**, 2.

[58] Madhankumar, A.B., Slagle-Webb, B., Wang, X., Yang, Q.X., Antonetti, D.A., Miller, P.A., ... Connor, J.R. Efficacy of interleukin-13 receptor-targeted liposomal doxorubicin in the intracranial brain tumor model. *Molecular Cancer Therapeutics*, **2009**, *8*(3), 648–654. Available from https://doi.org/10.1158/1535-7163.mct-08- 0853.

[59] Marziali, G., Signore, M., Buccarelli, M., Grande, S., Palma, A., Biffoni, M., ... Ricci-Vitiani, L. Metabolic/ proteomic signature defines two glioblastoma subtypes with different clinical outcome. *Scientific Reports*, **2016**, *6*, 21557. Available from https://doi.org/10.1038/srep21557. Available from http://www.nature.com/articles/srep21557#supplementary-information

[60] Fatehi, D., Baral, T.N., & Abulrob, A. *In vivo* imaging of brain cancer using epidermal growth factor single domain antibody bioconjugated to near-infrared quantum dots. *Journal of Nanoscience and Nanotechnology*, **2014**, *14*(7), 5355–5362.

[61] Shevtsov, M.A., Nikolaev, B.P., Ryzhov, V.A., Yakovleva, L.Y., Marchenko, Y.Y., Parr, M.A., ... Multhoff, G. Ionizing radiation improves glioma-specific targeting of superparamagnetic iron oxide nanoparticles conjugated with cmHsp70.1 monoclonal antibodies (SPION-cmHsp70.1). *Nanoscale*, **2015**, *7*(48), 20652–20664. Available from https://doi.org/10.1039/C5NR06521F

[62] Liu, H., Chen, X., Xue, W., Chu, C., Liu, Y., Tong, H., ... Zhang, W. Recombinant epidermal growth factor-like domain-1 from coagulation factor VII functionalized iron oxide nanoparticles for targeted glioma magnetic resonance imaging. *International Journal of Nanomedicine*, **2016**, *11*, 5099–5108. Available from https://doi. org/10.2147/IJN. S116980.

[63] Patil, R., Ljubimov, A.V., Gangalum, P.R., Ding, H., Portilla-Arias, J., Wagner, S., ... Ljubimova, J.Y. MRI virtual biopsy and treatment of brain metastatic tumors with targeted nanobioconjugates: Nanoclinic in the brain. *ACS Nano*, **2015**, *9*(5), 5594–5608. Available from https://doi. org/10.1021/acsnano.5b01872.

[64] Diaz, R.J., McVeigh, P.Z., O'Reilly, M.A., Burrell, K., Bebenek, M., Smith, C., ... Rutka, J.T. Focused ultrasound delivery of Raman nanoparticles across the blood-brain barrier: Potential for targeting experimental brain tumors. *Nanomedicine: Nanotechnology, Biology and Medicine*, **2014**, *10*(5), e1075–e1087. Available from https://doi.org/10.1016/j. nano.2013.12.006.

[65] Kircher, M.F., de la Zerda, A., Jokerst, J.V., Zavaleta, C.L., Kempen, P.J., Mittra, E., ... Gambhir, S.S. A brain tumor molecular imaging strategy using a new triple-modality MRI-photoacoustic-Raman nanoparticle. *Nature Medicine*, **2012**, *18*(5), 829–834. Available from https://doi. org/10.1038/nm.2721

[66] Shevtsov, M.A., Nikolaev, B.P., Yakovleva, L.Y., Marchenko, Y.Y., Dobrodumov, A.V., Mikhrina, A.L., ... Ischenko, A.M. Superparamagnetic iron oxide nanoparticles conjugated with epidermal growth factor (SPIONEGF) for targeting brain tumors. *International Journal of Nanomedicine*, **2014**, *9*, 273–287. Available from https://doi.org/10.2147/ IJN.S55118.

[67] Chertok, B., Moffat, B.A., David, A.E., Yu, F., Bergemann, C., Ross, B.D., & Yang, V.C. Iron oxide nanoparticles as a drug delivery vehicle for MRI monitored magnetic targeting of brain tumors. *Biomaterials*, **2008**, *29*(4), 487496. Available from https://doi. org/10.1016/j.biomaterials.2007.08.050.

[68] Khasraw, M., Ameratunga, M.S., Grant, R., Wheeler, H., & Pavlakis, N. Antiangiogenic therapy for high grade glioma. *Cochrane Database*

of Systematic Reviews, **2014**, 9. Available from https://doi.org/10.1002/14651858. CD008218.pub3, Cd008218.

[69] Yancopoulos, G.D., Davis, S., Gale, N.W., Rudge, J.S., Wiegand, S.J., & Holash, J. Vascular-specific growth factors and blood vessel formation. *Nature*, **2000**, *407*(6801), 242–248. Available from https://doi.org/10.1038/35025215.

[70] Schneider, S.W., Ludwig, T., Tatenhorst, L., Braune, S., Oberleithner, H., Senner, V., & Paulus, W. Glioblastoma cells release factors that disrupt blood-brain barrier features. *Acta Neuropathologica*, **2004**, 107(3), 272–276. Available from https://doi.org/10.1007/s00401-003-0810-2.

[71] Abakumov, M.A., Nukolova, N.V., Sokolsky-Papkov, M., Shein, S.A., Sandalova, T.O., Vishwasrao, H.M., ... Chekhonin, V.P. VEGF-targeted magnetic nanoparticles for MRI visualization of brain tumor. *Nanomedicine: Nanotechnology, Biology, and Medicine*, **2015**, *11*, 825–833

[72] Gaca, S., Reichert, S., Multhoff, G., Wacker, M., Hehlgans, S., Botzler, C., ... Rödel, F. Targeting by cmHsp70.1-antibody coated and survivin miRNA plasmid loaded nanoparticles to radiosensitize glioblastoma cells. *Journal of Controlled Release*, **2013**, *172*(1), 201–206. Available from https://doi.org/10.1016/j. jconrel.2013.08.020

[73] Bouras, A., Kaluzova, M., & Hadjipanayis, C.G. Radiosensitivity enhancement of radioresistant glioblastoma by epidermal growth factor receptor antibody-conjugated iron-oxide nanoparticles. *Journal of NeuroOncology*, **2015**, *124*(1), 13–22. Available from https://doi.org/10.1007/s11060-015-1807-0.

[74] Fan, Q.W., Cheng, C.K., Gustafson, W.C., Charron, E., Zipper, P., Wong, R.A., ... Weiss, W.A. EGFR phosphorylates tumor-derived EGFRvIII driving STAT3/5 and progression in glioblastoma. *Cancer Cell*, **2013**, *24*(4), 438–449. Available from https://doi.org/10.1016/j. ccr.2013.09.004

[75] Diaz Miqueli, A., Rolff, J., Lemm, M., Fichtner, I., Perez, R., & Montero, E. Radiosensitisation of U87MG brain Tumors by anti-epidermal growth factor receptor monoclonal antibodies. *British Journal of Cancer*, **2009**, *100*(6), 950–958. Available from https://doi.org/10.1038/sj.bjc.6604943.

[76] Maier-Hauff, K., Ulrich, F., Nestler, D., Niehoff, H., Wust, P., Thiesen, B., ... Jordan, A. Efficacy and safety of intratumoral thermotherapy using magnetic iron-oxide nanoparticles combined with external beam radiotherapy on patients with recurrent glioblastoma multiforme. *Journal of Neuro-Oncology*, **2011**, *103*(2), 317–324. Available from https://doi.org/10.1007/s11060-010-0389-0.

[77] Kaluzova, M., Bouras, A., Machaidze, R., & Hadjipanayis, C.G. Targeted therapy of glioblastoma stemlike cells and tumor non-stem cells using cetuximab-conjugated iron-oxide nanoparticles. *Oncotarget*, **2015**, *6*(11), 8788–8806. Available from https://doi.org/10.18632/oncotarget.3554.

[78] Barth, R.F., Wu, G., Meisen, W.H., Nakkula, R.J., Yang, W., Huo, T., ... Kaur, B. Design, synthesis, and evaluation of cisplatin-containing EGFR targeting bioconjugates as potential therapeutic agents for brain tumors. *OncoTargets and Therapy*, **2016**, *9*, 2769–2781.

[79] Li, A.J., Zheng, Y.H., Liu, G.D., Liu, W.S., Cao, P.C., & Bu, Z.F. Efficient delivery of docetaxel for the treatment of brain tumors by cyclic RGD-tagged polymeric micelles. *Molecular Medicine Reports*, **2015**, *11*(4), 3078–3086. Available from https://doi.org/10.3892/mmr.2014.3017

[80] Dahmani, F.Z., Xiao, Y., Zhang, J., Yu, Y., Zhou, J., & Yao, J. Multifunctional polymeric nanosystems for dual-targeted combinatorial chemo/angiogenesis therapy of tumors. *Advanced Healthcare Materials*, **2016**, *5*(12), 1447–1461. Available from https://doi.org/10.1002/adhm.201600169.

[81] Gao, H., Xiong, Y., Zhang, S., Yang, Z., Cao, S., & Jiang, X. RGD and interleukin-13 peptide functionalized nanoparticles for enhanced glioblastoma cells and neovasculature dual targeting delivery and elevated tumor penetration. *Molecular Pharmaceutics*, **2014**, *11*(3), 1042–1052. Available from https://doi.org/10.1021/mp400751g

[82] Shi, K., Long, Y., Xu, C., Wang, Y., Qiu, Y., Yu, Q., ... He, Q. Liposomes Combined an integrin alphavbeta3-specific vector with pH-responsible cell-penetrating property for highly effective antiglioma therapy through the blood-brain barrier. *ACS Applied Materials & Interfaces*, **2015a**, *7*(38), 21442–21454. Available from https://doi.org/10.1021/acsami.5b06429.

[83] Shi, K., Long, Y., Xu, C., Wang, Y., Qiu, Y., Yu, Q., ... He, Q. Liposomes Combined an integrin αvβ3 specific vector with pH-responsible cell-penetrating property for highly effective antiglioma therapy through the blood 2 brain barrier. *ACS Appl. Mater. Interfaces, A-M*, **2015b**, *7*(38), 21442–21454.

5

Solid-core Lipid Nanoparticles as a Vehicle for Brain Drug Delivery

Abstract

The blood–brain barrier is essential for preserving the homeostasis of the brain, but it also poses a significant challenge when it comes to effectively treating brain disorders. One of the most challenging problems in the area of cancer is the effective transport of drugs to the brain, which is hampered by several barriers. To overcome these limitations, targeted nanocarriers are employed through systemic administration. Solid lipid nanoparticles (SLNs), nanostructure lipid carriers, and lipid drug conjugates are a few examples of the several types of nanoparticles, which include nanocarriers with a diameter ranging from 10 to 1000 nm. They all have some potential for delivering medications and diagnostics to the brain, but spherical nanometer-sized solid lipid particles (SLNs) dispersed in water or an aqueous surfactant have the most potential. These nanoparticles have a number of benefits, including great physical stability, precision targeting to certain areas, and regulated drug release (which may be either protracted or quick, depending on the inclusion model). Nanoparticles represent a very promising pharmacological approach for treating illnesses of the central nervous system (CNS) by improving the drug's capacity to cross the blood–brain barrier.

5.1 Introduction

5.1.1 Physiological and anatomical dissection of the BBB

The blood–brain barrier (BBB) was initially described by Paul Ehrlich in 1885, and Edwin Goldman later validated Ehrlich's findings [1]. The BBB is one of the strongest constrictive barriers *in vivo* and is essential for maintaining brain homeostasis [2]. In the brain, a monolayer of endothelial cells lines the blood vessels, while three other types of cells surround the vessels, forming the BBB. The primary permeability barrier is a protein complex called zonulae occludentes, which is present in the foot processes of astrocytes [3]. The resistance to electrical current across the endothelial layer is used to measure the tightness of the junctions. As resistance increases, ion transport through paracellular pathways becomes more restricted, resulting in tighter junctions. Under healthy conditions, the endothelial electrical impedance exceeds $1000 \ \Omega/cm^2$ [4]. The BBB serves as a physiological and physical barrier that keeps drugs out of the brain. The central nervous system (CNS) is shielded from poisons and alterations in chemical concentrations by this process. This strategy also successfully excludes antibiotics and chemotherapy. The BBB's endothelial cells feature tight connections, few pinocytotic vesicles, and no fenestrations. The end foot of astrocytes, which are surrounded by a high concentration of pericytes covering 90% of brain capillaries, facilitates the close proximity of endothelial cells [5]. Beyond the astrocyte foot processes, there is an extracellular matrix that serves as an additional line of defense [6]. This layer contains multiple tight junctions, preventing agents from escaping brain capillaries between endothelial cells. Efflux transporters and high electrical resistance contribute to the BBB's physiological resistance to drug transport [7, 5]. Occludin and other organic anion and cation transporters are hypothesized to contribute to the electrical resistance by impeding the movement of polar and ionic molecules across the basolateral and luminal membranes. Numerous drug efflux receptors are present on the cell membranes of both cancer cells and brain capillary endothelial cells [8]. The most well-known MDR protein is probably P-glycoprotein (P-gp); however, the BBB expresses a variety of MDR proteins. This process is carried out by ABC transporters, a collection of receptors that cooperate to transport adenosine triphosphate (ATP) [5]. These membrane-bound proteins are produced in diverse types of healthy brain tissues and are in charge of reabsorption of anticancer medications into the circulation [5]. While ABC transporters are present in the healthy brain, they have been shown to be malignant brain tumors overexpress [8]. Additionally, therapies like chemotherapy and radiation therapy can improve their expression [9]. The extent to which ABC transporters are responsible for the typically subpar response of brain tumors to chemotherapy is still unknown, despite the fact that they have been identified as a barrier to drug delivery to the brain in several *in vitro* and animal studies. P-gp inhibitors have been shown to increase chemotherapy penetration and tumor response in animal models when used with P-gp substrate cytotoxic drugs [10]. Additionally, members of the ABCG2 family, such as MRP1 and BCRP (ABCG2), have shown similar outcomes [11]. The expression of several ABC transporters has been linked to decreased chemotherapeutic

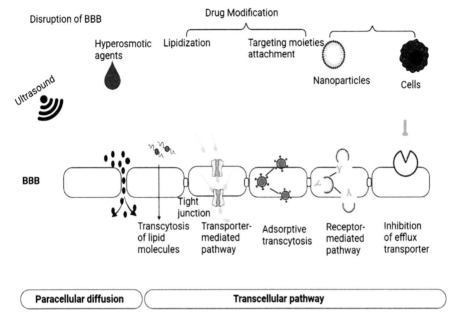

Figure 5.1 Receptor-specific ligands used to transport drugs over the BBB.

response and poor overall survival in systemic cancers [12]. In light of these findings, efflux transporter inhibitors used in combination with cytotoxic therapy are currently under investigation. However, the results of using this strategy to treat systemic cancers have been inconsistent, likely due to the higher toxicities associated with chemotherapies [12]. Although active drug efflux is not currently being evaluated in clinical trials, it is becoming increasingly clear that this issue must be resolved to advance both systemic and local therapy for brain cancers [6]. Indicators of restricted BBB penetration include high plasma protein binding and low serum concentrations in addition to size, water solubility, and charge. Despite the BBB's effective filtration mechanism, some chemicals can nevertheless get through it and endanger the CNS [6]. Low-molecular-weight, lipid-soluble, and neutral compounds can pass through the BBB by inactive dispersion. Their effectiveness, however, is limited by P-gp and other ABC proteins, which can lead to extrusion and rapid passage through the CNS [5]. Three new methods of delivering treatment for brain tumors have been developed to exploit the potential for their cargo to survive the initial rapid efflux and reach the tumor. These methods include absorptive endocytosis, receptor-mediated transcytosis, and carrier-mediated transport [5, 13] (Figure 5.1).

The free flow of chemicals like amino acids is crucial to maintaining healthy nerve cells, via carrier-mediated transport. Because carrier receptors are stereospecific and tiny, this delivery method can only be used to convey a small number of compounds [13].

A receptor-mediated method is used to transport bigger molecules like insulin and transferrin [5, 14]. Endothelial cells express an endothelial cell receptor, which is ligated by a molecule. When a "match" is found, it is endocytosed and transported to the basolateral membrane via vesicles, where it enters the central nervous system [13]. Medicines that cross the blood–brain barrier by attaching to a receptor there can "piggyback" through the BBB in the case of receptor-mediated anticancer medicines [15]. The amount of material that may cross cell membranes is severely constrained as a result of tight junctions, the lack of fenestrae, and the activity of pinocytotic processes. Therefore, molecules need to take the transcellular pathway to reach the brain, and solutes need to utilize either passive permeability or active transport to get across the brain endothelial barrier [2].

Drug uptake is affected not only by BBB transport capabilities but also by drug concentrations in circulation. Below is a simplified form of the pharmacokinetic rule that explains this observation (eqn (5.1)) [16].

$$\% \ ID/g = PS \times AUC \tag{5.1}$$

where %ID/g is the percentage of an administered dose absorbed by the brain; PS is the product of permeability × surface area; AUC is the area under the curve proportional to the blood concentration of the medication. For the most part, the pharmacokinetic rule, there are two ways in which medication absorption can be increased in the brain:

- Preserved blood concentrations (increased area under blood concentration curve) and stabilization.

- The drug's structure may need to be altered to improve its function as a transport substrate across the BBB.

Methods like drug tweaking, BBB opening, and BBB bypassing through different routes of administration are all used to successfully transport medications to the brain [2].

Neurotoxic chemicals (e.g., potassium, glycine, and glutamate) are protected from the brain by the BBB [1]. Because of the lack of fenestrations and the strong intracellular connections, molecular therapies such as anticancer medicines cannot pass this physical barrier (zona occludens). Due to weak metabolic capacity and the existence of pinocytic vesicles in brain endothelial cells, anticancer drugs cannot easily cross the blood–brain barrier and enter the central nervous system [17]. The BBB efficiently prevents the absorption of all large-molecule medications and more than 98% of small-molecule pharmaceuticals [18]. The BBB is selectively permeable to tiny molecules (<5000 Da), lipid-soluble compounds, chemicals with a neutral charge, and weak bases [19]. However, BBB disruption occurs often at the regional level due to tumor cell proliferation and invasion. Thromboxane B2, prostaglandin E, and arachidonic acid are a few of the many mediators produced by cancer cells, all of which increase the permeability of the capillary endothelium [1, 20].

Tumors encourage the development production of VEGF and bFGF (basic fibroblast growth factor) to promote angiogenesis (the development of new blood vessels) [21].

Blood–tumor interface permeability and medication penetration are both enhanced by these capillaries' numerous fenestrations. Anticancer drugs cannot get to the neighboring tumors in a healthy tissue since the BBB is not disrupted around them [22].

5.1.2 Statistics on brain tumors

Patients with brain tumors have a poor prognosis and a poor quality of life [23, 24, 25], making them a complex disease category. The World Health Organisation (WHO) uses the site, histological appearance, lineage markers, and probable cell of origin to classify CNS tumours [26]. Most adult brain tumors fall into one of three categories: astrocytomas, oligodendrogliomas, and oligoastrocytomas [27]. In the brain, glial cells known as astrocytes can develop into tumors known as astrocytomas. Each type of cancer has a spectrum of malignancies that are used to classify them. Anaplastic astrocytomas (grades III and IV) and glioblastomas (grades IV) stand out as the most prevalent and dangerous kinds of malignant gliomas in terms of incidence and risk. Despite advances in cancer therapy such as surgical resection, radiation, and chemotherapy over the past 30 years, the median survival time for cancer patients has not increased much [22]. Over the course of their lives, one in seven American men and one in five American women will receive a primary brain tumor diagnosis. This is 14.4 cases for every 100,000 persons annually [28]. Brain cancer is one of the most difficult types of cancer to treat [27]. Cancer in childhood ranks third among all cancers in terms of mortality rates among adolescents and young adults [23]. There is a 37% two-year survival rate and a 30% five-year survival rate for people who have primary malignant CNS tumors [28]. Despite having a lesser incidence than other malignancies (about 2%) and having a considerable morbidity and mortality rate, primary malignant brain tumors may be among the most severe human neoplastic disorders, according to these epidemiological statistics [23]. Gliomas are the most common primary tumor of the CNS in the United States, with an annual incidence rate of 6.42 per 100,000 individuals [23]. The four histological classifications of gliomas are ependymomas, mixed gliomas (which have both oligodendroglial and astrocytic characteristics), and oligodendrogliomas [23, 29]. The histological grade of gliomas, which is defined by the tumor's level of differentiation and anaplasia, relates to their prognosis [30]. High-grade gliomas such as glioblastomas, anaplastic astrocytomas, anaplastic oligodendrogliomas, and anaplastic oligoastrocytomas account for almost half of all adult gliomas and 78% of all primary malignant CNS tumors [23, 31].

The prognosis for patients with malignant gliomas varies with the histological subtype of the tumor and the patient's age at diagnosis [31]. There is a large variety in the United States, and the relative two-year survival probability ranges from 1.4% to 29.8% depending on histology and age at diagnosis; for anaplastic astrocytomas, it is 4.1%; for anaplastic oligodendrogliomas, it is 4.9%; and for mixed gliomas, it is 37.6% [28]. Methods of increasing a drug's concentration in the brain, whether via crossing the BBB or another means, are currently in development; employing alternate routes of administration is urgently needed due to the incidence of brain tumors and the BBB's inefficiency in transporting drugs to the brain.

To address present therapeutic constraints, one of the most promising options is to employ nanocarriers that are injected systemically and used for medication delivery [32].

The brain capillary endothelial cells are specifically targeted by these nanocarriers, triggering an internalization pathway (Figure 5.1). When exocytosed into the brain, the nanocarriers reach the cerebral parenchyma, which is where the medication is delivered into the brain. In comparison to medications that are connected to the direct binding of site-specific ligands, the main advantages of this method are that the packaged drug is less toxic while maintaining the same biological activity [22].

However, transport systems with poor affinity and capacity impede the delivery of big agents like antibodies and DNA, which may prevent them from binding to their intended targets [14]. Charged particle interactions are essential to the process of cellular absorption. Albumin and other plasma proteins appear to be transported into the CNS via electrostatic contact between cationized proteins and the BBB. Conjugated delivery of large-scale immunotherapies using nanoparticles is the subject of current investigation (such as gene therapy) [33].

5.2 Novel Drug Delivery System Approach: Nanoparticles

5.2.1 Definition and structural characteristics

Particles with sizes ranging from 10 to 1000 nm are classified as nanoparticles [34]. Lipid drug conjugates (LDCs), also known as lipid vesicles (LVs), and lipid nanoscopic spheres (SLNs) are particles that have a nanoscale-scaled lipid solid matrix [35]. Despite its benefits, such as BBB penetration, restrictions exist, particularly regarding toxicity and stability. SLNs are a feasible option to NLCs and LDCs for drug administration into the brain. Nanoscale lipid particles are uniformly dispersed in aqueous surfactant or water solutions and have a spherical shape. As a result, lipophilic or hydrophilic drugs or diagnostics might be delivered via them [36, 37, 38]. As a stabilizing agent, surfactants are included in the particle dispersions together with lipids and medicines. Excipients are either compounds that have been designated as GRAS (generally regarded as safe) or chemicals that are generally recognized as safe [39]. By using both synthetic and natural polymers, drug dispersion is improved while toxicity is minimized. Over the course of the last few decades, they have developed into a practical alternative to liposomes as drug carriers [34]. When employing nanoparticles for medication administration, they must be able to break past several barriers in the body, gradually release their payload over time, and keep their nanoscale size [34]. Due to their high price and the absence of secure polymers with regulatory approval, their medicinal usage is restricted. Lipids have been suggested as an alternative to polymeric nanoparticles as a delivery system for lipophilic medications. One of the most often utilized nanoparticles in formulation is the SLN, or lipid nanoparticle [40].

5.2.1.1 Nanoparticles composed of solid lipids

Emulsions, liposomes, and polymeric nanoparticles may all be replaced with the newer, more innovative colloidal carriers known as SLNs. The typical liquid lipid (oil) has been replaced with a solid lipid in modern submicron lipid emulsions. Due to their small size, large surface area, and high drug-loading capacity, SLNs may improve the effectiveness of medicines, nutraceuticals, and other items [41]. Due to the fact that SLNs are a novel colloidal drug carrier for intravenous delivery, they have attracted a lot of attention [34]. Physiological lipids create a colloidal submicroporous carrier when they are dispersed in water or an aqueous surfactant solution [42].

SLNs (i.e., lipids that are solid both at body and room temperatures) are nanoparticles composed of solid lipids that have been stabilized by a surfactant. There is a chance that they are extremely pure triglycerides or

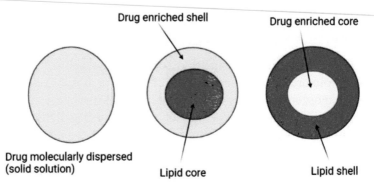

Figure 5.2   (A) Drug-enriched cell model, (B) a drug-enriched core model, and (C) a homogeneous matrix model of drug inclusion in solid lipid nanoparticles (solid solution).

complicated mixes of glycerides or even waxes by definition [43]. Para-acyl calix [4] arenes-based SLN has recently been produced and examined [44, 45].

SLNs may have one of the following three alternative morphologies (Figure 5.2) depending on where the drug molecule is inserted [46]: (i) a simulation of a drug-filled shell; (ii) enhanced central model for drugs; and (iii) modeling on a homogeneous matrix.

The carrier system SLN has been extensively studied by several research organizations [47, 48, 49]. Different methods of producing SLN were patented back in 1993 (M. R. Gasco, 1993) and 1996 (Westesen, Britta Siekmann) [43]. SLN is ideally suited for parenteral administration due to its better physical stability, capacity to retain integrated labile medicines drug stability, controlled release (fast or sustained), low toxicity, and targeted delivery to the intended organ system. Several potential drawbacks have been noted, including a high water content of the dispersions (70%–99.9%), drug ejection with polymorphism shift during storage, and a low loading capacity [35]. Due to the solubility, structure, and polymorphism of the lipid matrix, standard SLNs have a limited drug loading capacity (up to roughly 25% relative to the matrix, and up to 50% for unique actives like ubidecarenone) [50–57]. A defect-free crystal could form if the molecules in the lipid matrix are similar enough (such as tristearin or tripalmitin). SLNs may improve the drug's BBB-crossing capacity, making them effective pharmacological targets for CNS disorders [57]. Because the medications are wedged between fatty acid chains, lipid layers, and crystal defects, they cannot be incorporated in large quantities into a highly ordered crystal lattice [57]. Therefore, complex lipids (monoglycerides, diglycerides, and triglycerides of varied chain lengths) should be used because they enable increased drug loading [35].

A further consequence of this transition to highly organized lipid particles is the release of the drug. Almost immediately after synthesis, lipids crystallize in higher-energy variants with more defects in the crystal lattice [58, 59, 60]. For topical formulations, it has lately been explored whether or not it is possible to maintain the α- and β-modification throughout medications that need to be stored and altered (such as through temperature variations) [61]. Polymorphic shift during storage means that drugs cannot be safeguarded from degradation or released in regulated amounts once they exit the lipid matrix [35].

5.2.2 Comparative advantages of SLNs vs. polymeric nanoparticles (other delivery systems like liposomal drug delivery)

The benefits of polymeric nanoparticles, fat emulsions, and liposomes are all brought together in SLNs; they also have none of the downsides [62]. SLNs have the following advantages:

- Since the RES (reticuloendothelial system) cells do not readily take up the sub-100 nm nanoparticles and SLNs, the liver and spleen filtering organs are bypassed [63, 64].

- For up to a few weeks, the integrated medicine may be released in a controlled manner [48, 65]. Coating or adding ligands to SLNs may further enhance drug targeting [32].

- Ophthalmic, duodenal, percutaneous, and pulmonary methods may be used to give SLN, as can parenteral and intravenous routes. SLN can also achieve a brain–blood barrier (BBB) crossing [35, 36, 66].

- Lipid and surfactant types, particle sizes, and preparation processes all have an impact on how quickly a medication is released [36, 41, 67].

- High drug payload [68, 69].

- Long-lasting, new SLN formulations have been created; some of them can be stored for up to three years (longer than other NPs). This is critical in comparison to other colloidal carrier systems, which can be sterilized via lyophilization or steam [70–73].

- Supercritical fluid (SCF) and high-pressure homogenization (HPH) methods for sample pretreatment technique provide excellent repeatability and feasibility for large-scale manufacturing and sterilizing [42, 74, 75].

- The capacity to combine drugs that are hydrophilic and hydrophobic into a single formulation [36, 37, 38].

- Biodegradable and hence safe carrier lipids [76–78].

- To limit the danger of embolism caused by blood coagulation and aggregation, organic solvents should be avoided [79, 80].

- Adsorption on the capillary walls and improved concentration gradients in the BB are very important because of retention in brain blood capillaries [77, 81].

5.2.3 The downside of SLNs

The low solubility of pharmaceuticals in lipid melts in conventional SLNs affects their drug-loading capabilities and is one of the common problems associated with their specific structure and fabrication procedure:

- The capacity of certain lipids to construct flawless crystalline lattices with negligible imperfections contributes to drug ejection during storage [48].

- Observations have shown that the dispersions have a high water content (7099.9%) [50].

- Increased particle size and fluctuating gelation tendencies [79, 80].

However, traditional SLNs are unable to load many drugs because of the drugs' poor solubility following polymorphic transition, during the lipid melt, and the evacuation of drugs [58]. These problems were resolved by modifying the lipid matrix and the structure of the medications. Afterward, NLCs [82] and LDCs [83] were developed, which led to a huge boost in drug loading. PEG2000 is conjugated with phospholipids and glycerides to produce sterically stabilized SLN [84].

5.2.4 Factors to be considered in the formulation of SLNs

Lipid solids make up the bulk of SLNs, surfactants, cosurfactants (optional), and active substances (often medicines) [85].

5.2.4.1 Process of lipid selection

The building blocks for lipid nanoparticles are lipids extracted from human bodies. Triglycerides, fatty acids, fatty esters, and fatty alcohols are several types that can be distinguished based on their chemical makeup and molecular composition [86]. Using waxes to make lipid nanoparticles has been reported by a few researchers as well [87]. Lipid nanoparticles with attached surfactants provide additional stability to the colloidal solution. They may also be utilized with cosurfactants [86]. Drug loading capacity, stability, and sustained release behavior of lipid nanoparticles are impacted by the lipid. Nanoparticle dispersions of lipids have been studied. Lipids include things like fatty acids, glycerides, and waxes [88, 89, 90].

Cetyl palmitate is the only one of these lipids that has not been authorized by the FDA as generally regarded as safe (GRAS) [31]. Before using lipid nanoparticle dispersions, it is important to choose the right lipids. Despite the lack of defined guidelines, the drug's solubility in the lipid has been proposed as an important factor in making this choice [91]. Lipid nanoparticles' ability for encapsulation and loading is directly related to the drug's solubility in the lipid matrix, which determines how well the nanoparticles can deliver the medication [92]. UV-visible spectroscopy and chromatographic methods provide straightforward evaluations of a drug's solubility [93].

Mathematical equations may also be used to estimate medication separation into oily/fatty and watery components. Such forecasts are grounded in how various medications interact with lipids and water. A high drug loading in lipid nanoparticles requires either high solubility in lipids or a high partition coefficient for the drug. The apparent partition coefficient of a medicine in a lipid matrix depends on its solubility in that matrix. As a result, various lipid matrices have varying loading capabilities for the same medication. Since predictive models must deal with so much information, they are difficult to employ for anything other than screening and prediction [86].

In addition to lipid polymorphism, the characteristics of lipid nanoparticle systems are influenced by other factors. The structural information provided by solid lipids' many crystalline forms is of particular value flaws where medicinal molecules may fit. It is, nevertheless, more thermodynamically stable than the other lattice structures. To illustrate this point, consider the more stable β-forms of triglycerides [94]. As a rule, unstable forms that seem unstable at first often stabilize over time. As a result of the structural defects in solid lipids, transitions like this constitute a substantial difficulty when making nanoparticles out of solid lipids (SLNs). There is a risk of medication loss either during storage or after it has been given [86].

Another factor that plays a role in picking the best lipid is the lipid's metastable-to-stable transition rate or its ability to form flawless crystalline lattice structures. For this reason, there are no concrete guidelines for picking lipids [86]. Fats with longer fatty acid chains take longer to crystallize than those with shorter chains [95].

It has been reported that cationic lipids that go into making lipid nanoparticles are employed in the conveyance of genetic information. Positively charged lipids on the particle surface may increase transfection efficiency. Because of their greater toxicity to cells, unbranched cationic lipids are avoided by capillaries in favor of their branched counterparts [96].

Physically, lipid nanoparticles based on wax have greater stability, but their crystalline structure makes them more susceptible to drug ejection [97]. Non-crystallinity and polymorphism issues with lipids may be avoided by making dispersions of lipid nanoparticles known as "NLCs" from a binary combination of two lipid matrices, one solid and one liquid [98].

5.2.4.2 Choosing surfactants

In addition to lipids, surfactants (also known as emulsifiers or surface-active agents) play a crucial role in the production of lipid nanoparticles. Because they can be affected by both hydrophilicity and lipophilicity, amphipathic molecules like surfactants exhibit the characteristic head and tail of surfactants [86]. Surfactants adhere to the surface of a system or contact at low quantities. The stress between them can be alleviated by decreasing the surface or interfacial free energy [99]. If you take a look at the hydrophilic–lipophilic balance (HLB) value, you can see how much of each moiety is involved. Surfactants are used in the creation of lipid nanoparticles for two distinct and essential purposes:

- In the manufacturing process, surfactants distribute lipid melt in the aqueous phase.

- When the dispersions are cooled, the surfactants help keep the lipid nanoparticles from clumping together.

Depending on their charge, surfactants can be categorized into ionic, non-ionic, and amphoteric classes. The dispersion process, essential to the production of the final product, is aided by surfactants that reduce surface tension (first role). Some scientists believe that ionic surfactants imply electrostatic stability, whereas others believe that non-ionic surfactants imply steric-repulsion stability. However, many of the nonionic surfactants used are too tiny for the Gibbs–Marangoni effect to infer true steric stability [100]. Tween and pluronic are two of the most used nonionic surfactants. The hydrophilic (ethylene oxide) and hydrophobic (benzotriazole) moiety of most of these surfactants have been previously characterized (hydrocarbon chain). In the production of lipid nanoparticles, phospholipids and phosphatidylcholines are the most often employed amphoteric surfactants. In this context, surfactants feature functional groups that are both negatively and positively charged. At low and high pH, they display the characteristics of a cationic and an anionic surfactant, respectively.

A variety of criteria influence the choice of surfactants for the creation of nanoparticles, and among them are [86]:

- intended administration path;

- the surfactant's HLB value;

- impact on particle size and lipid alteration;

- participation in the lipid's *in vivo* breakdown.

Nonionic surfactants are preferred over ionic surfactants in oral and parenteral therapies because they are safer and less irritating [101].

5.2.4.3 Other agents

Lipid nanoparticle formulations may potentially include other ingredients like surface enhancers and counter-ions. The lipids used to create nanoparticles that will store cationic medications that are water-soluble may contain some organic anions and anionic polymers [102–104]. To reduce the absorption of RES, hydrophilic polymers and other surface modifiers may be utilized to modify the lipid nanoparticle surface. The drug's concentration in the blood is raised by stealth or long-circulating carriers because they linger there for longer [36, 105]. Numerous research works for the delivery and targeting of anticancer medications have focused on these "stealth" SLNs since they may be absorbed by tumor cells [106–108].

5.2.4.4 Drug lipid solubility

Triglycerides, diglycerides, and monoglycerides are frequently used as oil solvents in lipid-based medicinal products, along with fatty esters, fatty alcohols, and carboxylic fatty acids. The method of high-pressure homogenization (HPH) is commonly used to create lipid nanoparticles, where microemulsions, solvent emulsification–evaporation, and diffusion play crucial roles [109].

Glycerides with a medium chain length have the best properties for solubilizing medicines and forming microemulsions. The SLN production necessitates the use of long-chain glycerides with a higher melting point. In many circumstances, the amount of medication that can be dissolved in the lipid formulation is more than the amount of medication that can be dissolved in fat alone. A medicine may be present between the interface of lipid assemblies and the oil phase due to this higher solubility. Water-poor hydrophobic groups may thrive in the anisotropic environment provided by the interfacial regions. Entrapment efficiency and loading capacity may be improved by using lipid melts rather than lipid solids since the drug's solubility is greater in liquids than in solids [91].

As matrix material, lipids include monoglycerides and diglycerides, which facilitate drug solubilization. Azidothymidine palmitate and fluorouracil's stearic acid derivative both increase the drug's lipid solubility via the use of prodrugs [110, 111]. Complexation of the medication with lipid components and the creation of LDCs are further methods for creating SLNs for weakly lipid-soluble medicines [83, 104, 105].

5.2.5 Method of preparation of SLNs

Since the early 1990s, lipid nanoparticles have been described as carriers, and various fabrication techniques have been documented [42, 50, 76]. The efficacy of a colloidal composition is highly dependent on its preparation procedure. Several factors can influence lipid nanoparticle dispersions, including:

- the drug's physicochemical qualities that will be included;

- the drug's stability before incorporation;

- the lipid nanoparticle dispersion's desired particle properties;

- lipid nanoparticle dispersion stability;

- the production equipment is readily available.

This chapter provides a basic overview of several manufacturing methods. Table 5.1 lists the various techniques employed to produce lipid nanoparticles along with their benefits and drawbacks [86].

5.2.5.1 High-pressure homogenization

HPH has been established as the preferred method for producing lipid nanoparticle dispersions because of its reliability and influence. Muller, Schwarz, Mehnert, and Lucks (1993) [112], as well as Siekmann and Westesen (1992) [76], first described the technique, which was subsequently improved upon and patented by Muller and Lucks for the manufacturing of SLNs [113]. One of the two basic methods for producing SLNs using HPH is the hot and cold approaches to the process [86]. The procedure is simple and may be done on a large scale. The high-pressure homogenizers (100–2000 bar) used in this method drive liquids down to micrometer-sized gaps [114]. Figure 5.3 depicts the high-pressure homogenization.

Table 5.1 Mechanisms, benefits, and drawbacks of lipid nanoparticle preparation techniques.

Method of manufacturing	Formation mechanism	Pros	Cons
Homogenizing under intense pressure	There is a lot of shear force being applied, and it is all because of the turbulence	**Hot homogenization**	**Hot homogenization**
	Homogenizer pressure drop at the valves	Proven, time-tested methods	High levels of energy expenditures (heat and shear forces)
	High cavitation pressures	Optimal particle dispersal	The polydispersity was high
		Reproducible	Drugs deteriorate due to heat
		Excessive fat content	The crystallization process is complicated, resulting in several lipid changes and the formation of super-cooled melts
		Easy to expand upon	
		Cold homogenization	**Cold homogenization**
		Optimal particle dispersal	Power consumption that is through the roof
		Suitable for medications that are affected by heat	Discarding drugs due to their excessively large particle size and variability
		Not a lot of lipid tinkering needed	
		The decreased melting of lipids means less medication is lost, making them ideal for hydrophilic medicines	
		Easy to expand upon	

(Continued)

Table 5.1   *Continued.*

Method of manufacturing	Formation mechanism	Pros	Cons
Processing of microemulsions	Rapid solidification of the microemulsion causes the lipids to crystallize	No need for high-tech tools Inputs of little energy Larger temperature differences promote more rapid crystallization of lipids and inhibit particle aggregation Easy to expand upon	Reduced fat content
A microwave-assisted microemulsion method	Molecular microwave direct coupling Rapid solidification of the microemulsion causes the lipids to crystallize	Microwave cooking under the supervision Quickly and effectively warms up Inputs of little energy Less time spent on preliminary work Larger temperature differences accelerate lipid crystallization	Problems with scalability
Vaporization of the solvent	Removal of the solvent causes lipid crystallization in an antisolvent	No need for high-tech tools Extremely well-suited for temperature-sensitive medications Consisting primarily of particles with very small sizes Easy to expand upon	The use of organic solvents raises toxicological concerns Aggregation of particles in the absence of fast solvent evaporation Reduced fat content

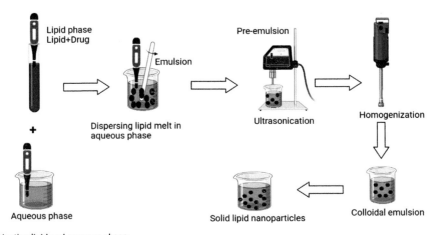

Lipid phase
Lipid+Drug

Emulsion

Pre-emulsion

Dispersing lipid melt in
aqueous phase

Ultrasonication

Homogenization

+

Aqueous phase

Solid lipid nanoparticles

Colloidal emulsion

Heating lipid and aqueous phase

Figure 5.3 Solid lipid nanoparticle production by high homogenization processes.

5.2.5.1.1 Hot homogenization

The hot homogenization approach is also known as "homogenization of emulsions" since lipid nanoparticle dispersions are created at temperatures above the lipids' melting points [49]. In a nutshell, heated HPH involves melting the lipid and medicine into a cold aqueous surfactant solution at a temperature that is around 5°C over the lipid's melting point.

5.2.5.1.2 Cool homogenization

Cold HPH may be used to process hydrophilic or treatments that are affected by temperature. Solid lipid microparticles are created after combining lipids and drugs before crushing them rapidly with liquid nitrogen [35]. When a cold aqueous surfactant solution is rapidly whirled, a presuspension is created. Homogenization of the presuspension must occur at or below room temperature for a minimum of five cycles at 500 bar to produce SLNs, NLCs, or LDCs [35].

5.2.5.2 Utilizing the microemulsions technique to produce SLN

Gasco described how to precipitate SLN dispersions from a heated microemulsion [42]. Microemulsions are thermodynamically stable and optically isotropic mixtures of water and oil. It is stabilized by a surfactant (and cosurfactant, if necessary). Precipitation from heated microemulsions can produce lipid nanoparticle dispersions, as demonstrated in Figure 5.4 [86]. The temperature of lipid and aqueous surfactant/cosurfactant systems is raised above the point at which solid lipids melt. To dissolve the medication in the lipid, heat is applied to both the drug and the lipid. Sludge-like substances (SLN) are created by dissolving the lipid melt in a creating a hot microemulsion by adding a hot surfactant/cosurfactant system and continuously swirling the mixture. Then, a machine is used to mechanically stir it into cold water (about 24°C) to disperse it. The ratio of the microemulsion to the aqueous phase is normally 1:25, although it can be as high as 1:50 [86].

5.2.5.3 Microwave-assisted microemulsion technique

Over the last several years, many studies have examined the potential of microwave radiation for chemical synthesis and processing [115]. Compound libraries may be synthesized via microwave-assisted synthesis for the creation and optimization of novel therapeutic candidates [116]. One of the most common uses of microwaves in the pharmaceutical industry is the drying and long-term stability of medication dispersions [117, 118]. According to a few studies, microwave radiation may be used to create polymeric nanoparticles in medicinal formulations [119, 120]. Microwave radiation may be used to create new SLNs [121].

The procedure of creating a microemulsion with the use of a microwave is depicted in Figure 5.4 [86]. A controlled microwave heating procedure is used to raise the temperature of the medicine, lipid, and aqueous surfactant/cosurfactant mixture over the point of melting for the solid lipid. Hot microemulsions can be made by stirring the ingredients in a microwave oven under controlled conditions. All components are heated in a single synthesis pot as opposed to using individual vessels for each ingredient as is done in the traditional microemulsion method. Consequently, this stage is characterized by the creation of microemulsion in a single vessel. The microemulsion is heated in a microwave and then redistributed in cold water to make SLNs (2–4°C) [86].

5.2.5.4 Solvent emulsification–evaporation method

The solvent emulsification–evaporation method was first created by Sjostrom and Bergenstahl to produce SLNs [122]. Figure 5.4 [86] depicts this solvent evaporation procedure. The solid lipid must first be dissolved in an organic solvent before a lipophilic drug may be taken. Lipid nanoparticle dispersions have changed since they were first created, necessitating the use of several organic solvents such as cyclohexane and chloroform [123, 122]. The organic phase is emulsified in an aqueous solution containing a surfactant to create an emulsion of an organic solvent in water [86]. To remove the organic phase, mechanical stirring or reduced pressure are used; the quicker evacuation of

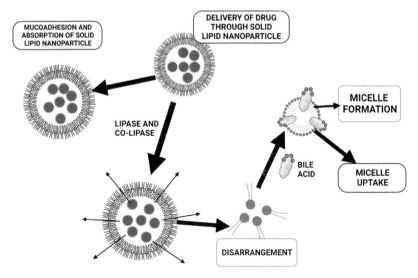

Figure 5.4 Solid lipid nanoparticles are generated by microemulsion and emulsification evaporation.

organic solvents reduces particle agglomeration. The medication is dissolved in the internal water phase of a w/o/w emulsion, allowing it to be included in the formulation [124]. A suspension of lipid nanoparticles is formed at low pressure created when the organic solvent has entirely evaporated [86]. This approach has the advantage of preventing pharmaceutical deterioration due to heat. The toxicity of the used organic solvents is this procedure's major downside [109].

5.3 Conclusion

Two distinct research teams separately suggested using solid lipid nanoparticles (SLNs) for targeted medication delivery to the brain in the late 1990s. This remark was made despite the original data showing that lipid particles can pass across the blood–brain barrier (BBB) having been published earlier. SLNs can be used to deliver medications that are not very soluble in water, such as peptides and proteins, as can other types of hydrophilic pharmaceuticals. In addition to their nanoscale size and protection against chemical and enzymatic destruction, nanoparticles provide several other benefits. While the BBB's tight endothelial cells cannot enable them to get through, their tiny size and limited size range (100–200 nm) allow them to get through. In addition, regardless of the mode of administration, SLNs are often used because of their improved bioavailability. It may be possible to target the delivery of the loaded medication by using SLNs, which alter pharmacokinetic and biodistribution patterns. Analgesics, antitubercular, anticancer, anti-agers, anti-anxiety, neuroleptics, antibiotics, and antivirals will all be delivered to the brain more efficiently using SLNs. Peptides, proteins, and medications with low water solubility are all examples of problematic pharmaceuticals that might be delivered using SLNs, which are straightforward distribution methods supported by solid lipids.

Cutaneous, transdermal, ocular, cutaneous, oral, intravenous, pulmonary, and rectal delivery SLNs have previously been used to deliver drugs. The researcher must have a thorough understanding of all BBB transport mechanisms, including those mediated by carriers and receptors. Drug distribution across the BBB using brain-targeted delivery techniques will be made possible, thanks to the discovery of this new knowledge. One rationale for using SLNs to deliver neuroactive medications is to modify the drug's pharmacokinetic profile, allowing for larger brain concentrations and thus better clinical outcomes. Pegylation and other covert changes will certainly be required to enhance CNS drug delivery.

Ineffective medicine administration in the brain can be attributed to two main factors:

- Inadequate drug molecule crossing of the BBB.

- Drug backflow (efflux) from the blood to the brain. Different researchers have experimented with a variety of colloidal delivery techniques to address, particularly, the first problem.

Chemotherapy diagnostics and therapeutics based on nanotechnology are the ultimate objectives of this field. As long as nanoparticle carrier technology retains the therapeutic drug molecule's original features, it can pass over the BBB. This is the key benefit for brain cancer patients. It is also possible that this mechanism reduces drug leaking in the brain and reduces the hazardous effects on the body. SLNs are a cost-effective and patient-friendly way to administer medications through a variety of channels. In the fight against cancer and TB, coating SLNs with hydrophilic chemicals is very promising. PEG-coated SLNs have received a lot of interest from researchers looking to boost the bioavailability of their drugs. As a colloidal drug delivery system, SLNs are becoming increasingly significant due to the idea of surface modification. The different barriers to medication absorption may be overcome by SLNs with a proper administration technique. Drugs administered by SLN may be a novel approach to intracranial dosing since it has the potential to circumvent or reduce the problems of solubility, permeability, and toxicity that are inherent to individual therapeutic compounds. The lipidic makeup of SLNs makes them readily absorbed by the brain. Even if the SLNs deliver a lot of medication to the brain, extrapyramidal adverse effects can still occur. One benefit of colloidal drug delivery systems, like SLNs, is their large surface areas. These systems can be customized by adding other charge modifiers, like stearic acid (SA) and stearyl amine. Low-toxicity, naturally occurring long-chain fatty acid saturated fatty acid (SA). It is safe to use on the human tissue and does not affect physiological fluids. A free carboxylic group is provided as well, which facilitates the conjugation of the target ligand to the SLN surface.

The lipid content and manufacturing mechanisms of SLNs may be modified to passively target them to the brain. SNN transport might be facilitated by active targeting, which would enhance the specificity of neoplastic cell population medication delivery. As it would address the many influx–flux transport mechanisms displayed by brain endothelial cells, this might be beneficial for actively targeting brain tumor cells. These include adsorptive-mediated endocytosis, carrier-mediated endocytosis (such as D-glucose), and receptor-mediated endocytosis (such as insulin, insulin-like growth factor (IGF), folic acid (FA), and transferrin (Tf)). The statistics demonstrate categorically that every site of the body where the medication may be administered is reached by even the most passively brain-targeted SLN. Additionally, therapeutic medicines are transported by non-actively focused SLNs into every part of the CNS, where they may be unwelcome or even detrimental after they cross the blood–brain barrier (BBB).

Because of their invasiveness, intrusive systems are not always appropriate. Thus, innovative drug delivery methods would be the primary method for attaining non-invasive delivery (NDDSs). Many different types of lipid microspheres and niosomal systems are included in this category. A successful delivery system must also have minimum toxicity, drug loading, and chemical and physical stability.

References

[1] Gururangan, S., & Friedman, H.S. Innovations in design and delivery of chemotherapy for brain tumors. *Neuroimaging Clinics of North America*, **2002**, *12*, 583–597.

[2] Koziara, J.M., Lockman, P.R., Allen, D.D., & Mumper, R.J. The blood-brain barrier and brain drug delivery. *Journal of Nanoscience and Nanotechnology*, **2006**, *6*, 2712–2735

[3] Bradbury, M.W.B. Introduction to the Blood-Brain Barrier. Methodology, Biology, and Pathology. *Journal of Anatomy*, **1999**, *194*, 153–157

[4] Butt, A. M., Jones, H.C., & Abbott, N.J. Electrical resistance across the blood-brain barrier in anaesthetized rats: A developmental study. *The Journal of Physiology*, **1990**, *429*, 47–62.

[5] Deeken, J.F., & Loscher, W. The blood-brain barrier and cancer: Transporters, treatment, and trojan horses. *Clinical Cancer Research*, **2007**, *13*, 1663–1674.

[6] Blakeley, J. Drug delivery to brain tumors. *Current neurology and Neuroscience Reports*, **2008**, *8*, 235–241

[7] Colgan, O.C., Collins, N.T., Ferguson, G., Murphy, R.P., Birney, Y.A., Cahill, P.A., & Cummins, P.M. Influence of basolateral condition on the regulation of brain microvascular endothelial tight junction properties and barrier function. *Brain Research*, **2008**, *1193*, 84–92.

[8] Calatozzolo, C., Gelati, M., Ciusani, E., Sciacca, F.L., Pollo, B., Cajola, L., ... Salmaggi, A. Expression of drug resistance proteins Pgp, MRP1, MRP3, MRP5 and GST-pi in human glioma. *J Neurooncol*, **2005**, *74*, 113–121.

[9] Szabo, D., Keyzer, H., Kaiser, H.E., & Molnar, J. Reversal of multidrug resistance of tumor cells. *Anticancer Research*, **2000**, *20*, 4261–4274

[10] Bihorel, S., Camenisch, G., Lemaire, M., & Scherrmann, J.-M. Modulation of the Brain Distribution of Imatinib and its Metabolites in Mice by Valspodar, Zosuquidar and Elacridar. *Pharmaceutical Research*, **2007**, *24*, 1720–1728

[11] De vries, N.A., Zhao, J., Kroon, E., Buckle, T., Beijnen, J.H., & Van tellingen, O. P-Glycoprotein and breast cancer resistance protein: Two dominant transporters working together in limiting the brain penetration of topotecan. *Clinical Cancer Research*, **2007**, *13*, 6440–6449

[12] Szakacs, G., Paterson, J.K., Ludwig, J.A., Booth-Genthe, C., & Gottesman, M.M. Targeting multidrug resistance in cancer. *Nature Reviews Drug Discovery*, **2006**, *5*, 219–234

[13] Jones, A.R., & Shusta, E.V. Blood-brain barrier transport of therapeutics via receptor-mediation. *Pharmaceutical Research*, **2007**, *24*, 1759–1771.

[14] Groothuis, D.R. The blood-brain and blood-tumor barriers: A review of strategies for increasing drug delivery. *Neuro-Oncology*, **2000**, *2*, 45–59

[15] Xia, C.F., Zhang, Y., Zhang, Y., Boado, R.J., & Pardridge, W.M. Intravenous siRNA of brain cancer with receptor targeting and avidin-biotin technology. *Pharm Res*, **2007**, *24*, 2309–2316.

[16] Kamphorst, W., De boer, A.G. & Gaillard, P.J. Brain Drug Targeting: The Future of Brain Drug Development.: Pardridge W.M. Cambridge University Press. *Journal of Clinical Pathology*, **2002**, *55*, 158–162.

[17] Reese, T.S., & Karnovsky, M.J. Fine structural localization of a blood-brain barrier to exogenous peroxidase. *Journal of Cell Biology*, **1967**, *34*, 207–217.

[18] Pardridge, W.M. BBB-Genomics: Creating new openings for brain-drug targeting. *Drug Discovery Today*, **2001**, *6*, 381–383.

[19] Abraham, M.H., Chadha, H.S., & Mitchell, R.C. Hydrogen bonding. 33. Factors that influence the distribution of solutes between blood and brain. *Journal of Pharmaceutical Sciences*, **1994**, *83*, 1257–1268

[20] Wahl, M., Schilling, L., Unterberg, A., & Baethmann, A. Mediators of vascular and parenchymal mechanisms in secondary brain damage. *Acta Neurochir Suppl (Wien)*, **1993**, *57*, 64–72.

[21] Folkman, J. Angiogenesis in cancer, vascular, rheumatoid and other disease. *Nature Medicine*, **1995**, *1*, 27–31

[22] Béduneau, A., Saulnier, P., & Benoit, J.-P. Active targeting of brain tumors using nanocarriers. *Biomaterials*, **2007**, *28*, 4947–4967.

[23] Buckner, J.C., Brown, P.D., O'neill, B.P., Meyer, F.B., Wetmore, C.J., & Uhm, J.H. Central nervous system tumors. *Mayo Clinic Proceedings*, **2007**, *82*, 1271–1286.

[24] Deangelis, L.M. Brain Tumors. *New England Journal of Medicine*, **2001**, *344*, 114-123

[25] Louis, D.N., Pomeroy, S.L., & Cairncross, J.G. Focus on central nervous system neoplasia. *Cancer Cell*, **2002**, *1*, 125–128.

[26] Louis, D.N., Ohgaki, H., Wiestler, O.D., Cavenee, W.K., Burger, P.C., Jouvet, A., ... Kleihues, P. The 2007 WHO classification of Tumors of the central nervous system. *Acta Neuropathologica*, **2007**, *114*, 97–109.

[27] Behin, A., Hoang-Xuan, K., Carpentier, A.F., & Delattre, J.Y. Primary brain Tumors in adults. *Lancet*, **2003**, *361*, 323–331

[28] Fisher, J.L., Schwartzbaum, J.A., Wrensch, M., & Wiemels, J.L. Epidemiology of brain tumors. *Neurol Clin*, **2007**, *25*, 867–890

[29] Norden, A.D., & Wen, P.Y. Glioma therapy in adults. *Neurologist*, **2006**, *12*, 279–292

[30] Brioschi, A.M., Calderoni, S., Zara, G.P., Priano, L., Gasco, M.R., & Mauro, A. Chapter 11 Solid lipid nanoparticles for brain tumors therapy: State of the art and novel challenges. *Progress in Brain Research*, **2009**, *180*, 193–223.

[31] Sathornsumetee, S., Rich, J.N., & Reardon, D.A. Diagnosis and treatment of high-grade astrocytoma. *Neurologic Clinics*, **2007**, *25*, 1111–1139

[32] Lockman, P.R., Mumper, R.J., Khan, M.A., & Allen, D.D. Nanoparticle Technology for Drug Delivery Across the Blood-Brain Barrier. *Drug Development and Industrial Pharmacy*, **2002**, *28*, 1–13.

[33] Lu, W., Zhang, Y., Tan, Y.-Z., Hu, K.-L., Jiang, X.-G., & Fu, S.-K. (2005). Cationic albumin-conjugated pegylated nanoparticles as novel drug carrier for brain delivery. *Journal of Controlled Release*, **2005**, *107*, 428–448.

[34] Scheffel, U., Rhodes, B.A., Natarajan, T.K., & Wagner, H.N., JR. Albumin microspheres for study of the reticuloendothelial system. *The Journal of Nuclear Medicine*, **1972**, *13*, 498–503.

[35] Wissing, S.A., Kayser, O., & Muller, R.H. Solid lipid nanoparticles for parenteral drug delivery. *Advanced Drug Delivery Reviews*, **2004**, *56*, 1257–1272.

[36] Fundarò, A., Cavalli, R., Bargoni, A., Vighetto, D., Zara, G.P., & Gasco, M.R. Non-stealth and stealth solid lipid nanoparticles (SLN) carrying doxorubicin: Pharmacokinetics and tissue distribution after i.v. administration to rats. *Pharmacological Research*, **2000**, *42*, 3–37

[37] Chen, D.-B., Yang, T.-Z., Lu, W.-L., & Zhang, Q. *In vitro* and *in vivo* study of two types of long-circulating solid lipid nanoparticles containing paclitaxel. *Chemical and Pharmaceutical Bulletin*, **2001**, *49*, 1444–1447.

[38] Suresh Reddy, J., & Venkateswarlu, V. Novel delivery systems for drug targeting to the brain. *Drugs of the Future*, **2004**, *29*, 63–83.

[39] Anon. Code of federal regulations. *Food Drugs*, **2001**, *21*, 1–70.

[40] Jumaa, M., & Müller, B.W. Lipid emulsions as a novel system to reduce the hemolytic activity of lytic agents: Mechanism of the protective effect. *European Journal of Pharmaceutical Sciences*, **2000**, *9*, 285–290.

[41] Cavalli, R., Caputo, O., & Gasco, M.R. Preparation and characterization of solid lipid nanospheres containing paclitaxel. *European Journal of Pharmaceutical Sciences*, **2000**, *10*, 305–309.

[42] Mr, G. Method for producing solid lipid microspheres having a narrow size distribution. *United states patent patent application*, **1993**.

[43] Müller, R., Maaben, S., Weyhers, H., Specht, F., & Lucks, J. Cytotoxicity of magnetite-loaded polylactide, polylactide/glycolide particles and solid lipid nanoparticles. *International Journal of Pharmaceutics*, **1996**, *138*, 85–94.

[44] Shahgaldian, P., Da silva, E., Coleman, A.W., Rather, B., & Zaworotko, M.J. Para-acyl-calix-arene based solid lipid nanoparticles (SLNs):

A detailed study of preparation and stability parameters. *International Journal of Pharmaceutics*, **2003**, *253*, 23–38

[45] Dubes, A., Parrot-Lopez, H., Abdelwahed, W., Degobert, G., Fessi, H., Shahgaldian, P., & Coleman, A.W. Scanning electron microscopy and atomic force microscopy imaging of solid lipid nanoparticles derived from amphiphilic cyclodextrins. European *Journal of Pharmaceutics and Biopharmaceutics*, **2003**, *55*, 279–282.

[46] Müller, R., Radtke, M., & Wissing, S. Nanostructured lipid matrices for improved microencapsulation of drugs. *International Journal of Pharmaceutics*, **2002a**, *242*, 121–128.

[47] Müller, R., Mehnert, W. Lucks, J.-S., Schwarz, C., Zur mühlen, A., Meyhers, H., ... Rühl, D. Solid lipid nanoparticles (SLN): An alternative colloidal carrier system for controlled drug delivery. *European Journal of Pharmaceutics and Biopharmaceutics*, **1995**, *41*, 62–69.

[48] Muller, R.H., Mader, K., & Gohla, S. Solid lipid nanoparticles (SLN) for controlled drug delivery a review of the state of the art. *European Journal of Pharmaceutics and Biopharmaceutics*, **2000**, *50*, 161–177.

[49] Mehnert, W., & Mader, K. Solid lipid nanoparticles: Production, characterization and applications. *Advanced Drug Delivery Reviews*, **2001**, *47*, 165–196.

[50] Schwarz, C., Mehnert, W., Lucks, J.S., & Müller, R. H. Solid lipid nanoparticles (SLN) for controlled drug delivery. I. Production, characterization and sterilization. *Journal of Controlled Release*, **1994**, *30*, 83–96

[51] Westesen, K., Sickmann, B., & Koch, M.H.J. Investigations on the physical state of lipid nanoparticles by synchrotron radiation X-ray diffraction. *International Journal of Pharmaceutics*, **1993**, *93*, 189–199

[52] Müller, R., Maassen, S., Schwarz, C., & Mehnert, W. Solid lipid nanoparticles (SLN) as potential carrier for human use: Interaction with human granulocytes. *Journal of Controlled Release*, **1997a**, *47*, 261–269

[53] Bunjes, H., Westesen, K., & Koch, M. Crystallization tendency and polymorphic transitions in triglyceride nanoparticles. *International Journal of Pharmaceutics*, **1996**, *129*, 159–173.

[54] Westesen, K., Bunjes, H., & Koch, M. H. J. Physicochemical characterization of lipid nanoparticles and evaluation of their drug loading capacity and sustained release potential. *Journal of Controlled Release*, **1997**, *48*, 223–236.

[55] Siekmann, B., & Westesen, K. Thermoanalysis of the recrystallization process of melt-homogenized glyceride nanoparticles. *Colloids and Surfaces B: Biointerfaces*, **1994**, *3*, 159–175.

[56] Westesen, K. Novel lipid-based colloidal dispersions as potential drug administration systems expectations and reality. *Colloid and Polymer Science*, **2000**, *278*, 608–618.

[57] Müller, R.H., Weyhers, H., Zur mühlen, A., & Mehnert, W. Solid lipid nanoparticles: A novel carrier system for cosmetics and pharmaceutics. 2nd communication: Properties, production and scaling up. *Die Pharmazeutische Industrie*, **1997b**, *59*, 614–619.

[58] Freitas, C., & Müller, R.H. Correlation between long-term stability of solid lipid nanoparticles (SLNt) and crystallinity of the lipid phase. *European Journal of Pharmaceutics and Biopharmaceutics*, **1999**, *47*, 125–132.

[59] Hagemann, J. W. Thermal behavior and polymorphism of acylglycerides. In N. Garti, & K. Sato (Eds.), Crystallization and polymorphism of fats and fatty acids,**1988**, 189–276. New York, Basel: Marcel Dekker.

[60] Hernqvist, L. Crystal structures of fats and fatty acids. In N. Garti, & K. Sato. (Eds.), Crystallization and polymorphism of fats and fatty acids, **1988**, 9–96, New York, Basel: Marcel Dekker.

[61] Jenning, V., Gysler, A., Schäfer-Korting, M., & Gohla, S.H. Vitamin A loaded solid lipid nanoparticles for topical use: Occlusive properties and drug targeting to the upper skin. *European Journal of Pharmaceutics and Biopharmaceutics*, **2000a**, *49*, 211–218.

[62] Polt, R., Porreca, F., Szabo, L.Z., Bilsky, E.J., Davis, P., Abbruscato, T.J., ... Hruby, V.J. Glycopeptide enkephalin analogues produce analgesia in mice: Evidence for penetration of the blood-brain barrier. *Proceedings of the National Academy of Sciences of the USA*, **1994**, *91*, 7114–7118.

[63] Chen, Y., Dalwadi, G., & Benson, H.A.E. Drug delivery across the blood-brain barrier. *Current Drug Delivery*, **2004**, *1*, 361–376.

[64] Saupe, A., Gordon, K.C., & Rades, T. Structural investigations on nanoemulsions, solid lipid nanoparticles and nanostructured lipid carriers by cryo-field emission scanning electron microscopy and Raman spectroscopy. *International Journal of Pharmaceutics*, **2006**, *314*, 56–62.

[65] Zur mühlen, A., & Mehnert, W. Drug release and release mechanism of prednisolone loaded solid lipid nanoparticles. *Pharmazie*, **1998**, *53*, 552–555

[66] Kreuter, J. Nanoparticulate systems for brain delivery of drugs. *Advanced Drug Delivery Reviews*, **2001**, *47*, 65–81.

[67] Scholer, N., Olbrich, C., Tabatt, K., Muller, R.H., Hahn, H., & Liesenfeld, O. Surfactant, but not the size of solid lipid nanoparticles (SLN) influences viability and cytokine production of macrophages. *International Journal of Pharmaceutics*, **2001**, *221*, 57–67.

[68] Fang, J.Y., Fang, C.L., Liu, C.H., & Su, Y.H. Lipid nanoparticles as vehicles for topical psoralen delivery: Solid lipid nanoparticles (SLN) versus nanostructured lipid carriers (NLC). *European Journal of Pharmaceutics and Biopharmaceutics*, **2008**, *70*, 633–640.

[69] Das, S., & Chaudhury, A. Recent advances in lipid nanoparticle formulations with solid matrix for oral drug delivery. *AAPS PharmSciTech*, **2011**, *12*, 62–76

[70] Diederichs, J., & Muller, R. Liposomes in cosmetics and pharmaceutical products. *Pharmazeutische Industrie*, **1994**, *56*, 267–275.

[71] Freitas, C., & Müller, R. H. Effect of light and temperature on zeta potential and physical stability in solid lipid nanoparticle (SLNt) dispersions. *International Journal of Pharmaceutics*, **1998a**, *168*, 221–229.

[72] Noack, A., Hause, G., & Mäder, K. Physicochemical characterization of curcuminoid-loaded solid lipid nanoparticles. *International Journal of Pharmaceutics*, **2012**, *423*, 440–451.

[73] Souto, E.B., & Müller, R.H. Lipid nanoparticles (SLN and NLC) for drug delivery. Nanoparticles for Pharmaceutical Applications. *Valencia, CA: American Scientific Publishers*, **2007**, 103–112.

[74] Dingler, A., & Gohla, S. Production of solid lipid nanoparticles (SLN): Scaling up feasibilities. *Journal of Microencapsulation*, **2002**, *19*, 11–16.

[75] Almeida, A.J., & Souto, E. Solid lipid nanoparticles as a drug delivery system for peptides and proteins. *Advanced Drug Delivery Reviews*, **2007**, *59*, 478–490.

[76] Siekmann, B., & Westesen, K. Submicron-sized parenteral carrier systems based on solid lipids. *Pharmaceutical and Pharmacological Letters*, **1992**, *1*, 123–126.

[77] Yang, S., Zhu, J., Lu, Y., Liang, B., & Yang, C. Body distribution of camptothecin solid lipid nanoparticles after oral administration. *Pharmaceutical Research*, **1999**, *16*, 751–757.

[78] Rupenagunta, A., Somasundaram, I., Ravichandiram, V., Kausalya, J., & Senthilnathan, B. Solid lipid nanoparticles-A versatile carrier system. *Journal of Pharmacy Research*, **2011**, *4*, 2069–2075.

[79] Jores, K., Mehnert, W., Drechsler, M., Bunjes, H., Johann, C., & Mäder, K. Investigations on the structure of solid lipid nanoparticles (SLN) and oil-loaded solid lipid nanoparticles by photon correlation spectroscopy, field-flow fractionation and transmission electron microscopy. *Journal of Controlled Release*, **2004**, *95*, 217–227.

[80] Shenoy, V., Vijay, I., & Murthy, R. Tumor targeting: Biological factors and formulation advances in injectable lipid nanoparticles. *Journal of Pharmacy and Pharmacology*, **2005**, *57*, 411–421.

[81] Kaur, I.P., Bhandari, R., Bhandari, S., & Kakkar, V. Potential of solid lipid nanoparticles in brain targeting. *Journal of Controlled Release*, **2008**, *127*, 97–109.

[82] Müller, R., Radtke, M., & Wissing, S. Nanostructured lipid matrices for improved microencapsulation of drugs. *International Journal of Pharmaceutics*, **2002a**, *242*, 121–128

[83] Olbrich, C., Gessner, A., Kayser, O., & Müller, R.H. Lipid-drug-conjugate (LDC) nanoparticles as novel carrier system for the hydrophilic antitrypanosomal drug diminazenediaceturate. *Journal of Drug Targeting*, **2002**, *10*, 387–396.

[84] Cavalli, R., Bocca, C., Miglietta, A., Caputo, O., & Gasco, M. Albumin adsorption on stealth and nonstealth solid lipid nanoparticles. *STP Pharma Sciences*, **1999**, *9*, 183–189.

[85] Weiss, J., Decker, E.A., Mcclements, D.J., Kristbergsson, K., Helgason, T., & Awad, T. Solid lipid nanoparticles as delivery systems for bioactive food components. *Food Biophysics*, **2008**, *3*, 146–154.

[86] Shah, R., Eldridge, D., Palombo, E., & Harding, I. Lipid nanoparticles: Production, characterization and stability, **2015**.

[87] Jenning, V., Mäder, K., & Gohla, S.H. Solid lipid nanoparticles (SLNt) based on binary mixtures of liquid and solid lipids: A 1 H-NMR study. *International Journal of Pharmaceutics*, **2002b**, *205*, 15–21.

[88] Blasi, P., Schoubben, A., Romano, G.V., Giovagnoli, S., Di michele, A., & Ricci, M. Lipid nanoparticles for brain targeting II. Technological characterization. *Colloids and Surfaces B: Biointerfaces*, **2013a**, *110*, 130–137.

[89] Doktorovova, S., Shegokar, R., Fernandes, L., Martins-Lopes, P., Silva, A.M., Müller, R.H., & Souto, E.B. Trehalose is not a universal solution for solid lipid nanoparticles freeze-drying. *Pharmaceutical Development and Technology*, **2014**, *19*, 922–929

[90] Dura´n-Lobato, M., Enguix-Gonza´lez, A., Ferna´ndez-Arévalo, M., & Martı´n-Banderas, L. Statistical analysis of solid lipid nanoparticles produced by high-pressure homogenization: A practical prediction approach. *Journal of Nanoparticle Research*, **2013**, *15*, 14–43.

[91] Bummer, P.M. Physical chemical considerations of lipid-based oral drug delivery—solid lipid nanoparticles. *Critical Reviewst in Therapeutic Drug Carrier Systems*, **2004**, 21.

[92] Kasongo, K.W., Pardeike, J., Müller, R.H., & Walker, R.B. Selection and characterization of suitable lipid excipients for use in the manufacture of didanosine-loaded solid lipid nanoparticles and nanostructured lipid carriers. *Journal of Pharmaceutical Sciences*, **2011**, *100*, 5185–5196.

[93] Joshi, M., Pathak, S., Sharma, S., & Patravale, V. Design and *in vivo* pharmacodynamic evaluation of nanostructured lipid carriers for parenteral delivery of artemether: Nanoject. *International Journal of Pharmaceutics*, **2008**, *364*, 119–126

[94] Chapman, D. The polymorphism of glycerides. *Chemical Reviews*, **1962**, *62*, 433–456.

[95] Wong, H.L., Li, Y., Bendayan, R., Rauth, M., & Wu, X. Solid lipid nanoparticles for anti-tumor drug delivery. In M. M. Amiji (Ed.), *Nanotechnology for cancer therapy*, **2007.**

[96] Tabatt, K., Kneuer, C., Sameti, M., Olbrich, C., Müller, R.H., Lehr, C.-M., & Bakowsky, U. Transfection with different colloidal systems: Comparison of solid lipid nanoparticles and liposomes. *Journal of Controlled Release*, **2004**, *97*, 321–332.

[97] Jenning, V., & Gohla, S. Comparison of wax and glyceride solid lipid nanoparticles (SLNs). *International Journal of Pharmaceutics*, **2000**, *196*, 219–222.

[98] Jenning, V., Thünemann, A.F., & Gohla, S.H. Characterisation of a novel solid lipid nanoparticle carrier system based on binary mixtures of liquid and solid lipids. *International Journal of Pharmaceutics*, **2000c**, *199*, 167–177.

[99] Corrigan O, H.A. Surfactants in pharmaceutical products and systems. *In: J, S. (ed.) Encyclopedia of pharmaceutical technology. NY, USA: Informa Health*, **2003**, *3.*

[100] Walstra, P. Principles of emulsion formation. *Chemical Engineering Science*, **1993**, *48*, 333–349

[101] Mcclements, D.J., & Rao, J. Food-grade nanoemulsions: Formulation, fabrication, properties, performance, biological fate, and potential toxicity. *Critical Reviews in Food Science and Nutrition*, **2011**, *51*, 285–330

[102] Cavalli, R., Morel, S., Gasco, M., & Chetoni, P. Preparation and evaluation *in vitro* of colloidal lipospheres containing pilocarpine as ion pair. *International Journal of Pharmaceutics*, **1995**, *117*, 243–246

[103] Cavalli, R., Gasco, M.R., Chetoni, P., Burgalassi, S., & Saettone, M.F. Solid lipid nanoparticles (SLN) as ocular delivery system for tobramycin. *International Journal of Pharmaceutics*, **2002**, *238*, 241–245.

[104] Cavalli, R., Bargoni, A., Podio, V., Muntoni, E., Zara, G.P., & Gasco, M.R. Duodenal administration of solid lipid nanoparticles loaded with different percentages of tobramycin. *Journal of Pharmaceutical Sciences*, **2003**, *92*, 1085–1094.

[105] Zara, G.P., Cavalli, R., Bargoni, A., Fundarò, A., Vighetto, D., & Gasco, M.R. Intravenous administration to rabbits of non-stealth and stealth doxorubicin-loaded solid lipid nanoparticles at increasing concentrations of stealth agent: Pharmacokinetics and distribution of doxorubicin in brain and other tissues. *Journal of Drug Targeting*, **2002**, *10*, 327–335

[106] Madan, J., Pandey, R.S., Jain, V., Katare, O.P., Chandra, R., & Katyal, A. Poly (ethylene)-glycol conjugated solid lipid nanoparticles of noscapine improve biological half-life, brain delivery and efficacy in glioblastoma cells. *Nanomedicine: Nanotechnology, Biology and Medicine*, **2013**, *9*, 492–503.

[107] Pignatello, R., Leonardi, A., Pellitteri, R., Carbone, C., Caggia, S., Graziano, A. C. E., & Cardile, V. Evaluation of new amphiphilic PEG derivatives for preparing stealth lipid nanoparticles. *Colloids and Surfaces A: Physicochemical and Engineering Aspects*, **2013**, *434*, 136–144.

[108] Priano, L., Zara, G.P., El-Assawy, N., Cattaldo, S., Muntoni, E., Milano, E., ... Gasco, M.R. Baclofenloaded solid lipid nanoparticles: Preparation, electrophysiological assessment of efficacy, pharmacokinetic and tissue distribution in rats after intraperitoneal administration. *European Journal of Pharmaceutics and Biopharmaceutics*, **2011**, *79*, 135–141.

[109] Manjunath, K., Reddy, J.S., & Venkateswarlu, V. Solid lipid nanoparticles as drug delivery systems. *Methods and Findings in Experimental and Clinical Pharmacology*, **2005**, *27*, 127–144.

[110] Yu, B.-T., Sun, X., & Zhang, Z.-R. Enhanced liver targeting by synthesis of N 1-stearyl-5-Fu and incorporation into solid lipid nanoparticles. *Archives of Pharmacal Research*, **2003**, *26*, 10, 96–110

[111] Heiati, H., Tawashi, R., & Phillips, N. Drug retention and stability of solid lipid nanopartiles containing azidothymidine palmitate after autoclaving, storage and lyophilization. *Journal of Microencapsulation*, **1998**, *15*, 173–184.

[112] Muller, R., Schwarz, C., Mehnert, W., & Lucks, J. Production of solid lipid nanoparticles (SLN) for controlled drug delivery. *Proceedings International Symposium Control Release Bioact Mater*, **1993**, 480–481.

[113] Müller, R., Maaben, S., Weyhers, H., Specht, F., & Lucks, J. Cytotoxicity of magnetite-loaded polylactide, polylactide/glycolide particles and solid lipid nanoparticles. *International Journal of Pharmaceutics*, **1996**, *138*, 85–94.

[114] Shah, M.R., Imran, M., & Ullah, S. Lipid-based nanocarriers for drug delivery and diagnosis, **2017**.

[115] Gawande, M.B., Shelke, S.N., Zboril, R., & Varma, R.S. Microwave-assisted chemistry: Synthetic applications for rapid assembly of nanomaterials and organics. *Accounts of Chemical Research*, **2014**, *47*, 1338–1348.

[116] Hayes, B. L. Recent advances in microwave-assisted synthesis. *Aldrichimica Acta*, **2004**, *37*, 66–77.

[117] Bergese, P., Colombo, I., Gervasoni, D., & Depero, L. Microwave generated nanocomposites for making insoluble drugs soluble. *Materials Science and Engineering: C*, **2003**, *23*, 791–795.

[118] Moneghini, M., Bellich, B., Baxa, P., & Princivalle, F. Microwave generated solid dispersions containing ibuprofen. *International Journal of Pharmaceutics*, **2008**, *361*, 125–130.

[119] An, Z., Tang, W., Hawker, C.J., & Stucky, G.D. One-step microwave preparation of well-defined and functionalized polymeric nanoparticles. *Journal of the American Chemical Society*, **2006**, *128*, 15054–15055

[120] Waters, L.J., Bedford, S., & Parkes, G.M. Controlled microwave processing applied to the pharmaceutical formulation of ibuprofen. *AAPS PharmSciTech*, **2011**, *12*, 1038–1043.

[121] Shah, R.M., Malherbe, F., Eldridge, D., Palombo, E.A., & Harding, I.H. Physicochemical characterization of solid lipid nanoparticles (SLNs) prepared by a novel microemulsion technique. *Journal of Colloid and Interface Science*, **2014**, *428*, 286–294.

[122] Sjöström, B., & Bergensta°hl, B. Preparation of submicron drug particles in lecithin-stabilized o/w emulsions I. Model studies of the precipitation of cholesteryl acetate. *International Journal of Pharmaceutics*, **1992**, *88*, 53–62

[123] Cortesi, R., Esposito, E., Luca, G., & Nastruzzi, C. Production of lipospheres as carriers for bioactive compounds. *Biomaterials*, **2002**, *23*, 2283–2294.

[124] Garcia-Fuentes, M., Torres, D., & Alonso, M. Design of lipid nanoparticles for the oral delivery of hydrophilic macromolecules. *Colloids and Surfaces B: Biointerfaces*, **2003**, *27*, 159–168.

6

Clinical Studies on the Efficacy and Safety of Nano-enabled Carriers for the Treatment of Brain Tumors

Abstract

Malignant brain tumor patients still have a terrible prognosis, with a survival rate of fewer than 15 months, despite substantial breakthroughs in tumor identification and treatment. The primary challenge in treating brain tumors lies in the limited ability of drugs or treatments to penetrate the BBB, or the blood–brain barrier. However, by promoting the movement of drugs and macromolecules over the BBB, nanotechnology-based therapies have showed promise in overcoming this obstacle, exploiting tumor biology, improving drug pharmacokinetics, and reducing off-target side effects. This chapter's main goal is to examine recent studies on nano-enabled therapeutics for brain tumor therapy, examining their efficacy and safety.

6.1 Introduction

Whether primary or metastatic, brain tumors have a dismal prognosis and much shorter post-diagnosis survival times. Glioblastoma multiforme (GBM), the most prevalent and dangerous kind of malignant glioma, is a tumor that is characterized by diffuse infiltrative growth, which makes complete surgical removal without causing significant cerebral damage nearly impossible [1]. The median survival time for GBM patients has not exceeded 15 months despite the adoption of multimodal treatments comprising tumor removal, radiation, and therapy [2]. The treatment of brain tumors poses specific challenges, including surgical excision, chemotherapy and radiation resistance, limited drug penetration into the tumor, limited medication absorption into the tumor, and potential damage to healthy cells since the blood–brain barrier (BBB) is still present in non-brain tissues. While certain cytotoxic drugs may

137

reach the tumor mass through a compromised or partial BBB, they often fail to traverse the protective barriers of the brain's vasculature [3], hindering their access to cancer cells located just centimeters away. Moreover, progress in understanding the brain tumor microenvironment and identifying targetable regulators of brain tumor cells has been slow, impeding the development of effective pharmacological treatments [4]. This stagnation can be attributed, in part, due to a lack of effective medication delivery methods [5].

Nanomedicine utilizes engineered nanostructures that are constructed from the ground up to achieve multifunctionality, spatial organization, and structural diversity. These nanostructures act at the molecular level to provide therapeutic or diagnostic effects. Nanoparticles (NPs) possess several desirable characteristics, including high mobility, the capacity to handle a high pharmacological load, and a vast surface area. Particles smaller than 1000 nm in at least one dimension are considered NPs. These unique material features can lead to improved drug targeting and absorption, reduced chemoresistance, and fewer unwanted side effects, such as bone marrow toxicity [5].

In the context of treating glioblastoma (GBM) and delivering medications across the blood–brain barrier or (BBB), only actively or passively targeted nanoparticles have shown potential. However, the application of rapid nanopharmaceuticals in neurosurgery and glioma treatments has garnered both interest and skepticism [3].

6.2 Nanoparticle Delivery and Glioma Targeting

Nanoparticulate accumulation in tumors has been linked to the EPR phenomenon since the 1980s, and in 1995, it was shown that NPs may cross the blood–brain barrier [6]. Tumor blood arteries may have a leaky endothelium due to fast and faulty angiogenesis, making their typical barrier function ineffective and enabling macromolecules to enter. Passive extravasation into tumor tissue occurs when NPs are injected intravenously, where they gather in the tumor bed and release their therapeutic payload close to tumor cells due to inadequate lymphatic outflow (EPR effect). EPR effect can be exploited with particles between 30 and 100 nm in size [6]. The kidneys readily excrete smaller NPs (10–20 nm), while larger NPs (150 nm or more) have a prolonged circulation time because they are absorbed by the reticuloendothelial system (RES) [7]. Appropriately sized nanoparticles can be accumulated in the nanoparticulate system or used for therapeutic blood–brain barrier crossing [8], although they have a long half-life in circulation (2–40 hours) before being taken up by the liver [9].

Table 6.1 The characteristics of nanoparticles and their observed effect on tumor location [13].

Size	Small				Large
	<10 nm	<20 nm	<70 nm	<100	>150 nm
	Rapid filtration by the glomerulus	Once absorbed, tumor cells are more readily expelled (decrease EPR)	Tumors and a healthy brain have better convection flow now	Permits tumor entry via EPR effect	Endocytosis is a difficult method of cell entrance, but RES cleared it
Hydrophobicity Charge	Hydrophilic Cationic Transcytosis of the BBB by adsorption-mediated cell membrane breakdown at high charge	Amphiphilic Uncharged The ECM of the tumor may be easier to spread if the charge is lower	Hydrophobic Anionic *In vivo*, reduced absorption of tumor cells by the brain		

The EPR effect is crucial to the "passive targeting" concept in cancer investigation into nanomedicine development. Additionally, it is possible that not all malignancies exhibit the EPR effect, and it is doubtful that this phenomenon will be the main factor influencing nanomedicine's effectiveness. How the medication is expelled from the delivery system, how quickly, and how much of the brain parenchyma is exposed to the drug are all important factors (assuming particles can breach BBB) that impact nanomedicine action, not only tumor formation and retention (EPR effect). Depending on the delivery method, drug/cargo, and tumor heterogeneity, the relative relevance of each of these components will change, and this must be considered while developing nanomedicine systems. In the case of brain tumours, EPR is unlikely to be useful. The dense brain matrix and high interstitial fluid pressure inhibit diffusion in the brain [10].

Tumor targeting in nanoparticulate delivery systems can be aided by adjusting variables including size, hydrophobicity, and surface charge (see Table 6.1). Additionally, the form of the particles matters since it affects their pharmacokinetics and, possibly, their permeability. It has been found that particles with a diameter bigger than 18 nm and smaller than 20 nm remain in circulation for longer than five days, which is beneficial for inhibiting macrophage uptake [11]. In the delivery of peptides utilizing long axial particles like carbon nanotubes and carbon nanofibers, where only 0.4% of the intravenously injected dose reaches the brain [8, 12, 13, 14], maintaining an intact blood–brain barrier (BBB) has shown promise. Preclinical evidence from mouse models supports the efficacy of peptide nanofibers, which exhibit minimal toxicity as they can be enzymatically converted into breakdown products already present in the body and brain parenchyma [14].

To counteract the detrimental effects of hydrophobic particle surfaces on prolonged circulation half-life, various polymeric surface modifications or coatings are employed. Polymers that are hydrophilic, such as poly(ethylene glycol) (PEG) (5 kDa), chitosan, albumin, and polysorbate 80 [6, 15, 16] are examples of materials used to mitigate this challenge.

Positively charged surfaces aid in making the BBB, or the blood–brain barrier, more permeable by physically adhering to endothelium. Cationic particles have shown greater ease in entering tumor cells at periphery compared to the most anionic particles [17]. Nanoparticles (NPs) offer potential benefits for glioma therapy, including their ability to remain at high concentrations in the blood plasma and exert a positive effect at the blood–tumor interface. Significant improvements in survival have been observed in orthotopic animal models with the use of various polymeric nanomedicines, including lipid-based formulations (refer to Table 6.2). Examples of such nanomedicines include dendrimers and peptide-based formulations (see Figure 6.1).

6.3 Lipid-based Nanomedicines

Liposomes and other lipid-based nanomedicines have been important in drug delivery technology since their development in the 1960s. One of the first nanomedicines to be approved for use in humans was liposome therapy, which is commonly used to treat malignant brain tumors. They have received the greatest attention from researchers and practitioners of lipid-based nanomedicine in this situation. However, ongoing studies are also looking at how exosomes and nanocapsules could be used to treat brain tumors (see Table 6.3). These newly developed nanomedicine platforms are promising, and their potential therapeutic uses are being investigated.

6.3.1 Liposomes

The first person to observe that aqueous phospholipid molecules from egg lecithin spontaneously organize into three-dimensional bilayers that may compartmentalize aqueous solutions and entrap any solutes dissolved therein

Table 6.2 Trials of liposomal nanomedicines in the treatment of GBM [13].

Description	Phase/status	Clinical trials gov. identifier
Ara-C (DepoCyt) encapsulated in liposomal atrioventricular delivery: in a phase II study for patients with recurrent GBM	The end of phases I and II	NCT01044966
Liposomal doxorubicin for the treatment of pediatric cancer with tumors that have become resistant to standard chemotherapy	Phase I/finished	NCT00019630
Newly diagnosed patients of GBM treated with pegylated lipid nanoparticle doxorubicin and prolonged temozolomide undergo radiation therapy	Both phases I and II have been finished	NCT00944801
This investigation evaluated the effectiveness, tolerance and safety of rhenium nanoliposomes when dealing with GBM that has come back after treatment	No longer accepting applications/phase I/II	NCT01906385
Nanoliposomal CPT-11 showed promising results in a phase I trial being tested on patients with recurrent high-grade gliomas (NL CPT-11)	Phase I/finished	NCT00734682
Liposomal irinotecan with image guiding was used to treat the recurrence of high-grade glioma	Invitation-only enrollment (phase I)	NCT02022644
Individuals with recurrent malignant gliomas or solid tumors and brain metastases are being studied when given 2B3-101	Participating in phases I and II but not yet recruiting	NCT01386580

was British hematologist Alec D. Bangham [18, 19]. The utilization of liposomes as enzyme carriers and the possibility of using them to transport other biological and therapeutic substances were then first mentioned [20, 21].

Hydrophilic and hydrophobic substances benefit from liposomes' bilayered structure, which makes them an ideal vehicle for their delivery. Liposomes are formed when the hydrophobic core of phospholipid bilayers binds hydrophilic molecules, enclosing them in the water-containing vesicles, which is what happens when they dissolve in water. However, generally speaking, hydrophilic chemicals have a lower loading efficiency than hydrophobic molecules. Vesicle diameters typically range from 50 to 5 nm. However, when exposed to extreme osmotic pressure and detergents, they can rupture or lyse. Liposomes can be utilized to build concentration ion gradients. Liposomes' early clinical translation was made possible thanks to

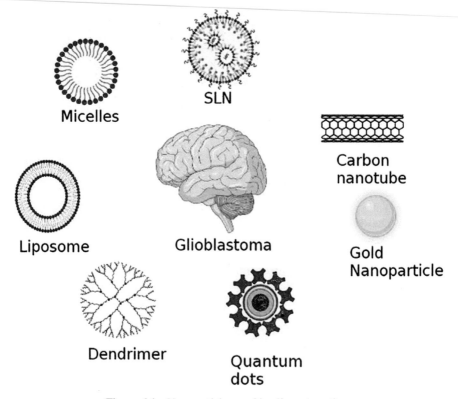

Figure 6.1   Nanoparticles used in glioma targeting.

their composition, which is largely composed of ingredients that are both biocompatible and biodegradable. A disadvantage of using liposomes is that the liposomal preparations are quickly removed from the circulation and predominantly absorbed by liver-based RES cells. PEG, an inert biocompatible polymer that forms a shield over the liposome surface and inhibits opsonins' detection of the liposomes and, consequently, their clearance, helped to overcome this problem in large part. Increased bioavailability and nonsaturable log-linear kinetics are demonstrated by long-circulating liposomes [22]. In order to provide a detachable method of attaching PEG, conditions such as low pH in the tumour microenvironment can be locally adverse.

Despite the high cost of high-purity lipids, the production technique for liposomal nanomedicines is scalable. Currently, clinical trials for liposomal nanomedicines are the only ones being conducted for glioblastoma multiforme (GBM), but the results and the preclinical stage of these studies are still pending (refer to Table 6.2). Since the mid-1990s, liposomal chemotherapeutics

Table 6.3 Investigation of nanomedicines for glioma in preclinical studies.

Nanoparticles	Drug/targeting moiety	Outcomes	Ref.
Passively transported			
Nanoparticles of PBCA coated with polysorbate 80	Low-density lipoprotein (LDL) with doxorubicin or temozolomide	The levels of TMZ increased in the liver, spleen, and lungs when NPs were connected to them. The usage of overcoated NPs significantly boosted the drug's accumulation in the brain, with a gain of a factor of 2.29 (1.10 0.19 g/g versus 0.48 0.11 g/g, 10 mg/kg temozolomide IV dose). In the 101/8 rat models, doxorubicin overcoated NPs (2.5 mg/kg) significantly increased survival at 2, 5, and 8 days after implantation (24.5, 27, and 35 days, respectively). Doxorubicin PBCA NPs demonstrated superior effectiveness to either saline or doxorubicin alone.	77
N-palmitoyl-N-monomethyl-N,N-dimethyl-N,N,Ntrimethyl-6-O-glycol	Lomustine	Brain/bone $AUC_{0\text{-}4h}$ ratios of 0.90 for MET and 0.53 for ethanolic lomustine values in the brain/liver $AUC_{0\text{-}4h}$ ratio of 0.24 and 0.15 indicate that moderate brain targeting was accomplished with the MET formulation. The median and interquartile range (IQR) survival rates of MET lomustine-, ethanolic lomustine-, and undiagnosed mice (U-87 MG tumors) were 33.2, 22.5, and 21.3 days, respectively. Compared to liposomes, MET NPs had a reduced absorption rate in macrophages.	5
Transportation of liposomal nanomedicines			
Dequalinium-coupled liposomes containing p-aminophenyl—D-mannopyranoside-D—tocopherol	Artemether/glucose transporter 1 (GLUT-1) and paclitaxel (and adsorption endocytosis)	When apoptotic enzymes and proapoptotic proteins are increased and antiapoptotic proteins are downregulated, brain cancer cells and brain cancer stem cell s undergo apoptosis. Physiological saline (17 days), taxol (22 days), paclitaxel liposomes (24 days), paclitaxel plus artemether (25 days), or MAN-targeting paclitaxel plus artemether liposomes (27 days) were administered to rats with C6 orthotopic tumors. The median survival time was significantly longer in the latter group ($n = 35$) than in the other groups ($n = 17$) after treatment.	23

(Continued)

Table 6.3 *Continued.*

Nanoparticles	Drug/targeting moiety	Outcomes	Ref.
Adsorption in the endocyte			
Liposomes conjugated with combined wheat germ agglutinin (WGA) with tamoxifen	Because tamoxifen blocks ABC transporters, daunomycin and quinacrine	Through *in vitro* studies, it was found that multifunctional liposomes (uncharged, B100 nm) may penetrate the BBB via an adsorption endocytosis pathway. Survival in a GSC ICR mouse model was extended from 26 to 30.83 to 36.33 days when 5 mg/kg of liposomal WGA-tamoxifen, daunorubicin, quinacrine, or saline were administered intravenously on days 10, 14, and 12 following tumor implantation.	23
Dendrimer transportation in action			
CTX-PEG-PAMAM (G5)	Gene encoding trail	Fluorescence imaging biodistribution studies showed that CTXPEG-PAMAM was less concentrated in the liver and kidneys than it was in tumors. CX-PEGPAMAM (50 g DNA per IV dose, three treatments) resulted in a median survival period of 59.5 days, compared to temozolomide (50 mg/kg per dosage, five doses).	55
CREKA-PEG-PAMAM (G5)	Gene-encoding TRAIL	U-87 MG orthotropic mice showed enhanced dendrimer fluorescence in the brain (IV:0.6 mol/kg).	62

(such as doxorubicin, vincristine, daunorubicin, and cytarabine) have received the FDA and European Medicines Agency approval, which has accelerated the development of liposomal nanomedicines for GBM. However, there is currently no approved liposomal therapy specifically for GBM.

PEG chain lengths of 2–5 kDa are ideal for liposomal formulations to ensure acceptable stability and steric hindrance of the liposome, concealment of the surface charge, and enhanced circulation half-life for liposomes. When liposomes are synthesized with cationic phospholipids like adsorptive endocytosis, 1,2-distearoylsn-glycero-3-phosphoethanolamine of the particles is made possible [23]. Liposomes can only cross the BBB if they are adorned with a BBB-expressed carrier protein or receptor as the vector or substrate if their charge is sufficient to facilitate their endocytosis (Table 6.3). In some situations, the liposomes can be effectively targeted to cancer cells via a cleavable PEG linker. The epidermal growth receptor, folic acid, neuropilin, and insulin are all examples of these vectors (Table 6.3). The tumor-to-plasma ratio can be improved, and the toxicity can be minimized by functionalized or cationic liposomes loaded with chemotherapy agents. When compared to traditional anthracyclines, favorable toxicity profiles were observed with both liposomal and PEGylated liposomal doxorubicin, with less cardiac toxicity and fewer adverse effects like hair loss, nausea, and vomiting. Because of this, they are favored over conventional anthracyclines in patients who are elderly, at risk for myelosuppression, or who have gastrointestinal problems [24].

6.3.2 Exosomes

There are many different types of GBM, and each has a unique capability of interacting with and influencing other cells in the tumor microenvironment. Mesenchymal cells influence the surrounding cells via miRNA to create an invasive microenvironment [25, 26]. Extracellular vesicles (EVs) are structures that contain secreted chemicals utilized in EVs for cell-to-cell communication. In terms of size and origin, EVs can be broken down into three groups, depending on their diameter between 30 and 2000 nm [27]. MVB-derived vesicles known as exosomes are called vesicles in this context (microvesicles are micro-sized vesicles that originate from the plasma membrane) [28].

Sucrose density gradient ultracentrifugation (110,000 g at a concentration of 1.13–1.19 g/mL) has been shown to sediment exosomes, which are typically 40–120 nm in size. They contain a variety of proteins, receptors, and nucleic acids, all of which are extremely dependent on other proteins and receptors indigenous to the producing cell, either in their watery core or as receptors embedded in the membrane bilayer. Originating as ILVs within MVBs, exosomes can carry out their duties either alone or with the help of the endosomal sorting complex, even if the mechanism governing exosome regulation and its contents is not fully known [27]. The initial stage in the process of making exosomes is endocytosis. The membrane proteins are carried into the early endosomes by vesicles covered with clathrin. ILVs and MVBs are formed as a result of the membrane budding inward and the creation of MVBs. Exosome MVBs are either degraded in lysosomes or membrane-bound or membrane-fused for secretion upon cellular maturity [27].

Histones [29], oncogenic species (EGFRvIII) [30], noncoding microRNAs [31], and tumor suppressors (PTEN) [32] are all demonstrated to be transported by exosomes in glioma cells. Among the four molecular subtypes of GBM, there is a notable difference in the transcripts of known exosome formation markers (i.e., mesenchymal, classical, neural, and proneural) [33]. Extracellularly released exosomes affect angiogenesis, functional RNA transcript transfer, proliferation resulting from paracrine stimulation, promigratory factor dissemination, and immunological triggering normal cell tolerance or malignancy [27]. Immune cells (macrophages and microglia) have been shown to lose their phagocytotic ability when exposed to exosomes [34, 35].

It has been shown that both brain tumor and glioblastoma multiforme (GBM) cells isolated from human tissue samples can form invadopodia, which are extracellular substrates that attach to and are degraded by multiple transmembrane and secreted extracellular proteases and are dynamic, and actin-rich protrusions on the cell membrane [36], which are involved in migration. Matrix-degrading proteinases of invadopodia may be synthesized, stabilized, and exocytosed by the exosome, according to recent studies [37]. It has also been found to be beneficial for tumor advancement to incubate mesenchymal exosomes with normal cells like astrocytes [34].

Better diagnostics and tailored therapeutics for glioblastoma can be created if the role exosomes play in the progression of the disease is better understood. Due to their capacity to transport both hydrophilic (proteins, DNA, and RNA) and hydrophobic (lipids, fatty acids, and cytokines) cargo, exosomes can be used as a delivery vehicle for a range of therapies and diagnostics. Paclitaxel and doxorubicin, two biotherapeutic drugs, were successfully transported over the BBB using exosomes made by brain endothelial cells [38].

The progression of tumors in xenograft animals was caused by the uptake of anticancer medications and the cytotoxicity of exosomes expressing CD63 tetraspanin transmembrane proteins [38]. Some exosomes may be able to get into the brain via the circulation and bind to their designated acceptor cells once they are there if they are made from genetically modified cells that express on their cell surface ligands that are supplied to the exosome's surface. The endogenous Lamp2b protein, which is a part of the exosomal membrane, and the rabies virus glycoprotein (RVG), which is known to bind the cholinergic receptors on neurons, were fused and transfected into dendritic cells. This fusion was then used to transport siRNA to the targeted neurons [39, 40].

Studies have shown vesicle formation-related gene expression is inversely correlated with tumor cell chemosensitivity in terms of exosomes, which is worth mentioning. Transmembrane transporter P-glycoprotein for drug efflux is overexpressed in GBM cells that have acquired resistance to temozolomide (miR-9 gene expression). Treating within cells that had become resistant to temozolomide, its expression was re-established by administering exosomal-anti-miR-9. Temozolomide is the medicine of choice for treating GBM along with radiotherapy and surgery (Stupp regimen) [41]. The therapy inhibited the multidrug transporter's expression. This is achieved by increasing the GBM cell production of exosomes and promoting their absorption by acceptor cells; exosome treatments for GBM therapy can be improved [42].

6.4 Polymeric Nanomedicines

In the encapsulation of hydrophilic as well as hydrophobic medicines, polymeric nanocarriers are often used. Polymeric NPs often have a larger drug loading compared to lipidic NPs, and this is true for both hydrophobic poorly soluble medicines and hydrophilic biomacromolecules and gene treatments. They resist enzymatic metabolism and are more stable in the body's fluids (pH, osmolarity, dilution, etc.) than lipidic nanomedicines, which vary depending on the polymer used.

By engaging with a range of receptors expressed on or produced by GBM cells or involved in BBB crossing, polymeric nanocarriers can be altered to precisely target cancer cells, in addition to functioning as passive smart delivery vehicles [5] (Table 6.3). Triblock polymers, which include PEG, polyglycolic acid, and polylactic acid, are the most studied (Table 6.3). Over the recent decade, more and more effective animal tests have been conducted on mice and rats, increasing the median survival time by as much as ~20 days [43]. However, because of the wide variety of animal models used and the small number of studies that included pharmacokinetic analyses, caution is warranted when comparing the results of these investigations. In comparison to xenografts made from chemically induced models or regular glioma cell lines kept in serum-supplemented medium, neurosphere and biopsy spheroid culture xenografts more faithfully depict the aggressive infiltrative development of human gliomas [13, 44]. An in-depth investigation of large-animal models for biodistribution is required prior to the therapeutic use of polymeric nanocarriers [45]. Currently, protocols for the large-scale formulation of functionalized and loaded NPs that uphold their target molecules are under development.

6.5 Dendrimers

In preclinical animal studies, dendrimers have gained attention as potential delivery systems for cancer drugs, despite limited evidence of their efficacy in GBM. Polymers with remarkable new characteristics may be made from commercially available monomers in a stepwise fashion to make dendrimers, which are little, uniformly sized macromolecules [46]. Structured like an onion's inner and outer layers, dendrimers (typically 110 nm) vary structurally from other polymers in that they begin with a hub surrounded by radial layers of branched monomers that are produced and anchored back to the core (i.e., generations) [46]. Dendrimer synthesis may be accomplished in two ways: either by a convergent or divergent approach, where the dendrimer is synthesized from the peripheral to the center [47] or by adding monomers one at a time from the core outwards [48]. The central part, the offshoots/next generation, and the many-sided exterior of dendrimers are the three structural domains that can be altered. When it comes to hydrophobic medications, drug loading rises as the number of generations grows [49]. The complexation of genetic material and absorption by cells is made possible by dendrimers with strong cationic surface charges [50].

As medication and gene delivery systems, dendrimers have shown a lot of potentials. Dedrimers prepared using Poly(glycerol-co-succinic acid), poly(lactic acid), poly(glycerol), poly(2,2 bis(hydroxymethyl)-poly(AMAM) and propionic acid) have been used to deliver therapeutic agents [51]. Both types of dendrimers have received a lot of research interest since they were commercially accessible, although Tomalia's PAMAM dendrimers were the first to be characterized, in 1985, while the PPI dendrimers were the first to be synthesized, in 1993. Dendrimers come in a wide range of sizes (e.g., 10–100 kDa), molecular weights (e.g., 10–100 kDa), and functional end-groups (e.g., amine, thiol, phosphate, carboxylic acid, and hydroxyl). The potential of PAMAM and PPI dendrimers should be studied in the context of passive and active targeted techniques for the treatment of brain tumors (Table 6.3).

There is evidence to suggest that dendrimers, which can be as small as 10–20 nm, have the potential to passively transport drugs to tumors [52]. Dendrimers exhibit a longer half-life in circulation [53] because they can bind to biomolecules such as plasma proteins and other high molecular weight substances. In a research by Zhang et al. (2015), the intracranial tumor biodistribution of hydroxyl-terminated PAMAM dendrimers (G4) was examined [54] using a model of intracranial tumor (9 L gliosarcoma). The study showed a 48-hour retention of dendrimers in the tumor and the accompanying microglia/macrophages, demonstrating their preferred retention within the solid tumor (6 mm) and their accumulation (15 minutes).

Due to the presence of the reactive functional groups on "dendrimers," various ligands with activity against brain cancer can be attached to their outer surface. Examples of such ligands include short peptides (angiopep [55], T7 [56, 57, 58], RGD [59, 60, 61], and CREKA [62]), proteins (transferrin [63]), antibodies [64, 65], and sugars (D-glucosamine [66]). Zhao et al. reported the successful utilization of the fibrin-binding peptide CREKA, linked to PAMAM dendrimers, as a therapy for glioblastoma [62]. In this study, PEGylated PAMAM dendrimers, known for their small size and ability to penetrate tumors, were used as carriers, and CREKA, a peptide that specifically targets tumors, was employed due to its high affinity for fibrin protein, which is abundant in glioblastoma. Fluorescence imaging demonstrated that CREKA-modified PAMAM dendrimers accumulated 1.75-fold more in tumor tissue compared to unmodified dendrimers in glioblastoma-bearing nude mice.

These results emphasize the potential of dendrimers as nanocarriers for precise medication delivery to brain tumors, and the capacity to target tumors by altering their surface with certain ligands.

Utilizing dendrimers to transport drugs and the genes to tumors of the brain has unquestionably sparked a medical revolution. This is because dendrimers and cell membranes both have negative charges and the rupture and lysis of cells are well-known to occur when they are the right size, i.e., between 1 and 100 nm in size, and the nanometric components of cells (membrane, organelles, proteins, etc.) [51, 67]. *In vitro* tests on dendrimer toxicity (based on cell viability) show that dendrimers, (particularly PAMAM, PPII, and PLL nanocarriers), are cytotoxic and hemolytic [68-73]. PAMAM and PPL dendrimers were highly concentrated after just 1 hour of exposure, and Malik et al. saw that, even at modest concentrations (10 g/mL), generation-dependent hemolysis and red blood cell dysfunction problems occur in cancer cell lines [73]. The cytotoxicity of cationic dendrimers ranged from 50 to 300 μg/mL, and this value was highly dependent on the dendrimer type, the cells, and the concentration. Using Caco-2 cell lines, Jevprasesphant et al. [71] tested the cytotoxicity of cationic PAMAM dendrimers at varying concentrations (G4 < 2 µM; G3 < 10 µM; G2 < 1000 µM) ($-NH_2$ and $-OH$). When evaluated on human RBCs, the IC50 values for PAMAM G2, G3, and G4 dendrimers are 735, 77, and 28 M, respectively [70]. The hemolytic toxicity of a PPI dendrimer (G5) after 1, 2, and 4 hours of incubation at 1 mg/ mL was determined to be 34.2% ± 0.2%, 51.6% ± 0.3%, and 86.2% ± 0.6%, respectively [68]. The G4 factor hemolysis was also elicited by PLL dendrimers (14.1% ± 1.02%) [69]. The safety of dendrimers has only been tested in a small number of *in vivo* toxicity investigations [74–76]. The initial *in vivo* toxicological investigation showed that only generation 7 PAMAM dendrimers were dangerous at 10 mg/kg [75] when tested on Swiss Webster mice. Recent studies in immune-competent CD-1 mice found that dendrimers often exhibited little toxicity following oral administration, with the exception of G7-NH2 and G7-OH (maximum tolerated dosage, 200 mg/kg). Wistar rats treated to PPI dendrimers (G5) (2.5 mg/kg) showed anorexia, lethargy, and sleepiness, as well as a decline in red blood cell count and hemoglobin content and a lack of immunogenicity [68, 75]. To lessen or completely remove their cytotoxicity and hemolytic toxicity, dendrimers have been proposed using a range of biocompatible (peptide, polyester, polyether, polyether imine, phosphate, citric acid, triazine, melamine, and peptide) or surface-engineered alterations (tuftsin, folate, acetylated, and PEGylated dendrimers) [67].

6.6 Nanomedicines Constructed from Amino Acids and Nucleic Acids

Nanomedicines based on amino acids and nucleic acids have gotten a lot of attention because of the advantages they provide in terms of biocompatibility and safety. Despite the absence of clinical trials, lipidic nanomedicines show significant potential due to their exceptional effectiveness in the realm of brain drug administration, levels of specificity, and targeting, as well as their low risk to the body.

6.6.1 Spherical nucleic acids

New nucleic acid structures known as round nucleic acids (SNAs) are increasingly important in biological systems construction that overcomes the constraints of classic nucleic acids. Because of their unmodified oligonucleotides, they are swiftly eliminated by the kidneys and cleaved by DNA and

RNA enzymes in the bloodstream, which prevents them from passing across both the blood–brain and the blood–tumor barriers [78].

Single-entity agents (SNAs) consist of oligonucleotides on the surface of a nucleic acid particle that has been extensively modified and oriented in a specific way (NP). An SNA is composed of an inorganic or hollow core, typically between 10 and 50 nm in diameter, and an oligonucleotide, which can also be an inorganic compound. The inorganic center's chemistry and physics (such as plasmons, scattering, or catalysis) and the role of the scaffold it plays in the assembly and orientation of the oligonucleotides, which give birth to many of the functional qualities, have been shown in studies [79]. The element for affixing particles (SH, N3, NH2, COO, and Tocopherol) is one of the three primary components of an SNA's oligonucleotide. The recognition area is separated from the NP's surface, thanks to a spacer, which can be a synthetic polymer or a DNA base (T10 or A10) (PEG). Based on the biological use, the recognition area may be modified, although it is usually the active segment that can be paired combined with a variety of different threads (strands with sticky ends used as linkers, strands used as targets in detection assays, complementary strands used to make siRNA, etc.) [80, 81].

Detection of caveolae-mediated endocytosis, which is initiated by the fast uptake of SNAs, may be facilitated when transfection reagents are not employed [79,82]. The binding affinity [83] constants of SNAs for their complements are higher than those of unbound strands of the same sequence, making SNAs more stable than free oligonucleotides [84]. SNAs have shown that the doses necessary to regulate genes effectively have minimal destruction of cells (cytotoxicity) [85, 86]. For 48 hours, SNAs containing nonsense siRNA sequences cultured with primary human keratinocytes were indistinguishable from untreated cells in terms of morphology [86]. Although the same keratinocytes treated with the same quantity of siRNA given by the same 427 genes were found to be upregulated or downregulated by the transfection agent, only seven were found to be increased in the genome-wide expression profile [87]. Tumor-bearing mice were given seven injections of 10 mg/kg siRNA each to see whether this induced an inflammatory response. No changes were seen between the tumor-bearing animals and the controls. Sprague–Dawley rats were given an intravenous injection of 10 mg/kg once siRNA SNAs, with no alterations at therapeutic doses, as evidenced by no changes in histology, body weight, or blood counts on days 1 or 14, indicating that SNAs had no acute or long-term damage. Research has shown that SNAs barely affect the immune system (relative to distribution via cationic carriers, the effect is 25 times less) [88].

The Bcl2L12 oncogene is the target of SNAs (siRNAs), which are being employed to treat malignant brain tumors. In contrast to nontumor brain regions, intravenous treatment with Cy5- or gadolinium (GdIII)-labeled SNAs revealed a 10-fold increase in SNA concentration in the tumor. Mice with orthotopic tumors were given an intravenous injection of the miRNA miR-182-SNA at a level of 1.4 mg/kg RNA, and the mice had an average survival time of 42–55 days (after being given high doses of the RTK c-Met and the hypoxia-inducible factor 2) [89]. SNAs have demonstrated potential as a technique for delivering genetic material to brain tumors. However, more investigation is necessary to completely comprehend the *in vivo* mechanics of penetration.

6.6.2 Nanomedicines that rely on amino acids

Amphiphiles are man-made peptides that, if necessary, have hydrophobic tails linked via a linker or spacer [14]. Micelles, vesicles, nanotubes, nanofibers, and nanosheets all have fundamental structural properties that can be altered, and these alterations can have profound effects on the morphology, surface chemistry, and possibly the entire function of the material [90, 91]. Amino acid block copolymers have peptide backbones with 8–30 amino acids; the hydrophilic block is composed of polar amino acids and the hydrophobic block is composed of nonpolar amino acids with grafted alkyl, anhydride, or acrylic tails [92, 93]. Thirty-nine Nonpolar amino acids or 12–16 carbons in an acyl or alkyl chain are commonly found in hydrophobic blocks [93]. Between the two blocks of peptide amphiphiles, a linker or spacer such as poly(ethylene glycol) [94] or glycine may be present [95]. Stacking, hydrogen bonding, electrostatic interactions, and hydrophobic contacts drive amphiphile self-assembly [91]. The peptide's lipid tail interacts hydrophobically with the peptide's nonpolar amino acid portion necessary for loading hydrophobic medicines such as paclitaxel [96], camptothecin [97], and carmustine [98] into well-defined nanostructures. This results in the creation of a hydrophobic core. There are two primary nonselective driving factors for self-assembly: hydrophilic block amino acids are involved in electrostatic interactions with hydrophobic contacts.

For the treatment of brain tumors, medication and gene delivery systems based on peptide amphiphiles have been studied (Table 6.4). The R3V6 peptide is an amphiphilic amphiphile that self-assembles into micelles; Yi et al. harnessed this property to deliver VEGF siRNA and carmustine to C6 glioma cells. The hydrophobic core of the micelles efficiently gathered carmustine, and a stable combination was established between VEGF siRNA

Table 6.4 Studies on peptide-based nanomedicines for glioma in preclinical studies.

Nanoparticles	Drug/targeting moiety	Outcomes	Ref.
CGKRKD [KLAKLAK] 2-Iron oxide	D[KLAKLAK]2	In mice with orthotopic GBM, CGKRKD[KLAKLAK]2 accumulates in vascular structures (80% tumor vs. 4% normal arteries) (IV: 200 g of rhodamine-labeled CGKRK). The median survival of mice given systemic injections every other day for three weeks rose dramatically from 32 to 52 days, while the median survival of mice given the peptide plus iRGD (4 mmol/kg) therapy significantly increased to 95 days.	99
CREKA-PEG-Cy7	Cy7/CREKA	Injection of Cy7-CREKA-micelles (IV 100 L of 1 mM of micelles) was followed by 1 hour of immunohistochemistry, *in vivo* imaging, and *ex vivo* imaging showing enhanced tumor homing via active targeting). Research into biodistribution highlighted a pronounced accumulation in certain tissues. After seven days, micellar concentrations dropped in the blood but remained in the liver.	94

and the positively charged R3V6. Cytotoxicity assays utilizing C6 glioma cells showed that complexes were more toxic than either siRNA/carmustine or carmustine alone (20% loss of glioblastoma cell viability vs. 50% for R3V6carmustine) [98]. Several types of research on illnesses, such as brain tumors, have shown that the treatment is effective *in vivo* [94, 99] (Table 6.4). Chung and colleagues [94] examined if the tumor-homing CREKA peptide is bound to fibrin in glioblastoma blood vessels. Cy7-PEGCREKA micelles rapidly aggregated at the tumor site within 1 hour after intravenous administration to a mouse model of intracranial GL261 glioma and were entirely cleared from the brain by day 7. After seven days, when most of the micelles had been eliminated and only the liver remained, histological images demonstrated that there was no tissue damage and that the morphologies of the liver and kidney were similar to the control. So far, *in vivo* studies of self-assembled peptide amphiphiles have produced encouraging findings. Low cytotoxicity and immunogenicity have been found in the vast majority of investigations [100–103]. The hydrogels of peptide Q11 (QKFQFEQQ) coupled with ligands for RGD and IKVAV [103] were studied by Jung et al. It was discovered that at the lowest concentration tested (0.011 mg/mL), the peptides in the HUVEC culture, Q11, RGDS-Q11, and IKVAV-Q11, showed no cytotoxicity. RGDS-Q11 and Q11 peptides (2 mM) were given subcutaneously to the C57BL/6 mice, although neither strain responded favorably. When injected into the heart of rats [102] and mice [100], RAD16 peptide fibers elicited no inflammatory response and were not recognized by the immune system. Peptide amphiphiles with nonimmunogenic epitopes are useful for medication delivery against brain tumors due to their low toxicity and immunogenicity. Recent research has shown that peptide nanofibers, in addition to peptide micelles, can cross the blood–brain barrier [13, 104]; therefore, peptide-based nanomedicines are becoming trustworthy and focused on the treatments for GBM.

6.7 Drug Conjugates

Clinical trials using chemotherapeutic agent carrier ligand conjugates for the treatment of malignant brain tumors have made significant strides in recent years (Table 6.5).

Targeting receptors expressed in cancer cells with peptide drug conjugates has been extensively investigated in solid tumors using small peptides such as RGD [105], gonadotropin-releasing hormone (GnRH) [106], somatostatin [107], bombesin [108], and angiopep-2 [109, 110]. Phase I, II, and III clinical trials have been conducted with the cyclic RGD-containing

Table 6.5 Research on glioma drug conjugates in preclinical and clinical settings.

Nanoparticles	Phase	Drug/targeting moiety	Outcomes	Ref.
Conjugates of drugs with peptides				
ANG1005	II	Paclitaxel/angiopep-2	There is a 4.5-fold increase in brain absorption of the ANG1005 compound compared to no-cost paclitaxel. Intraperitoneal administration of ANG1005 to U87MG mice (40 mg/kg once daily for five days, followed by 100 mg/kg every third day for two doses) significantly reduced tumor development (107%).	110
Cilengitide (Merck KGaA), a cyclic RGDfV inhibitor	III	$-/\alpha\nu\beta3$ $\alpha\nu\beta5$	Intravenous infusions of cilengitide were administered twice weekly during the first stage, lasting for 1 hour each time. With doses up to 2400 mg/m^2, no dose-limiting toxicity was seen. There was no increased toxicity in a phase II pilot study of cilengitide (500 mg) paired with standard chemoradiotherapy.	105
ANG1007	Preclinical	Doxorubicin/angiopep-2	When compared with doxorubicin, ANG1007's IV bolus injection penetration was three times greater in normal tissue and two times greater in brain tumors.	109
AN-152 (D-Lys6) GnRH-doxorubic	Preclinical	Doxorubicin/ (D-Lys6)-GnRH	Tumor volume was significantly reduced in AN-152 (413 nmol/20 g) treated groups of U87 MG-carrying nude mice tumors compared to doxorubicin alone after six weeks of treatment (B1.5-fold decrease).	106

(Continued)

Table 6.5   *Continued.*

Nanoparticles	Phase	Drug/targeting moiety	Outcomes	Ref.
Drug-antibody fusions				
AMG 595	I	DM1/anti-EGFRvIII antibody	17 mg/kg (or 250 g DM1/kg) AMG 595 treatment effectively reduced tumor development in mouse models of U251vIII xenografts compared to vehicle-treated controls (1375 mm^3).	117
ABT-414	I/II	Monomethyl auristatin F/anti-EGFR antibody ABT-806	ABT-414, when given at a dose of 4 mg/kg, totally reversed an exogenously increased EGFRvIII GBM mouse model.	118
Transfusion proteins				
Aflibercept	II	IgG1/VEGF PlGF	IV dosing of 4 mg/kg given on cycle day 1 in patients with anaplastic glioma and glioblastoma (5.7%) had a 25% progression-free survival rate at six months.	119
TNF-alpha cyclic CDCRGDCFC	Preclinical	TNF / v 3	Although U87MG was more highly expressed than MDA-MB-435 or C6, all three glioma lines showed a negative correlation between uptake and integrin expression. Uptake of 64Cu-DOTA-RGD4C-TNF by tumors was increased by a factor of B2 compared to B1.5 significant liver buildup at early time points in a U-87 MG cancer model, which diminished over time.	120

pentapeptide cilengitide (EMD 121974, Merck) for the treatment of glioblastoma [105]. Ciligitide doses between 120 and 2400 milligrams per square meter (mg/m²) went over well in phase I investigations [111, 112]. Phase II trials suggested that cilengitide (500–2000 mg) or chemoradiotherapy with temozolomide might have an anticancer effect in patients with recurrent or newly diagnosed GBM. This was notably true for tumors where methylation of the MGMT promoter was prevalent. Positive findings from earlier clinical studies led to the initiation of a randomized phase III investigation of MGMT promoter methylation in glioblastoma patients [113]. Median overall survival was 26.3 months in both the cilengitide and control groups, which was not a particularly encouraging result. Angiochem Inc. (Montreal, Canada) has developed peptide drug conjugates utilizing a vector consisting of a 19-amino acid peptide designed to bind to the abundant LDL receptors on BBB and GBM cells. Angiopep-2 conjugates are utilized to transport cytotoxic medications that eliminate cancer cells to the brain. ANG1005 (paclitaxel), ANG1007 (doxorubicin), ANG1009 (etoposide), and ANG4043 (anti-HER2 monoclonal antibodies mAb) are a few examples of such medications. Phase I and phase II clinical trials have examined tri-paclitaxel-coupled angiopep-2. In two phase I, multicenter, sequential cohort studies, patients with glioblastoma [114] and brain metastases [115] were observed to tolerate dosages of a chemical ranging from 30 to 700 mg/m² well. The clinical efficacy of ANG1005 was demonstrated in phase II, multicenter, open-label trial in patients with recurrent high-grade glioma related to breast cancer (NCT01967810).

Monoclonal antibodies linked to cytotoxic chemicals are known as antibody-drug conjugates, and they provide a level of selectivity and efficacy not possible with standard medicines alone [116]. IC50 values in the subnanomolar range have been seen in antibody conjugates tested *in vitro*, indicating strong receptor selectivity [117, 118]. Clinical trials involving AMG 595 [117] and ABT-414 [118] to treat glioblastoma have recently begun. ABT-414, an MMAF-conjugated ABT-806, is effective against wild-type or EGFR variant III-expressing patient-derived xenograft models of glioblastoma (humanized monoclonal antibody 806). Clinical trials for the ABT-414 conjugate are now ongoing in phases I and II (NCT01800695, NCT02573324, NCT02573324, and NCT02343406) based on preclinical data.

6.8 Conclusion

To the extent that they can be used in combination, nanomedicines offer the potential for diverse and multifaceted therapeutic approaches. While iron oxide may be used to detect the tumor's margins, it may also include a drug that can cross the BBB to reach tumor cells where they reside. NPs may also be used to augment ionizing-beam treatment or to deliver entrapped or conjugated medicines concurrently after resection. CED of the nanoparticulate formulation can be used if resection is not required and may be performed simultaneously with stereotactic biopsy, and imaging may also be employed to verify that the nanoparticles do not diffuse off-target. Preclinical and clinical data suggest that lipidic nanomedicines and drug conjugates will be the easiest to bring to market in the coming decade, followed by those based on peptides and nucleic acids, which are more difficult. Because nanomedicines will be used as an adjuvant to surgical treatment rather than a replacement, they will enhance resection and work noninvasively toward tumor elimination to facilitate the targeting of biomolecular pathways that contribute to GBM's untreatable nature.

References

[1] Sanai, N., & Berger, M.S. Glioma extent of resection and its impact on patient outcome. *Neurosurgery*, **2008**, *62* (4), 753–764. Available from https://doi.org/10.1227/01.neu.0000318159.21731.cf, discussion 264–756.

[2] Stupp, R., Mason, W.P., van den Bent, M.J., Weller, M., Fisher, B., Taphoorn, M.J., ... National Cancer Institute of Canada Clinical Trials, G. (2005). Radiotherapy plus concomitant and adjuvant temozolomide for glioblastoma. *New England Journal of Medicine*, **2005**, *352*(10), 987–996. Available from https://doi.org/10.1056/ NEJMoa043330.

[3] Lalatsa, A., Leite, D.M., & Pilkington, G.J. Nanomedicines and the future of glioma. *Neuro-oncology News*, **2015**, *10*(2), 51–57

[4] Karathanasis, E., & Ghaghada, K.B. Crossing the barrier: Treatment of brain tumors using nanochain particles. *Wiley Interdisciplinary Reviews: Nanomedicine and Nanobiotechnology*, **2016**, *8*(5), 678–695. Available from https://doi.org/10.1002/wnan.1387

[5] Fisusi, F.A., Siew, A., Chooi, K.W., Okubanjo, O., Garrett, N., Lalatsa, K., ... Uchegbu, I.F. Lomustine nanoparticles enable both bone marrow sparing and high brain drug levels - a strategy for brain cancer treatments. *Pharmaceutical Research*, **2016**, *33*(5), 1289–1303. Available from https://doi.org/10.1007/s11095-016-1872-x

[6] Serrano Lopez, D.R., & Lalatsa, A. Peptide pills for brain diseases? Reality and future perspectives. *Ther Deliv*, **2013**, *4*(4), 479–501. Available from https://doi.org/10.4155/tde.13.5

[7] Jiang, W., Kim, B.Y., Rutka, J.T., & Chan, W.C. Nanoparticle-mediated cellular response is sizedependent. *Nature Nanotechnology*, **2008**, *3*(3), 145–150. Available from https://doi.org/10.1038/nnano.200

[8] Lalatsa, A., Schatzlein, A.G., & Uchegbu, I.F. Strategies to deliver peptide drugs to the brain. *Molecular Pharmaceutics*, **2014**, *11*(4), 1081–1093. Available from https://doi.org/10.1021/mp400680d.

[9] Owens, D.E., 3rd, & Peppas, N.A. Opsonization, biodistribution, and pharmacokinetics of polymeric nanoparticles. *International Journal of Pharmaceutics*, **2006**, *307*(1), 93–102. Available from https://doi.org/10.1016/j. ijpharm.2005.10.010.

[10] Sehedic, D., Cikankowitz, A., Hindre, F., Davodeau, F., & Garcion, E. Nanomedicine to overcome radioresistance in glioblastoma stem-like cells and surviving clones. *Trends in Pharmacological Sciences*, **2015**, *36*(4), 236–252. Available from https://doi.org/10.1016/j.tips.2015.02.002

[11] Geng, Y., Dalhaimer, P., Cai, S., Tsai, R., Tewari, M., Minko, T., & Discher, D.E. Shape effects of filaments versus spherical particles in flow and drug delivery. *Nature Nanotechnology*, **2007**, *2*(4), 249–255. Available from https://doi.org/10.1038/nnano.2007.70.

[12] Lalatsa, A., Lee, V., Malkinson, J.P., Zloh, M., Schatzlein, A.G., & Uchegbu, I.F. A prodrug nanoparticle approach for the oral delivery of a hydrophilic peptide, leucine(5)-enkephalin, to the brain. *Molecular Pharmaceutics*, **2012**, *9*(6), 1665–1680. Available from https://doi.org/10.1021/mp300009u.

[13] Lalatsa, A., Schatzlein, A.G., Garrett, N.L., Moger, J., Briggs, M., Godfrey, L., ... Uchegbu, I.F. Chitosan amphiphile coating of peptide nanofibres reduces liver uptake and delivers the peptide to the brain on intravenous administration. *Journal of Controlled Release*, **2015**, 197, 87–96. Available from https://doi.org/10.1016/j. jconrel.2014.10.028.

[14] Lalatsa, A., Schatzlein, A.G., Mazza, M., Le, T.B., & Uchegbu, I.F. Amphiphilic poly(L-amino acids) - new materials for drug delivery. *Journal of Controlled Release*, **2012**, *161*(2), 523–536. Available from https://doi.org/ 10.1016/j.jconrel.2012.04.046.

[15] Lu, W., Zhang, Y., Tan, Y.Z., Hu, K.L., Jiang, X.G., & Fu, S.K. Cationic albumin-conjugated pegylated nanoparticles as novel drug carrier for brain delivery. *Journal of Controlled Release*, **2005**, *107*(3), 428–448. Available from https://doi.org/10.1016/j.jconrel.2005.03.027.

[16] Wang, C. X., Huang, L.S., Hou, L.B., Jiang, L., Yan, Z.T., Wang, Y.L., & Chen, Z.L. Antitumor effects of polysorbate-80 coated gemcitabine polybutylcyanoacrylate nanoparticles *in vitro* and its pharmacodynamics

in vivo on C6 glioma cells of a brain tumor model. *Brain Research*, **2009**, *1261*, 91–99. Available from https://doi.org/10.1016/j.brainres. 2009.01.011.

[17] Kim, B., Han, G., Toley, B.J., Kim, C.K., Rotello, V.M., & Forbes, N.S. Tuning payload delivery in Tumor cylindroids using gold nanoparticles. *Nature Nanotechnology*, **2010**, *5*(6), 465–472. Available from https:// doi.org/10.1038/nnano.2010.58.

[18] Bangham, A.D. Properties and uses of lipid vesicles: An overview. *Annals of the New York Academy of Sciences*, **1978**, *308*, 2–7.

[19] Bangham, J.A., & Lea, E.J. The interaction of detergents with bilayer lipid membranes. *Biochimica et Biophysica Acta*, **1978**, *511*(3), 388–396.

[20] Gregoriadis, G., Leathwood, P.D., & Ryman, B.E. Enzyme entrapment in liposomes. *FEBS Letters*, **1971**, *14*(2), 95–99.

[21] Gregoriadis, G., & Ryman, B.E. Liposomes as carriers of enzymes or drugs: A new approach to the treatment of storage diseases. *Biochemical Journal*, **1971**, *124*(5), 58P.

[22] Torchilin, V.P. Recent advances with liposomes as pharmaceutical carriers. *Nature Reviews Drug Discovery*, **2005**, *4*(2), 145–160. Available from https://doi.org/10.1038/nrd1632.

[23] Li, X.-T., Ju, R.-J., Li, X.-Y., Zeng, F., Shi, J.-F., Liu, L., ... Lu, W.-L. Multifunctional targeting daunorubicin plus quinacrine liposomes, modified by wheat germ agglutinin and tamoxifen, for treating brain glioma and glioma stem cells. *Oncotarget*, **2014**, *5*(15), 6497–6511.

[24] Rafiyath, S.M., Rasul, M., Lee, B., Wei, G., Lamba, G., & Liu, D. Comparison of safety and toxicity of liposomal doxorubicin vs. conventional anthracyclines: A meta-analysis. *Experimental Hematology & Oncology*, **2012**, *1*(1), 10. Available from https://doi.org/10.1186/2162-3619-1-10.

[25] Moller, H.G., Rasmussen, A.P., Andersen, H.H., Johnsen, K.B., Henriksen, M., & Duroux, M. A systematic review of microRNA in glioblastoma multiforme: Micro-modulators in the mesenchymal mode of migration and invasion. *Molecular Neurobiology*, **2013**, *47*(1), 131–144. Available from https://doi.org/10.1007/ s12035-012-8349-7

[26] Siegal, T., Charbit, H., Paldor, I., Zelikovitch, B., Canello, T., Benis, A., ... Lavon, I. Dynamics of circulating hypoxia-mediated miRNAs and tumor response in patients with high-grade glioma treated with bevacizumab. *Journal of Neurosurgery*, **2016**, *125*(4), 1008–1015. Available from https://doi.org/10.3171/2015.8.JNS15437.

[27] Gourlay, J., Morokoff, A.P., Luwor, R.B., Zhu, H.J., Kaye, A.H., & Stylli, S.S. The emergent role of exosomes in glioma. *Journal of*

Clinical Neuroscience, **2017**, *35*, 13–23. Available from https://doi. org/10.1016/j. jocn.2016.09.021

[28] Raposo, G., & Stoorvogel, W. Extracellular vesicles: Exosomes, microvesicles, and friends. *Journal of Cell Biology*, **2013**, *200*(4), 373–383. Available from https://doi.org/10.1083/jcb.201211138

[29] Schiera, G., Di Liegro, C.M., Saladino, P., Pitti, R., Savettieri, G., Proia, P., & Di Liegro, I. Oligodendroglioma cells synthesize the differentiation-specific linker histone H1 and release it into the extracellular environment through shed vesicles. *International Journal of Oncology*, **2013**, *43*(6), 1771–1776. Available from https://doi.org/10.3892/ ijo.2013.2115.

[30] Al-Nedawi, K., Meehan, B., Micallef, J., Lhotak, V., May, L., Guha, A., & Rak, J. Intercellular transfer of the oncogenic receptor EGFRvIII by microvesicles derived from Tumor cells. *Nature Cell Biology*, **2008**, *10*(5), 619–624. Available from https://doi.org/10.1038/ ncb1725.

[31] Li, C.C., Eaton, S.A., Young, P.E., Lee, M., Shuttleworth, R., Humphreys, D.T., ... Suter, C.M. Glioma microvesicles carry selectively packaged coding and non-coding RNAs which alter gene expression in recipient cells. *RNA Biology*, **2013**, *10*(8), 1333–1344. Available from https://doi.org/10.4161/rna.252

[32] Putz, U., Howitt, J., Doan, A., Goh, C.P., Low, L.H., Silke, J., & Tan, S.S. The tumor suppressor PTEN is exported in exosomes and has phosphatase activity in recipient cells. *Sci Signal*, **2012**, *5*(243), ra70. Available from https://doi.org/10.1126/scisignal.2003084.

[33] Verhaak, R.G., Hoadley, K.A., Purdom, E., Wang, V., Qi, Y., Wilkerson, M.D., ... Cancer Genome Atlas Research, N. Integrated genomic analysis identifies clinically relevant subtypes of glioblastoma characterized by abnormalities in PDGFRA, IDH1, EGFR, and NF1. *Cancer Cell*, **2010**, *17*(1), 98–110. Available from https://doi. org/10.1016/j.ccr.2009.12.020.

[34] de Vrij, J., Maas, S.L., Kwappenberg, K.M., Schnoor, R., Kleijn, A., Dekker, L., ... Broekman, M.L. Glioblastoma-derived extracellular vesicles modify the phenotype of monocytic cells. *International Journal of Cancer*, **2015**, *137*(7), 1630–1642. Available from https://doi. org/10.1002/ijc.29521.

[35] Ge, R., Tan, E., Sharghi-Namini, S., & Asada, H.H. Exosomes in cancer microenvironment and beyond: Have we overlooked these extracellular messengers? *Cancer Microenviron*, **2012**, *5*(3), 323–332. Available from https://doi.org/10.1007/s12307-012-0110-2.

[36] Stylli, S.S., Kaye, A.H., & Lock, P. Invadopodia: At the cutting edge of Tumor invasion. *Journal of Clinical Neuroscience*, **2008**, *15*(7), 725–737. Available from https://doi.org/10.1016/j.jocn.2008.03.003.

[37] Hoshino, D., Kirkbride, K.C., Costello, K., Clark, E.S., Sinha, S., Grega-Larson, N., ... Weaver, A.M. Exosome secretion is enhanced by invadopodia and drives invasive behavior. *Cell Reports*, **2013**, *5*(5), 1159–1168. Available from https://doi.org/10.1016/j.celrep.2013.10.050

[38] Yang, T., Martin, P., Fogarty, B., Brown, A., Schurman, K., Phipps, R., ... Bai, S. Exosome delivered anticancer drugs across the blood-brain barrier for brain cancer therapy in Danio rerio. *Pharmaceutical Research*, **2015**, *32* (6), 2003–2014. Available from https://doi.org/10.1007/s11095-014-1593-y

[39] Alvarez-Erviti, L., Seow, Y., Yin, H., Betts, C., Lakhal, S., & Wood, M.J. Delivery of siRNA to the mouse brain by systemic injection of targeted exosomes. *Nature Biotechnology*, **2011**, *29*(4), 341–345. Available from https:// doi.org/10.1038/nbt.1807.

[40] Lakhal, S., & Wood, M.J. Exosome nanotechnology: An emerging paradigm shift in drug delivery: Exploitation of exosome nanovesicles for systemic *in vivo* delivery of RNAi heralds new horizons for drug delivery across biological barriers. *Bioessays*, **2011**, *33*(10), 737–741. Available from https://doi.org/

[41] Munoz, J. L., Bliss, S.A., Greco, S.J., Ramkissoon, S.H., Ligon, K.L., & Rameshwar, P. Delivery of functional anti-miR-9 by mesenchymal stem cell-derived exosomes to glioblastoma multiforme cells conferred chemosensitivity. *Molecular Therapy—Nucleic Acids*, **2013**, *2*, e126. Available from https://doi.org/10.1038/mtna.

[42] Arscott, W.T., Tandle, A.T., Zhao, S., Shabason, J.E., Gordon, I.K., Schlaff, C.D., ... Camphausen, K.A. Ionizing radiation and glioblastoma exosomes: Implications in tumor biology and cell migration. *Translational Oncology*, **2013**, *6*(6), 638–648

[43] Cheng, Y., Morshed, R.A., Auffinger, B., Tobias, A.L., & Lesniak, M.S. (2014). Multifunctional nanoparticles for brain tumor imaging and therapy. *Advanced Drug Delivery Reviews*, **2014**, *66*, 42–57. Available from https://doi.org/ 10.1016/j.addr.2013.09.006.

[44] Huszthy, P.C., Daphu, I., Niclou, S.P., Stieber, D., Nigro, J.M., Sakariassen, P.O., ... Bjerkvig, R. *In vivo* models of primary brain tumors: Pitfalls and perspectives. *Neuro Oncol*, **2012**, 14(8), 979–993. Available from https://doi.org/10.1093/neuonc/nos135.

[45] Simon, L.C., & Sabliov, C.M. The effect of nanoparticle properties, detection method, delivery route and animal model on poly(lactic-co-glycolic)

acid nanoparticles biodistribution in mice and rats. *Drug Metabolism Reviews*, **2014**, *46*, 128–141.

[46] Tomalia, D.A., & Khanna, S.N. A systematic framework and nanoperiodic concept for unifying nanoscience: Hard/soft nanoelements, superatoms, meta-atoms, new emerging properties, periodic property patterns, and predictive mendeleev-like nanoperiodic tables. *Chemical Reviews*, **2016**, *116*(4), 2705–2774. Available from https://doi.org/10.1021/acs.chemrev.5b00367.

[47] Fréchet, J.M.J., & Hawker, C.J. Preparation of polymers with controlled molecular architecture a new convergent approach to dendritic macromolecules. *Journal of the American Chemical Society*, **1990**, *112*, 7638–7647.

[48] Esfand, R., & Tomalia, D.A. Poly(amidoamine) (PAMAM) dendrimers: From biomimicry to drug delivery and biomedical applications. *Drug Discovery Today*, **2001**, *6*, 427–436.

[49] Shao, N., Su, Y., Hu, J., Zhang, J., Zhang, H., & Cheng, Y. Comparison of generation 3 polyamidoamine dendrimer and generation 4 polypropylenimine dendrimer on drug loading, complex structure, release behavior, and cytotoxicity. *International Journal of Nanomedicine*, **2011**, *6*, 3361–3372.

[50] Dufes, C., Uchegbu, I.F., & Schatzlein, A.G. Dendrimers in gene delivery. *Advanced Drug Delivery Reviews*, **2005**, *57*(15), 2177–2202. Available from https://doi.org/10.1016/j.addr.2005.09.017.

[51] Madaan, K., Kumar, S., Poonia, N., Lather, V., & Pandita, D. Dendrimers in drug delivery and targeting: Drug-dendrimer interactions and toxicity issues. *Journal of Pharmacy & Bioallied Sciences*, **2014**, *6*(3), 139–150. Available from https://doi.org/10.4103/0975-7406.130965

[52] Kaminskas, L.M., Boyd, B.J., & Porter, C.J.H. Dendrimer pharmacokinetics: The effect of size, structure and surface characteristics on ADME properties. *Nanomedicine*, **2011**, *6*, 1063–1084.

[53] Patel, S.K., Gajbhiye, V., & Jain, N.K. Synthesis, characterization and brain targeting potential of paclitaxel loaded thiamine-PPI nanoconjugates. *Journal of Drug Targeting*, **2012**, *20*(10), 84.

[54] Zhang, F., Mastorakos, P., Mishra, M.K., Mangraviti, A., Hwang, L., Zhou, J., ... Kannan, R.M. Uniform brain tumor distribution and tumor associated macrophage targeting of systemically administered dendrimers. *Biomaterials*, **2015**, *52*, 507–516.

[55] Huang, S., Li, J., Han, L., Liu, S., Ma, H., Huang, R., & Jiang, C. Dual targeting effect of Angiopep-2- modified, DNA-loaded nanoparticles for glioma. Biomaterials, **2011**, *32*, 6832–6838

[56] Han, L., Li, J., Huang, S., Huang, R., Liu, S., Hu, X., ... Jiang, C. Peptide-conjugated polyamidoamine dendrimer as a nanoscale tumor-targeted T1 magnetic resonance imaging contrast agent. *Biomaterials*, **2011**, *32*, 2989–2998.

[57] Kuang, Y., An, S., Guo, Y., Huang, S., Shao, K., Liu, Y., ... Jiang, C. T7 peptide-functionalised nanoparticles utilizing RNA interference for glioma dual targeting. *International Journal of Pharmaceutics*, **2013**, 454, 11–20

[58] Liu, S., Guo, Y., Huang, R., Li, J., Huang, S., Kuang, Y., ... Jiang, C. Gene and doxorubicin co-delivery system for targeting therapy of glioma. *Biomaterials*, **2012**, *33*, 4907–4916.

[59] Kaneshiro, T.L., & Lu, Z.-R. Targeted intracellular codelivery of chemotherapeutics and nucleic acid with well-defined dendrimer-based nanoglobular carrier. *Biomaterials*, **2009**, *30*, 5660–5666

[60] Zhang, L., Zhu, S., Qian, L., Pei, Y., Qiu, Y., & Jiang, Y. RGD-modified PEG-PAMAM-DOX conjugates: *In vitro* and *in vivo* studies for glioma. *European Journal of Pharmaceutics and Biopharmaceutics*, **2011**, *79*, 232–240

[61] Zhu, S., Qian, L., Hong, M., Zhang, L., Pei, Y., & Jiang, Y. RGD-modified PEG-PAMAM-DOX conjugate: *In vitro* and *in vivo* targeting of both tumor neovascular endothelial cells and tumor cells. *Advanced Materials*, **2011**, *23*, H84-H89.

[62] Zhao, J., Zhang, B., Shen, S., Chen, J., Zhang, Q., Jiang, X., & Pang, Z. CREKA peptide-conjugated dendrimer nanoparticles for glioblastoma multiforme delivery. *Journal of Colloid and Interface Science*, **2015**, *450*, 396–403

[63] Li, Y., He, H., Jia, X., Lu, W.-L., Lou, J., & Wei, Y. A dual-targeting nanocarrier based on poly(amidoamine) dendrimers conjugated with transferrin and tamoxifen for treating brain gliomas. *Biomaterials*, **2012**, *33*, 3899–3908.

[64] Wu, G., Barth, R.F., Yang, W., Kawabata, S., Zhang, L., & Green-Church, K. Targeted delivery of methotrexate to epidermal growth factor receptor-positive brain tumors by means of cetuximab (IMC-C225) dendrimer bioconjugates. *Molecular Cancer Therapeutics*, **2006**, *5*(1), 52–59.

[65] Wu, G., Yang, W., Barth, R.F., Kawabata, S., Swindall, M., Bandyopadhyaya, A.K., ... Fenstermaker, R.A. Molecular targeting and treatment of an epidermal growth factor receptorpositive glioma using boronated cetuximab. *Clinical Cancer Research*, **2007**, *13*(4), 12–60

[66] Dhanikula, R.S., Argaw, A., Bouchard, J.F., & Hildgen, P. Methotrexate loaded polyether-copolyester dendrimers for the treatment of gliomas: Enhanced efficacy and intratumoral transport capability. *Molecular Pharmaceutics*, **2008**, *5*, 105–116.

[67] Jain, K., Kesharwani, P., Gupta, U., & Jain, N.K. Dendrimer toxicity: Let's face the challenge. *International Journal of Pharmaceutics*, **2010**, *394*, 122–142.

[68] Agashe, H.B., Dutta, T.D., Garg, M., & Jain, N.K. Investigations on the toxicological profile of functionalized fifth-generation poly (propylene imine) dendrimer. *Journal of Pharmacy and Pharmacology*, **2006**, *58*(11), 1491–1498

[69] Agrawal, P., Gupta, U., & Jain, N.K. Glycoconjugated peptide dendrimers-based nanoparticulate system for the delivery of chloroquine phosphate. *Biomaterials*, **2007**, *28*, 3349–3359.

[70] Domanski, D.M., Klajnert, B., & Bryszewska, M. Influence of PAMAM dendrimers on human red blood cells. *Bioelectrochemistry*, **2004**, *63*, 189–191.

[71] Jevprasesphant, R., Penny, J., Jalal, R., Attwood, D., McKeown, N.B., & D'Emanuele, A. The influence of surface modification on the cytotoxicity of PAMAM dendrimers. *International Journal of Pharmaceutics*, **2003**, *252*, 263–266

[72] Jones, C.F., Campbell, R.A., Franks, Z., Gibson, C.C., Thiagarajan, G., Vieira-de-Abreu, A., ... Grainger, D.W. Cationic PAMAM dendrimers disrupt key platelet functions. *Molecular Pharmaceutics*, **2012**, *9*, 1599–1611.

[73] Malik, N., Wiwattanapatapee, R., Klopsch, R., Lorenz, K., Frey, H., Weener, J.W., ... Duncan, R. Dendrimers: Relationship between structure and biocompatibility *in vitro*, and preliminary studies on the biodistribution of 125I-labelled polyamidoamine dendrimers *in vivo*. *Journal of Controlled Release*, **2000**, *65*, 133–148

[74] Dutta, T., Garg, M., Dubey, V., Mishra, D., Singh, K.,Pandita, D., ... Jain, N.K. Toxicological investigation of surface engineered fifth generation poly (propyleneimine) dendrimers *in vivo*. *Nanotoxicology*, **2008**, *2*(2), 62–70.

[75] Roberts, J.C., Bhalgat, M.K., & Zera, R.T. Preliminary biological evaluation of polyamidoamine (PAMAM) StarburstTM dendrimers. *Journal of Biomedical Materials Research*, **1996**, *30*, 53–65.

[76] Thiagarajan, G., Greish, K., & Ghandehari, H. Charge affects the oral toxicity of poly(amidoamine) dendrimers. *European Journal of Pharmaceutics and Biopharmaceutics*, **2013**, 84, 330–334.

[77] Tian, X.H., Lin, X.N., Wei, F., Feng, W., Huang, Z.C., Wang, P., ... Diao, Y. Enhanced brain targeting of temozolomide in polysorbate-80 coated polybutylcyanoacrylate nanoparticles. *Int J Nanomedicine*, **2011**, *6*, 445–452. Available from https://doi.org/10.2147/IJN.S16570

[78] Barbany, S.N., Sita, T.L., Petrosko, S.H., Stegh, A.H., & Mirkin, C.A. Therapeutic applications of spherical nucleic acids. In C. A. Mirkin, T. J. Meade, S. H. Petrosko, & A. H. Stegh (Eds.), Nanotechnology-based precision tools for the detection and treatment of cancer, *Cancer treatment and research*, **2015**, 23–50.

[79] Cutler, J.I., Auyeung, E., & Mirkin, C.A. Spherical nucleic acids. *Journal of the American Chemical Society*, **2012**, *134*, 1376–1391.

[80] Choi, C.H., Hao, L., Narayan, S.P., Auyeung, E., & Mirkin, C.A. Mechanism for the endocytosis of spherical nucleic acid nanoparticle conjugates. *Proceedings of the National Academy of Sciences*, **2013**, *10*(19), 7625–7630.

[81] Narayan, S.P., Choi, C.H., Hao, L., Calabrese, C.M., Auyeung, E., Zhang, C., ... Mirkin, C. A. The sequence-specific cellular uptake of spherical nucleic acid nanoparticle conjugates. *Small*, **2015**, *11*(33), 4173–4182.

[82] Giljoham, D.A., Seferos, D.S., Daniel, W.L., Massich, M.D., Patel, P.C., & Mirkin, C.A. Gold nanoparticles for biology and medicine. *Angewandte Chemie International Edition England*, **2010**, *49*(19), 3280–3294.

[83] Seferos, D.S., Prigodich, A.E., Giljoham, D.A., Patel, P.C., & Mirkin, C.A. (2009). Polyvalent DNA nanoparticle conjugates stabilize nucleic acids. *Nano Letters*, **2009**, *9*(1), 308–311.

[84] Lytton-Jean, A.K.R., & Mirkin, C.A. A thermodynamic investigation into the binding properties of DNA functionalized gold nanoparticle probes and molecular fluorophore probes. *Journal of the American Chemical Society*, **2005**, *127*(37), 12754–12755.

[85] Rosi, N.L., Giljoham, D.A., Thaxton, C.S., Lytton-Jean, A.K.R., Han, M.S., & Mirkin, C.A. Oligonucleotide-modified gold nanoparticles for intracellular gene regulation. *Science*, **2006**, *312*, 1027–1030.

[86] Zheng, D., Giljoham, D.A., Chen, D.L., Massich, M.D., Wang, X.-Q., Iordanov, H., ... Paller, A.S. Topical delivery of siRNA-based spherical nucleic acid nanoparticle conjugates for gene regulation. *Proceedings of the National Academy of Sciences*, **2012**, *109*(30), 11975–11980

[87] Jensen, S.A., Day, E.S., Ko, C.H., Hurley, L.A., Luciano, J.P., Kouri, F.M., ... Stegh, A.H. Spherical nucleic acid nanoparticle conjugates as an RNAi-based therapy for glioblastoma. *Science Translational*

Medicine, **2013**, *5*(209). Available from https://doi.org/10.1126/scitranslmed.3006839, 209ra152-209ra152.

[88] Massich, M.D., Giljoham, D.A., Seferos, D.S., Ludlow, L.E., Horvath, C.M., & Mirkin, C.A. Regulating immune response using polyvalent nucleic acid-gold nanoparticle conjugates. *Molecular Pharmaceutics*, **2009**, *6*(6), 1934–1940.

[89] Kouri, F.M., Hurley, L.A., Daniel, W.L., Day, E.S., Hua, Y., Hao, L., ... Stegh, A.H. miR-182 integrates apoptosis, growth, and differentiation programs in glioblastoma. *Genes & Development*, **2015**, *29*(7), 732–745. Available from https://doi.org/10.1101/gad.257394.114

[90] Rouge, J.L., Sita, T.L., Hao, L., Kouri, F.M., Briley, W.E., Stegh, A.H., & Mirkin, C.A. Ribozymespherical nucleic acids. *Journal of the American Chemical Society*, **2015**, *137*(33), 10528–10531.

[91] Leite, D.M., Barbu, E., Pilkington, G.J., & Lalatsa, A. Peptide self-assemblies for drug delivery. *Current Topics in Medicinal Chemistry*, **2015**, *15*(22), 2277–2289.

[92] Lowik, D.W., & van Hest, J.C. Peptide based amphiphiles. *Chemical Society Reviews*, **2004**, *33*(4), 234–245

[93] Zhao, X., Pan, F., Xu, H., Yaseen, M., Shan, H., Hauser, C.A., ... Lu, J.R. Molecular self-assembly and applications of designer peptide amphiphiles. *Chemical Society Reviews*, **2010**, *39*(9), 3480–3498

[94] Chung, E.J., Cheng, Y., Morshed, R., Nord, K., Han, Y., Wegscheid, M.L., ... Tirrell, M.V. Fibrin-binding, peptide amphiphiles micelles for targeting glioblastoma. *Biomaterials*, **2014**, *35*, 1249–1256.

[95] Tan, A., Rajadas, J., & Seifalian, A.M. Biochemical engineering nerve conduits using peptide amphiphiles. *Journal of Controlled Release*, **2012**, *163*(3), 342–352.

[96] Zhang, P., Cheetham, A.G., Lin, Y., & Cui, H. Self-assembled Tat nanofibers as effective drug carrier and transporter. *ACS Nano*, **2013**, *7*(7), 5965–5977.

[97] Soukasene, S., Toft, D.J., Moyer, T.J., Lu, H., Lee, H.-K., Standley, S.M., ... Stupp, S.I. Antitumor activity of peptide amphiphile nanofiber-encapsulated camptothecin. *ACS Nano*, **2011**, *5*(11), 9113–9121

[98] Yi, N., Oh, B., Kim, H.A., & Lee, M. Combined delivery of BCNU and VEGF siRNA using amphiphilic peptides for glioblastoma. *Journal of Drug Targeting*, **2014**, *22*(2), 156–164.

[99] Agemy, L., Friedmann-Morvinski, D., Kotamraju, V.R., Roth, L., Sugahara, K.N., Girard, O.M., ... Ruoslahti, E. Targeted nanoparticle enhanced proapoptotic peptide as potential therapy for glioblastoma. *Proceedings of the National Academy of Sciences*, **2011**, *108*(42), 17450–17455

[100] Davis,M.E.,Motion,J.P.M.,Narmoneva,D.A.,Takahashi,T.,Hakuno,D., Kamm, R.D., ... Lee, R.T. Injectable self-assembling peptide nanofibers create intramyocardial microenvironments for endothelial cells. *Circulation*, **2005**, *111*, 442–450.

[101] Holmes, T.C., Lacalle, S., Su, X., Liu, G., Rich, A., & Zhang, S. Extensive neurite outgrowth and active synapse formation on self-assembling peptide scaffolds. *Proceedings of the National Academy of Sciences*, **2000**, *97*(12), 6728–6733.

[102] Hsieh, P.C.H., Davis, M.E., Gannon, J., MacGillivray, C., & Lee, R.T. Controlled delivery of PDGF-BB for myocardial protection using injectable self-assembling peptide nanofibers. *The Journal of Clinical Investigation*, **2006**, *116*(1), 237–248

[103] Jung, J.P., Nagaraj, A.K., Fox, E.K., Rudra, J.S., Devgun, J.M., & Collier, J.H. Co-assembling peptides as defined matrices for endothelial cells. *Biomaterials*, **2009**, *30*, 2400–2410.

[104] Mazza, M., Notman, R., Anwar, J., Rodger, A., Hicks, M., Parkinson, G., ... Uchegbu, I.F. Nanofiberbased delivery of therapeutic peptides to the brain. *ACS Nano*, **2013**, *7*(2), 1016–1026. Available from https://doi. org/10.1021/nn305193d

[105] Tabatabai, G., Weller, M., Nabors, B., Picard, M., Reardon, D., Mikkelsen, T., ... Stupp, R. Targeting integrins in malignant glioma. *Targeted Oncology*, **2010**, *5*, 175–181

[106] Jaszberenyi, M., Schally, A.V., Block, N.L., Nadji, M., Vidaurre, I., Szalontay, L., & Rick, F.G. Inhibition of U-87 MG glioblastoma by AN-152 (AEZS-108), a targeted cytotoxic analog of luteinizing hormone-releasing hormone. *Oncotarget*, **2013**, *4*(3), 422–432

[107] Kiaris, H., Schally, A.V., Nagy, A., Sun, B., Szepeshazi, K., & Halmos, G. Regression of U-87 MG human glioblastomas in nude mice after treatment with a cytotoxic somatostatin analog AN-238. *Clinical Cancer Research*, **2000**, *6*, 709–717

[108] Szereday, Z., Schally, A.V., Nagy, A., Plonowski, A., Bajo, A.M., Halmos, G., ... Groot, K. Effective treatment of experimental U-87MG human glioblastoma in nude mice with a targeted cytotoxic bombesin analogue, AN-215. *British Journal of Cancer*, **2012**, *86*, 1322–1327.

[109] Ché, C., Yang, G., Thiot, C., Lacoste, M.-C., Currie, J.-C., Demeule, M., ... Castaigne, J.-P. New angiopepmodified doxorubicin (ANG1007) and etoposide (ANG1009) chemotherapeutics with increased brain penetration. *Journal of Medicinal Chemistry*, **2010**, *53*, 2814–2824.

[110] Régina, A., Demeule, M., Ché, C., Lavallée, I., Poirier, J., Gabathuler, R., ... Castaigne, J.-P. AntiTumor activity of ANG1005, a conjugate between paclitaxel and the new brain delivery vector Angiopep-2. *British Journal of Pharmacology*, **2008**, *155*, 185–197

[111] MacDonald, T.J., Stewart, C.F., Kocak, M., Goldman, S., Ellenbogen, R.G., Phillips, P., ... Kun, L.E. Phase I clinical trial of cilengitide in children with refractory brain tumors: Pediatric brain tumor consortium study PBTC-012. *Journal of Clinical Oncology*, **2008**, *26*(6), 919–924. Available from https://doi.org/10.1200/JCO.2007.14.1812.

[112] Nabors, L.B., Mikkelsen, T., Rosenfeld, S.S., Hochberg, F., Akella, N.S., Fisher, J.D., ... Grossman, S.A. Phase I and correlative biology study of cilengitide in patients with recurrent malignant glioma. *Journal of Clinical Oncology*, **2007**, *25*(13), 1651–1657. Available from https://doi.org/10.1200/JCO.2006.06.6514

[113] Stupp, R., Hegi, M.E., Gorlia, T., Erridge, S.C., Perry, J., Hong, Y.-K., ... Weller, M. Cilengitide combined with standard treatment for patients with newly diagnosed glioblastoma with methylated MGMT promoter (CENTRIC EORTC 26071–22072 study): A multicentre, randomised, open-label, phase 3 trial. *The Lancet Oncology*, **2014**, *15*(10), 1100–1108. Available from https://doi.org/10.1016/S1470-2045(14)70379-1

[114] Drappatz, J., Brenner, A., Wong, E.T., Eichler, A., Schiff, D., Groves, M.D., ... Wen, P.Y. Phase I study of GRN1005 in recurrent malignant glioma. *Clinical Cancer Research*, **2013**, *19*(6), 1567–1576

[115] Kurzrock, R., Gabrail, N., Chandhasin, C., Moulder, S., Smith, C., Brenner, A., ... Sarantopoulos, J. Safety, pharmacokinetics, and activity of GRN1005, a novel conjugate of angiopep-2, a peptide facilitating brain penetration, and paclitaxel, in patients with advanced solid tumors. *Molecular Cancer Therapeutics*, **2012**, *11*(2), 308

[116] Thomas, A., Teicher, B.A., & Hassan, R. Antibody-drug conjugates for cancer therapy. *Lancet Oncology*, **2016**, *17*, e254262.

[117] Hamblett, K.J., Kozlosky, C.J., Siu, S., Chang, W.S., Liu, H., Foltz, I.N., ... Fanslow, W.C. AMG 595, an anti-EGFRvIII antibody-drug conjugate, induces potent antitumor activity against EGFRvIII-expressing glioblastoma. *Molecular Cancer Therapeutics*, **2015**, *14*(7), 1614–1624.

[118] Phillips, A.C., Boghaert, E.R., Vaidya, K.S., Mitten, M.J., Norvell, S., Falls, H.D., ... Reilly, E.B. ABT414, an antibody drug

conjugate targeting a tumor-selective EGFR epitope. *Molecular Cancer Therapeutics*, **2016**, *15*(4), 661–669.

[119] Groot, J.F., Lamborn, K.R., Chang, S.M., Gilbert, M.R., Cloughesy, T.F., Aldape, K., ... Wen, P.Y. Phase II Study of aflibercept in recurrent malignant glioma: A north american brain tumor consortium study. *Journal of Clinical Oncology*, **2011**, *29*(19), 2689–2695. Available from https://doi.org/ 10.1200/JCO.2010.34.1636.

[120] Wang, H., Chen, K., Cai, W., Li, Z., He, L., Kashefi, A., & Chen, X. Integrin-targeted imaging and therapy with RGD4C-TNF fusion protein. *Molecular Cancer Therapeutics*, **2008**, *7*(5), 1044–1053.

7

Degenerative Diseases Treated with Brain-directed Lipid/Polymeric (Hybrid) Nanoparticles

Abstract

A central nervous system's (CNS) state of health depends on barriers separating it from the body's remainder. Endothelium, which makes up the BBB, or blood–brain barrier, functions as a thick network of cells to control what chemicals are permitted to enter the blood arteries of the brain. Neurodegenerative diseases like Parkinson's and Alzheimer's are now treated only through symptom relief. Developing drugs capable of penetrating the BBB without causing irreversible neuronal damage or disrupting the delicate balance of the CNS is an enormous challenge. One significant barrier to the creation of novel pharmacological treatments for brain diseases is effectively delivering therapeutic drugs across the BBB, while excluding potentially harmful neurotoxins. Drugs' pharmacokinetic qualities are being improved through nanotechnology, which also makes it easier for them to cross the blood–brain barrier. The trafficking of medicines across the BBB is crucial in treating neurodegenerative illnesses and nanoparticle (NP) formulations capable of encapsulating therapeutic compounds and increasing drug delivery by focusing on particular metabolic mechanisms in the brain. This chapter explores the potential uses of nanotechnology-based drug delivery systems for the treatment of neurodegenerative diseases, with a focus on the challenges that must be overcome to enhance drug delivery to the central nervous system.

7.1 Introduction

The global life expectancy has grown as a result of the growing prevalence of neurodegenerative illnesses like Alzheimer's and Parkinson's brought about by medical and pharmacological improvements. These ailments, along with other brain and spinal cord problems, can significantly affect a person's life and frequently necessitate protracted hospital admissions [1]. These circumstances may have significant social and economic repercussions [2, 3, 4]. The quality of life of patients is only little improved by the central nervous system (CNS) issues that are currently treated, which are often symptomatic rather than curative. In the search for innovative treatments, it is thought to be essential to overcome the problem of drug distribution, whether it includes developing new compounds or optimizing ones that already exist [5].

Since the beginning of the 21st century, there has been steady progress in medication development. In 2012, the FDA approved 39 new drugs in the United States, but only two of them were for the treatment of CNS disorders [6]. Discovering new drugs for brain diseases is a challenging and costly endeavor for pharmaceutical companies. Despite significant advancements in the pharmaceutical and biotechnology industries, a new generation of pharmacological treatments for CNS disorders has yet to materialize. The research and development of novel CNS drugs typically takes around 12–16 years and costs between USD 0.8 and 1.7 billion before they reach the market [7]. The stringent requirements for novel pharmaceutical preparations also apply to CNS-targeting drugs, including high activity levels, selectivity, and bioavailability, with the added complexity of crossing the blood–brain barrier (BBB). In the past few decades, only 3%–5% of brain-targeted medications have successfully reached the market due to the difficulty of penetrating the BBB [8].

The complex anatomy and physiology of the BBB present numerous challenges that new approaches to CNS drug delivery must overcome. This intricate cellular architecture regulates the exchange of nutrients and metabolites between the peripheral and brain circulatory systems, supporting the prevention of damage to the brain, spinal cord, and neurons [9]. Brain infections, neurodegenerative diseases, and strokes are examples of conditions that alter the BBB, allowing chemicals to enter the brain [10]. However, developing novel pharmaceutical options for treating brain diseases is challenging due to the need to deliver therapeutic drugs across the BBB without permitting harmful neurotoxins to enter. Various drug delivery techniques and modifications to the existing drug efflux mechanism have been developed to address this issue [11].

Advancements in nanomedicine have led to the development of several promising platforms that enhance drug distribution across the BBB, making them potential candidates for CNS pharmacological therapy [8, 12, 13, 14]. Among these, nanoparticles (NPs) have emerged as one of the most versatile and promising methods of drug delivery. NPs effectively protect therapeutic compounds while targeting and delivering them to damaged areas, particularly difficult-to-reach regions like the brain. In healthy animal models, various NP formulations can cross the BBB after intravenous injection, demonstrating their potential [15]. Understanding the morphology, physiological changes, and pathogen physiology of the BBB is essential for developing NP formulations that can effectively target injured brain regions and comprehend their physicochemical and toxicological profiles.

The pros and cons of using nanotechnology for CNS medication delivery in the management of neurodegenerative illnesses will be covered in this chapter. Based on current research findings, it will summarize the best nanosystems for brain drug delivery and examine the most recent developments in nano-delivery technology help combat neurodegenerative conditions including MS, Parkinson's, Alzheimer's, and Huntington's disease.

7.2 Blood–Brain Barrier Crossing with Brain Targeting

Several barriers in the central nervous system stop neurotoxic chemicals, blood cells, and invading pathogens from penetrating and spreading throughout the nervous system. Instances of such barriers include the blood–brain barrier (BBB), the blood–retinal barrier (BRB), and the blood–cerebrospinal-fluid barrier [16]. The BBB is the most conspicuous and widespread circulatory system in the brain and is composed primarily of endothelial cells and pericytes (Figure 7.1). The BBB's durability and the angiogenic capacity of the cerebral endothelium allow for revascularization if necessary [17]. As a means of keeping the extracellular matrix (EC) barrier intact, ECs express the protein's tight junctions (TJs) and adherent junctions (AJs). The BBB uses a strict cellular architecture to regulate the selective entry of cells and small substances into the brain [18].

For effective pharmaceutical formulations that may reach the brain and central nervous system, it is essential to comprehend the morphological makeup and biological operation of the BBB.

7.2.1 Anatomy and role of the BBB

Endothelial cells (ECs) shield the blood vessels in the brain and spinal cord, while smooth muscle cells, microglia, astrocytes, and pericytes surround them [19, 20]. The brain's blood vessel lining consists of two membranes, the apical and basolateral, each of which performs a unique function. This asymmetry belongs to the organization's core values of membrane-bound transport networks [9].

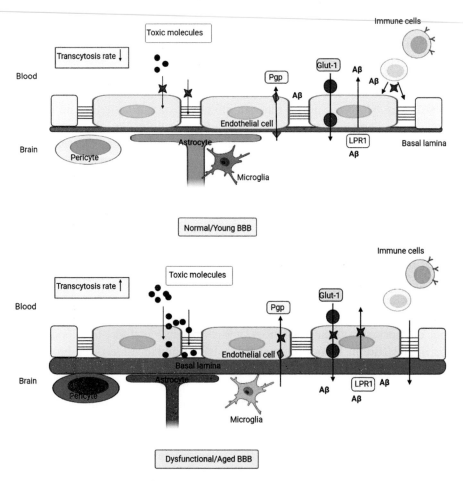

Figure 7.1   The BBB in normal and abnormal states.

The physical barrier alone is insufficient to provide a complete picture of the BBB's effectiveness and also its metabolic, immunological, and transport functions. If there are TJs and AJs between neighboring ECs, there is a physical barrier (Figure 7.1).

Tight junctions (TJs) are found in the apical region of the paracellular space, and they are composed of the transmembrane proteins occludin and claudin, as well as the junctional adhesion molecule-1 (JAM-1) and cingulin [21, 22]. The paracellular space is where proteins like cadherin and integrin come together to create adhesion junctions (AJs) at the cell's basal lamina [22]. Intracellular and external enzymes work together to allow the BBB to serve as a metabolic barrier [23]. Lymphocytes and other immune cells are stopped at this barrier made up of microglia [24], perivascular macrophages, and mast cells [10]. Trans and paracellular pathways are part of the barrier. Various chemicals penetrate the BBB through the transcellular pathway, which is critical. Cell-mediated transcytosis and adsorptive transcytosis are both included in this pathway as well as transport through carriers and receptors [25]. Xenobiotics and endogenic substances (metabolites, hormones, and mediators) that may be hazardous to the nervous system are also blocked from passing over this barrier [8]. The paracellular transport of ions and solutes is one of the most common methods for crossing cells [26]. Passive diffusion of lipophilic compounds via specialized receptors to transport molecules is the most common mode of administration in the transcellular pathway [23]. Proteins and peptides are hydrophilic molecules that cannot enter the brain without the help of a specialized transport or receptor. The invaginations of cells known as caveolae are still another kind of transportation [16]. They form vesicles to carry the chemical both into and out of the brain. Some medications may not be able to enter the brain parenchyma due to a family of active efflux pumps termed ATP-binding cassette (ABC) transporters [27]. ABC transporters are responsible for the intravenous delivery of lipid-soluble but potentially toxic substances, such as some pharmaceutical medications. Some examples include P-gp (permeability glycoprotein) and MDR1 (multidrug resistance protein 1). Solute carrier (SLC) transporters play a significant role in ECs' organic anion efflux transport mechanism. This polypeptide is composed of two different proteins called organic anion transporter (OAT)/solute carrier polypeptide (SLC22A) and organic anion transporter (OAT)/solute carrier protein (SLC22B) (SLCO). These transporters, together with MRPs and MRPAPs, help the brain flush out medicines by efflux [28].

As a result of the BBB's selective solute permeability, which is controlled by many transporters, it can maintain brain homeostasis. Transport mechanisms and channels in the endothelium membrane of endothelial cells stabilize the ionic content of the interstitial fluid and preserve synaptic transmission [13]. The BBB is useful for transporting nutrients to cells and also plays a role in regulating intracellular pH. Hydrophilic nutrients cannot be passively transported across the BBB.

Several distinct transport mechanisms are required for nutrient distribution to be carried out effectively [29]. Lipophilic compounds or substrates for active transport can only permeate the BBB [30]. Amino acids can be transported via cationic, anionic, or neutral transporters in the BBB [31]. N-amino acid (NAA) transporters are found on both EC membranes [32], delivering critical amino acids to the brain. Multiple SLC2 transport systems (glucose transporters [GLUTs]) are involved in the transfer of carbohydrates to cells in mammalian animals. Rather than relying on glucose buildup, these systems rely on assisted diffusion, an energy-independent transport method [33].

7.2.2 The improvement of brain drug delivery

7.2.2.1 BBB morphological modulation

A time- and reversible-controlled BBB opening has been created, and modulating BBB morphology may improve the distribution of active pharmacological formulations. While TJs prevent medications from crossing the BBB, this barrier is compromised when their structure is compromised. When TJ structures are disrupted, drugs can be transported paracellularly. Injections of osmotic solutions, bioactive compounds, and physical stimulation are all often employed to improve vascular paracellular transport in the brain [34]. The BBB's osmosis was used to combat malignant brain tumors. Hyperosmolar formulations of antitumor medicines including cyclophosphamide, procarbazine, and methotrexate may improve their tumor penetration (mannitol). After being exposed to a hypertonic solution, the ECs changed their morphology and the rate of paracellular transport increased [35]. Several biologically active chemicals, including histamine and bradykinin, have the potential to increase the blood–brain barrier (BBB) permeability. Actin restructuring, claudin and occludin remodeling, and enhanced absorption of Ca21 ions are all caused by bradykinin's action on the endothelium of brain arteries, which is mediated by B2 receptor activation [36]. Physical manipulation of TJs has been used to disrupt the BBB in other ways. Ultrasound is a popular technique to increase the penetration of drug through BBB [37, 38]. The paracellular space was likewise enlarged by ultrasound, but the efflux transporter's ability to inhibit the active transport of hydrophobic drugs was reduced. Physically opening TJs using electromagnetic radiation is an interesting yet uncommon procedure [39].

A larger number of medications that work for neurological disorders need to be developed, and the BBB alteration has several drawbacks. These include a high level of complexity and a lack of selectivity.

7.2.2.2 Modulation of the BBB transport system

Various chemicals have the ability to accumulate in the expression of the brain transport mechanisms on the surface of ECs. Lipophilic compounds can cross the apical membrane and enter the EC cytoplasm, where they can be efficiently expelled through ABC transport pathways [40]. Also, pathological conditions might increase P-gp and other ABC transporter activities. The anti-epileptic medications phenytoin, levetiracetam, lamotrigine, and pheno-barbital may be less effective if P-gp activity is elevated. Endothelial cell per-meability has been increased with the help of ABC transporter substrates and efflux inhibitors [41]. Verapamil and diltiazem are examples of P-gp modu-lators and facilitate the transport of antiviral and anticancer medicines to the brain. Some polymers may inhibit ABC transporter function by decreasing membrane fluidity. Several drugs have been demonstrated to be more able to enter cells *in vitro* after being treated with Pluronic P85 because of their potential to inhibit P-gp [42]. Low P-gp affinity, dangerous side effects at high doses, and simultaneous inhibition of CYP3A enzymes were some of the problems with the initial generation of P-gp inhibitors like verapamil and cyclosporine. The second-generation P-glycoprotein (P-gp) inhibitor val-spodar 10, which is structurally similar to cyclosporine, has a high affinity for the transporter and is less toxic and less detrimental to liver microsomal enzymes than cyclosporine. In contrast to the previous one, the new P-gp inhibitor generation, elacridar 11, does not affect CYP3A. The idea of "zones of responsibility" with P-gp mutually overlapping makes the modulation of BCRP/ABCG2 activity an important therapeutic consideration [43]. BCRP is known to be inhibited by the proton pump inhibitor pantoprazole and elacri-dar 11 [44]. There may be some drawbacks to blocking P-gp, such as expos-ing the BBB to potentially hazardous chemicals [45].

7.3 Nano-engineered Colloid Drug Delivery Systems

There are a variety of natural and manufactured colloidal nanocarriers, rang-ing in size from one nanometer (nm) to more than a thousand nanometers (nm). Dendrimers, solid lipid nanoparticles, polymeric nanoparticles, poly-meric micelles, and liposomes are examples of noninvasive methods being researched to penetrate the BBB [46]. Medicines and large molecules could be transported to the brain by these colloid transporters.

Due to the BBB's poor direct permeability, the capacity of these nano-systems to carry medications to the brain is constrained. Nanosystems' versatility in design and engineering, however, suggests that other modes of transport via the BBB, such as EC receptors and endocytosis, may be explored. Although nanocarriers may be destroyed by lysosomes in endothe-lial cells (EC), their drug load is still released and carried effectively to the ultimate destination in the brain [41].

Chitosan and alginate are examples of polysaccharides; poly(lysine) and poly(aspartic acid) (PASA) are examples of polypeptides and amino acids; and proteins are examples of polypeptides (gelatine and albumin), which may all be used to make natural nanocarriers [47]. Because of their inherent batch-to-batch unpredictability, limited ability to be modified in a controlled manner, and poor imaging platform tracking, natural NPs offer certain distinct advantages over synthetic ones. Nanocarriers made from inorganic substances, including gold, silicon dioxide (silica), and others, may also be used to make synthetic nanocarriers. These carriers can carry medicines through adsorption, entrapment, or covalent attachment [8, 14].

When compared to polymeric nanosystems, inorganic nanosystems excel due to their superior size and shape control, simplicity of manufacture, and amenability to functionalization. Optical microscopy and other microscopy techniques, as well as analytical tools (e.g., MRI and TEM), make it much easier to keep tabs on inorganic NPs (e.g., magnetic resonance imaging and transmission electron microscopy) (such as ICP-MS).

Carbon nanotubes and fullerenes, for example, may induce lipid peroxidation and oxygen radical production, which makes them difficult to degrade. They may also be harmful in other ways [48].

Particle size, hydrophobicity, coating, chemistry, and surface charge are only a few of the modifiable form variables of NPs, in particular, which make them attractive delivery vehicles for brain drugs. Controlling these qualities is necessary for increasing the NP stability in circulation, regulating drug release at the target location, increasing BBB penetration efficacy, and evading the reticuloendothelial system [12, 14].

A better understanding of how NPs travel through the BBB may help researchers identify potential target areas. It has been established that the following transport mechanisms exist: the blood–brain barrier can be penetrated by drugs in free form or when combined with NPs (BBB) because (i) NPs can cause localized permeabilization of the BBB through the opening of TJs between ECs or the generation of local toxic effects [27, 49], (ii) NPs can enter cells via transcytosis [50], (iii) NPs can be conveyed through endocytosis through ECs, with their contents exocytosed on the abluminal side of the endothelium after being discharged into the cytoplasm [51], and (iv) any strategy that utilizes more than one of the above. Several studies have suggested that mechanisms 2, 3, and 4 are the primary means by which NPs are transported. Among the receptors that NPs aim for in the mechanism are transferrin and low-density lipoprotein receptors [52, 53]. Proteins [52], peptides [53], and antibodies [38] deposited on top of nanoparticles (NPs) have all been used to target cells.

Several physicochemical variables influence cellular delivery, BBB penetration, and NP systemic circulation. Numerous investigations have revealed that as the NP size grows, BBB penetration decreases [54, 55]. In most of the studies done so far, nanoparticles (NPs) between 50 and 100 nm in size were used to examine their effects on neuronal cells and animal models. Absorption and distribution in the body may also be affected by NPs, in addition to their physical shape [56]. NPs can be of any shape, including spherical, cubic, or rod-like. Due to their convenience in manufacturing, spherical NPs have been used in the great majority of investigations. The surface adhesion of antibody-coated nanorods has been reported to be higher than that of their spherical counterparts [57]. Furthermore, the zeta potential of NPs is a crucial factor in their capacity to penetrate the BBB. High zeta potential NPs are responsible for BBB toxicity (high positive surface charge) [14]. That is why most NP formulations for brain administration have zeta potentials between −1 and −45 mV in the literature [13, 27, 50, 56, 59].

7.3.1 Liposomes

Liposomes have long been recognized as conventional transport mechanisms, with various phospholipids forming mono- and multi-lamellar structures under different technical conditions, extensively studied in liposome production. Systems with high bioavailability and low toxicity provide benefits such as simplicity of preparation, low toxicity, and cost efficiency. They are desirable for treatments that target the brain because they can effectively encapsulate both lipophilic and hydrophilic substances. They can only be used temporarily since they are swiftly absorbed by reticuloendothelial system (RES) cells [60]. To address this issue, reducing liposome size to the nanometric range and surface modifying them with polyethylene glycol (PEG) can extend their circulation time.

Functionalizing the surface of liposomes with viruses and specific ligands enables the targeting of specific tissues or cells in the body. For example, conjugating antibodies to liposome surfaces enhances their recognition by endothelial cells (ECs) [61].

7.3.2 Nanoparticles of polymeric materials

These polymeric nanoparticles, which make up these solid colloidal nanosystems, are biocompatible copolymers with low water solubility [62, 63]. At the moment, a wide variety of polymers are being employed as nanoparticle matrices. This includes plasma albumins as well as PLA and PLGA. Nanoparticles (NPs) may carry chemicals that have been adsorbent, covalently bonded, integrated within a polymer matrix, or enclosed on their surface [41]. For example, these polymers have minimal toxicity and biodegradability, contain active pharmaceutical ingredients (APIs), are pharmacologically stable, and have precise control over drug release, which are all examples of desirable properties of these particles [8]. The development of polymers has caused an increase in medication delivery vectors capable of crossing the BBB. RES cells, like liposomes, rapidly engulf intact nanoparticles in circulation. It has been found that the absorption of surfactants on NPs' surfaces is more effective in extending the time they spend in the blood than shrinking NPs to make them last longer. PEG, polysorbate 80, and polysaccharides may be absorbed or covalently linked onto NP surfaces to improve blood flow while compounds that identify biological determinants can be included to allow the blood–brain barrier or BBB by nanoparticles [13].

7.3.3 Solid nanoparticles

SLNs, or solid nanoparticles, are another smart drug delivery method. High-pressure homogenization or microemulsion technologies may be used to easily create these particles for use. An SLN typically has a phospholipid coating on top of its hydrophobic core. For targeting, including BBB penetration, transcytosis mediated by receptors or the inhibition of efflux transport are both crucial. SLNs outperform polymer nanoparticles and liposomes in several important ways, including drug loading capacity, stability, cytotoxicity, controlled release, and cost. However, SLNs could be able to move substances that are both hydrophilic and lipophilic [5]. Numerous drugs have been transported to the brain via SLNs, including camptothecin [64], piperine [65], docetaxel [66], small interfering RNA [67], curcumin [68], quercetin [69], idebenone [70], apomorphine [71], risperidone [72], and quinine [73]. Recently, the use of SLNs as drug delivery vehicles has been the subject of controversy and discussion, with advocates and opponents on both sides of the issue [5, 74].

7.3.4 Ligands

One of the many advantages of nanocarriers, especially NPs, is the possibility to introduce specific molecules or ligands onto the surfaces. It has been found that ligand-conjugated NPs may cross the blood–brain barrier rather easily. For instance, (i) blood protein absorption-promoting ligands that interact with BBB receptors or transporters [75, 76, 77]; (ii) apolipoprotein E and/or A-I-anchoring poly(sorbate 80) (Tween 80), which improves their ability to interact with lipoprotein receptors expressed in brain endothelium and, consequently, to cross the blood–brain barrier (BBB); (iii) PEGylated NPs;

and (iv) PEG, a 5 kDa polymer with 0.16 to 0.64 PEG molecules per nm^2, is added to NPs to slow down their clearance and lessen the quantity of protein adsorption [78]. PEGylated NPs also aggregate in the brain with greater efficiency due to their longer half-life in the blood [79].

NP trafficking through the BBB is influenced by receptor affinity, ligand abundance, and ligand specificity (avidity). The ligand density is influenced by both the ligand size and the NP surface area due to the ligand's decreased affinity for its receptor following conjugation to NPs. The resemblance and selectivity of NPs are enhanced by the attachment of several ligands [27]. Transcytosis across the BBB is similarly reliant on NP avidity. Receptor-bound NPs with a high avidity were found to be less likely to leave the brain parenchyma [50].

7.4 Neurodegenerative Diseases: New Advances in Nanomedicine

Alzheimer's, Parkinson's, and Huntington's diseases are just a few of the illnesses whose prevalence has grown as life expectancy has risen (HDs).

Although some treatments may help reduce symptoms or even slow the progression of some diseases, there are presently no drugs available that may cure or prevent them. Numerous neurodegenerative diseases can be diagnosed and treated with the help of nanotechnology today, with a focus on amyloid-β [Aβ] and vascular endothelial cell (EC) targeting and oxidative stress.

7.4.1 Alzheimer's disease

Alzheimer's disease accounts for a staggering 9 out of 10 cases of dementia in those over the age of 65 (AD). Dementia with Alzheimer's disease is characterized by a progressive decline in mental faculties over time. A breakdown in cholinergic signaling is suspected to be at the root of this deterioration, which may also lead to later physiological impairment. In addition, neurofibrillary tangles and amyloid-β (Aβ) peptides (or senile plaques) (also known as microtubule-stabilizing proteins) are found in both the extracellular and intracellular environments [80]. In addition to reducing the A-induced toxicity of the condition, these nanoparticles could be used to encapsulate physiologically active medicines for direct brain delivery. Noncompetitive and reversible cholinesterase inhibitors like tacrine and rivastigmine have been used to treat Alzheimer's disease (AD) since they were respectively cleared by the FDA in 1991 and 2000 [80, 81, 82]. Because of their low brain translocation, these medicines have limited effectiveness in the clinic; they must be administered often, and they trigger harmful cholinergic effects in the body's periphery [83]. Rat *in vivo* investigations indicated that drug concentrations in the brain were dramatically increased after the nanoparticles were coated with polysorbate-80 and poly(n-butyl cyanoacrylate) [82]. Rivastigmine tartrate was loaded onto polysorbate-80-coated human serum albumin (HSA) nanoparticles for enhanced brain targeting via endocytosis and a sustained release of the medication. Recently, there has been a lot of interest in delivering rivastigmine through nasal spray directly to the brain. After being loaded into NLCs by an ethanol injection method involving Lecithin (L), glyceryl monostearate (GMS), Capmul MCM C8, and Tween 80, the therapeutic efficacy of rivastigmine was boosted by a factor of 3, and mucosa permeability was improved by a factor of 2 (TWE) [84]. These steps can increase the drug's effectiveness and safety, but they only address the symptoms of Alzheimer's disease (AD), not its underlying cause.

7.4.2 Parkinson's disorder

As the condition advances, the brain's dopamine concentration decreases, making it harder to govern movement. There is also an accumulation of a protein inclusion known as α-synuclein in cells called neurons, which is a symptom of Parkinson's disease (PD), a neurological condition with degenerative symptoms. Muscle rigidity, tremors, and irregularities in speech and movement are all symptoms experienced by people with Parkinson's disease (PD). Symptoms can only be alleviated by therapy after diagnosis [85].

L-dopa is used to treat Parkinson's disease; however, it has been shown to cause further damage by generating free radicals, hastening the death of nigrostriatal dopaminergic neurons [86]. Researchers have constructed to increase the therapeutic potential of these medicines, which are not well soluble in water; several other L-dopa codrugs have been developed and packaged in nanostructured lipid carriers (NLCs) [87]. These include lipoic acid dopamine (PDB), lipoic acid-3,4-acetoxy-dopamine (PDC), and 3,4-diacetyl oxy-LD-caffeic acid (PDA) [89]. Dopamine agonist medications such as ropinirole, bromocriptine (Parlodel), and apomorphine are effective in treating PD symptoms in both *in vitro* and *in vivo* trials [88].

7.4.3 Huntington's disease

In the middle of life, repeats of the Huntingtin gene's cytosine–adenine–guanine (CAG) triplet that are unstable lead to polyglutamine expansion at NH2-tetraphosphate, which in turn causes the protein manifestations of Huntington's disease, including involuntary movement abnormalities, mental symptoms, and cognitive decline [89, 90]. Aggregation of mutant HTT to toxic levels disrupts mitochondrial function and causes energy depletion, both of which are detrimental to neuronal function and survival [91]. Glial cell and cortical neuron degeneration have a profound effect on striatal neurons, especially moderately spiny neurons (MSN; GABAergic neurons) [89]. There are now no treatments that can stop the progression of this disease, and the only option is to manage the symptoms [92]. Numerous methods have been used to study the possibility of cell therapy, including the generation of pluripotent stem cells, the replacement of injured neurons with new neurons, and the stimulation of neurotrophic factor concentrations and activities (e.g., BDNF) [89,93]. Through coordinating life and death pathways, the proteins of the brain-derived neurotrophic factor (BDNF) family are crucial for neuronal survival, function, proliferation, differentiation, maintenance, and plasticity. Neuroprotection and cell treatment are two of the many applications for nanocarriers in this area.

7.4.4 Multiple sclerosis

T-cell and macrophage infiltration are hallmarks of the chronic inflammatory condition known as multiple sclerosis (MS), which affects the central nervous system and leads to widespread axonal and oligodendrocyte loss [94]. To give just one example, glucocorticosteroids may require multiple intravenous injections, each of which can be a hassle and take a significant amount of time [95]. There has been extensive research on whether or not long-term circulating liposomes can safely reduce glucocorticoid dosage or frequency of treatment. In 2003, Schmidt and coworkers found that prednisolone loaded onto liposomes (PL) was more efficacious than methylprednisolone at five times the dose [96]. Additionally, it was shown that PL can reduce the number of inflammatory macrophages and T-cell infiltration in the spinal cord, demonstrating the system's selectivity [96]. In a study using rats as a disease model, researchers compared PEGylated liposomal formulations of methylprednisolone (LM) and methylprednisolone (PL) to free methylprednisolone [97].

Reactive oxygen species (ROS) production is important in multiple sclerosis pathogenesis [98].

ROS scavengers may be able to alleviate the symptoms of the condition. PEGylated liposomes enclosing the antioxidant tempamine (TMN) were used to achieve systemic delivery and selective tissue anti-inflammatory effects [99]. In rats with experimental autoimmune encephalomyelitis (EAE), clinical symptoms were alleviated following a systemic treatment of TMN-containing PEGylated liposomes [100], reduced T-cell proliferation, and, consequently, the production of inflammatory cytokines like IFN and TNF by scavenging free radicals. Nanoparticles of cerium oxide whose structure is maintained by citrate/EDTA were administered to EAE mice had their motor impairment and MS symptoms reduced, and ROS was associated with CNS illness [101].

Many disorders, including multiple sclerosis (MS), have seen considerable improvements in therapy because of recent developments in utilizing nanoparticles for the transport of genes (e.g., SLN) [102]. An adapter protein called STING stimulates the genes that produce interferon (IFN) activated when cytosolic DNA is detected, resulting in the generation of IFN type I (IFN-α,β). Systemic DNA therapy might reduce autoimmune processes by triggering strong immune regulatory responses through STING signaling [103]. For gene therapy, DNA nanoparticles may be made by condensing DNA with cationic polymers or polyamine analogs [104]. When given intravenously to EAE mice, synthesized DNA nanoparticles were found to have beneficial therapeutic effects, including a decrease in CNS T-cell infiltration, which was linked to the nanoparticles' ability to regulate the immunomodulatory enzyme indoleamine 2,3-dioxygenase (IDO) [103].

7.5 Conclusion

In conclusion, the growing prevalence of central nervous system (CNS) disorders in an aging global population necessitates further exploration of novel drug delivery technologies and formulations. To bring new treatment medications to patients, it is crucial to develop biological models that take advantage of the anomalies in the BBB, or blood–brain barrier, observed in various conditions. This will enable the development of safer and more effective noninvasive treatments targeting the brain. BBB is critical to the proper functioning of the central nervous system. Impaired BBB aggravates the brain disease. Multiple receptors are overexpressed on endothelial cells (ECs) in neurological disorders, offering prospective therapeutic targets.

A very promising application for CNS medication delivery is colloidal nanocarriers, offering several advantages over conventional approaches. Their small size allows for encapsulation and controlled, targeted transport of drugs to the desired site while providing some degree of protection for the transported medications. Recent studies have uncovered fundamental rules guiding the movement of nanoparticle (NP) formulations through the blood–brain barrier, including elements that can affect the structure of nanocarriers and the permeation procedure, such as ligand type, ligand density, and NP shape. These results can serve as a basis for NP changes catered to certain brain diseases or drug chemistry and can direct the creation of superior formulations. Additionally intriguing evidence of the therapeutic benefits of NPs on neurological illnesses has come from animal research. To comprehend the differences in NP transport between healthy and ill animals, additional study is necessary, considering the limitations of current experimental models in accurately representing specific human diseases. Addressing nanotoxicological concerns will also be crucial for future therapeutic approaches.

Future breakthroughs in the realm of NP delivery systems for the brain might include nanoparticles that can target just certain brain cells and remotely controlled nanoformulations that only release medications after they reach the brain. Neurodegenerative illnesses like Parkinson's disease (PD), where microglia and neuroinflammation play major roles, may respond particularly well to treatment by certain types of brain cells, such as dopaminergic neurons, microglia, or neural stem cells. Preclinical NP research should soon lead to clinical trials, even though there is still considerable work to be done in this area.

References

[1] Pan, A., Sun, Q., Okereke, O.I., Rexrode, K.M., & Hu, F.B. Depression and risk of stroke morbidity and mortality a meta-analysis and systematic review. *JAMA-Journal of the American Medical Association*, **2011**, *306*(11), 1241–1249. Available from https://doi.org/10.1001/jama.2011.1282

[2] Assoc, A. Alzheimer's Association Report 2015 Alzheimer's disease facts and figures. *Alzheimer's & Dementia*, **2015**, *11*(3), 332–384. Available from https://doi.org/10.1016/j.jalz.2015.02.003.

[3] Jimenez-Jimenez, F.J., Alonso-Navarro, H., Garcia-Martin, E., & Agundez, J.A.G. Advances in understanding genomic markers and pharmacogenetics of Parkinson's disease. *Expert Opinion on Drug Metabolism & Toxicology*, **2016**, *12*(4), 433–448. Available from https://doi.org/10.1517/17425255.2016.1158250.

[4] Mozaffarian. Heart disease and stroke statistics-2016 update: A report from the American Heart Association (vol 133, pg e38, 2016). *Circulation*, **2016**, *133*(15), E599. Available from https://doi.org/10.1161/ Cir.0000000000000409, E599

[5] Patel, M., Souto, E.B., & Singh, K.K. Advances in brain drug targeting and delivery: Limitations and challenges of solid lipid nanoparticles. *Expert Opinion on Drug Delivery*, **2013**, *10*(7), 889–905. Available from https:// doi.org/10.1517/17425247.2013.784742.

[6] Mullard, A. 2012 FDA drug approvals. *Nature Reviews Drug Discovery*, **2013**, *12*(2), 87–90

[7] Matschay, A., Nowakowska, E., Hertmanowska, H., Kus, K., & Czubak, A. Cost analysis of therapy for patients with multiple sclerosis (MS) in Poland. *Pharmacological Reports*, **2008**, *60*(5), 632–644.

[8] Cupaioli, F.A., Zucca, F.A., Boraschi, D., & Zecca, L. Engineered nanoparticles. How brain friendly is this new guest? *Progress in Neurobiology*, **2014**, *119*, 20–38. Available from https://doi.org/10.1016/j. pneurobio.2014.05.002.

[9] Patel, M.M., Goyal, B.R., Bhadada, S.V., Bhatt, J.S., & Amin, A.F. Getting into the brain approaches to enhance brain drug delivery. *Cns Drugs*, **2009**, *23*(1), 35–58. Available from https://doi.org/10.2165/0023210- 200923010-00003

[10] Obermeier, B., Daneman, R., & Ransohoff, R.M. Development, maintenance and disruption of the blood-brain barrier. *Nature Medicine*, **2013**, *19*(12), 1584–1596. Available from https://doi.org/10.1038/nm.3407

[11] Alyautdin, R., Khalin, I., Nafeeza, M.I., Haron, M.H., & Kuznetsov, D. Nanoscale drug delivery systems and the blood-brain barrier. *International Journal of Nanomedicine*, **2014**, *9*, 795–811. Available from https://doi.org/ 10.2147/Ijn.S52236.

[12] Goldsmith, M., Abramovitz, L., & Peer, D. Precision nanomedicine in neurodegenerative diseases. *ACS Nano*, **2014**, *8*(3), 1958–1965. Available from https://doi.org/10.1021/nn501292z

[13] Kreuter, J. Nanoparticulate systems for brain delivery of drugs. *Advanced Drug Delivery Reviews*, **2012**, *64*, 213–222. Available from https://doi.org/10.1016/j.addr.2012.09.015.

[14] Lockman, P.R., Koziara, J.M., Mumper, R.J., & Allen, D.D. Nanoparticle surface charges alter blood-brain barrier integrity and permeability. *Journal of Drug Targeting*, **2004**, *12*(9-10), 635–641. Available from https:// doi.org/10.1080/10611860400015936.

[15] Saraiva, C., Praca, C., Ferreira, R., Santos, T., Ferreira, L., & Bernardino, L. Nanoparticle-mediated brain drug delivery: Overcoming blood-brain barrier to treat neurodegenerative diseases. *Journal of Controlled Release*, **2016**, *235*, 34–47. Available from https://doi.org/10.1016/j. jconrel.2016.05.044.

[16] Persidsky, Y., Ramirez, S.H., Haorah, J., & Kanmogne, G.D. Blood-brain barrier: Structural components and function under physiologic

and pathologic conditions. *Journal of Neuroimmune Pharmacology*, **2006**, *1*(3), 223–236. Available from https://doi.org/10.1007/s11481-006-9025-3.

[17] Boyer-Di Ponio, J., El-Ayoubi, F., Glacial, F., Ganeshamoorthy, K., Driancourt, C., Godet, M., ... Uzan, G. Instruction of circulating endothelial progenitors *in vitro* towards specialized blood-brain barrier and arterial phenotypes. *PLoS One*, **2014**, *9*(1). Available from https://doi.org/10.1371/journal.pone.0084179, ARTN e84179.

[18] Huber, J.D., Witt, K.A., Hom, S., Egleton, R.D., Mark, K.S., & Davis, T.P. Inflammatory pain alters blood-brain barrier permeability and tight junctional protein expression. *American Journal of Physiology-Heart and Circulatory Physiology*, **2011**, *280*(3), H1241–H1248.

[19] Begley, D.J. Delivery of therapeutic agents to the central nervous system: The problems and the possibilities. *Pharmacology & Therapeutics*, **2004**, *104*(1), 29–45. Available from https://doi.org/10.1016/j.pharmthera.2004.08.001.

[20] Bernacki, J., Dobrowolska, A., Nierwinska, K., & Malecki, A. Physiology and pharmacological role of the blood-brain barrier. *Pharmacological Reports*, **2008**, *60*(5), 600–622.

[21] Matter, K., & Balda, M.S. Signalling to and from tight junctions. *Nature Reviews Molecular Cell Biology*, **2003**, *4*(3), 225–236. Available from https://doi.org/10.1038/nrm1055.

[22] Hawkins, B.T., & Davis, T.P. The blood-brain barrier/neurovascular unit in health and disease. *Pharmacological Reviews*, **2005**, *57*(2), 173–185. Available from https://doi.org/10.1124/pr.57.2.4.

[23] Abbott, N.J., Ronnback, L., & Hansson, E. Astrocyte-endothelial interactions at the blood-brain barrier. *Nature Reviews Neuroscience*, **2006**, *7*(1), 41–53. Available from https://doi.org/10.1038/nrn1824.

[24] Aguzzi, A., Barres, B., & Bennett, M.L. Microglia: Scapegoat, Saboteur, or Something Else? *Science*, **2013**, *339*(6116), 156–161. Available from https://doi.org/10.1126/science.1227901.

[25] Chen, Y., & Liu, L.H. Modern methods for delivery of drugs across the blood-brain barrier. *Advanced Drug Delivery Reviews*, **2012**, *64*(7), 640–665. Available from https://doi.org/10.1016/j.addr.2011.11.010.

[26] Wolburg, H., & Lippoldt, A. Tight junctions of the blood-brain barrier: Development, composition and regulation. *Vascular Pharmacology*, **2002**, *38*(6), 323–337. Available from https://doi.org/10.1016/S1537-1891(02) 00200-8.

[27] Choi, Y.K., & Kim, K.W. Blood-neural barrier: Its diversity and coordinated cell-to-cell communication. *Bmb Reports*, **2008**, *41*(5), 345–352.

[28] Tamai, I., & Tsuji, A. Transporter-mediated permeation of drugs across the blood-brain barrier. *Journal of Pharmaceutical Sciences*, **2000**, *89*(11), 1371–1388. Available from http://dx.doi.org/10.1002/1520-6017(200011) 89:11.201371::Aid-Jps1%203.0.Co;2-D.

[29] Gingrich, M.B., & Traynelis, S.F. Serine proteases and brain damage is there a link? *Trends in Neurosciences*, **2000**, *23*(9), 399–407. Available from https://doi.org/10.1016/S0166-2236(00)01617-9.

[30] Reiber, H. Dynamics of brain-derived proteins in cerebrospinal fluid. *Clinica Chimica Acta*, **2001**, *310*(2), 173–186. Available from https://doi.org/10.1016/S0009-8981(01)00573-3.

[31] Wolburg, H., Noell, S., Mack, A., Wolburg-Buchholz, K., & Fallier-Becker, P. Brain endothelial cells and the glio-vascular complex. *Cell and Tissue Research*, **2009**, *335*(1), 75–96. Available from https://doi.org/10.1007/ s00441-008-0658-9.

[32] Vorbrodt, A.W., Dobrogowska, D.H., Tarnawski, M., Meeker, H.C., & Carp, R.I. Immunogold study of altered expression of some interendothelial junctional molecules in the brain blood microvessels of diabetic scrapie-infected mice. *Journal of Molecular Histology*, **2006**, *37*(1-2), 27–35. Available from https://doi.org/10.1007/ s10735-006-9026-9.

[33] Farrell, C.L., & Pardridge, W.M. Blood-brain-barrier glucose transporter is asymmetrically distributed on brain capillary endothelial lumenal and ablumenal membranes - an electron-microscopic immunogold study. *Proceedings of the National Academy of Sciences of the United States of America*, **1991**, *88*(13), 5779–5783. Available from https://doi.org/10.1073/pnas.88.13.5779.

[34] Shilo, M., Motiei, M., Hana, P., & Popovtzer, R. Transport of nanoparticles through the blood-brain barrier for imaging and therapeutic applications. *Nanoscale*, **2014**, *6*(4), 2146–2152. Available from https://doi.org/10.1039/ c3nr04878k.

[35] Gabathuler, R. Approaches to transport therapeutic drugs across the blood-brain barrier to treat brain diseases. *Neurobiology of Disease*, **2010**, *37*(1), 48–57. Available from https://doi.org/10.1016/j.nbd.2009.07.028.

[36] Regoli, D., & Barabe, J. Pharmacology of bradykinin and related kinins. *Pharmacological Reviews*, **1980**, *32*(1), 1–46.

[37] Sheikov, N., McDannold, N., Vykhodtseva, N., Jolesz, F., & Hynynen, K. Cellular mechanisms of the blood-brain barrier opening induced by ultrasound in presence of microbubbles. *Ultrasound in Medicine and Biology*, **2004**, *30*(7), 979–989. Available from https://doi.org/10.1016/j.ultrasmedbio.2004.04.010.

[38] Yemisci,M.,Caban,S.,Gursoy-Ozdemir,Y.,Lule,S.,Novoa-Carballal,R., Riguera, R., ... Dalkara, T. Systemically administered brain-targeted nanoparticles transport peptides across the blood-brain barrier and provide neuroprotection. *Journal of Cerebral Blood Flow and Metabolism*, **2015**, *35*(3), 469–475. Available from https:// doi.org/10.1038/ jcbfm.2014.220

[39] Tang, J., Zhang, Y., Yang, L.M., Chen, Q.W., Tan, L., Zuo, S.L., ... Zhu, G. Exposure to 900 MHz electromagnetic fields activates the mkp-1/ERK pathway and causes blood-brain barrier damage and cognitive impairment in rats. *Brain Research*, **2015**, *1601*, 92–101. Available from https://doi.org/10.1016/j. brainres.2015.01.019.

[40] Pardridge, W.M. A morphological approach to the analysis of blood-brain barrier transport function. *Brain Barrier Systems*, **1999**, *45*, 19–42

[41] Denora, N., Trapani, A., Laquintana, V., Lopedota, A., & Trapani, G. (2009). Recent advances in medicinal chemistry and pharmaceutical technology-strategies for drug delivery to the brain. *Current Topics in Medicinal Chemistry*, **2009**, *9*(2), 182–196.

[42] Kabanov, A.V., Batrakova, E.V., & Miller, D.W. Pluronic((R)) block copolymers as modulators of drug efflux transporter activity in the blood-brain barrier. *Advanced Drug Delivery Reviews*, **2003**, *55*(1), 151–164. Available from https://doi.org/10.1016/S0169-409x(02)00176-X.

[43] Laquintana, V., Trapani, A., Denora, N., Wang, F., Gallo, J.M., & Trapani, G. New strategies to deliver anticancer drugs to brain tumors. *Expert Opinion on Drug Delivery*, **2009**, *6*(10), 1017–1032. Available from https:// doi.org/10.1517/17425240903167942.

[44] Litman, T., Brangi, M., Hudson, E., Fetsch, P., Abati, A., Ross, D.D., ... Bates, S.E. The multidrug-resistant phenotype associated with overexpression of the new ABC half-transporter, MXR (ABCG2). *Journal of Cell Science*, **2000**, *113*(11), 2011–2021.

[45] Malmo, J., Sandvig, A., Varum, K.M., & Strand, S.P. Nanoparticle mediated P-glycoprotein silencing for improved drug delivery across the blood-brain barrier: A siRNA-chitosan approach. *PLoS One*, **2013**, *8*(1). Available from https://doi.org/10.1371/journal.pone.0054182, ARTN e54182.

[46] Moghimi, S.M., Hunter, A.C., & Murray, J.C. Long-circulating and target-specific nanoparticles: Theory to practice. *Pharmacological Reviews*, **2001**, *53*(2), 283–318

[47] Karatas, H., Aktas, Y., Gursoy-Ozdemir, Y., Bodur, E., Yemisci, M., Caban, S., ... Dalkara, T. A nanomedicine transports a peptide caspase-3 inhibitor across the blood-brain barrier and provides neuroprotection.

Journal of Neuroscience, **2009**, *29*(44), 13761–13769. Available from https://doi.org/10.1523/Jneurosci.4246- 09.2009.

[48] Rai, M., Ingle, A.P., Gupta, I., & Brandelli, A. (2015). Bioactivity of noble metal nanoparticles decorated with biopolymers and their application in drug delivery. *International Journal of Pharmaceutics*, **2015**, *496*(2), 159–172. Available from https://doi.org/10.1016/j.ijpharm.2015.10.059.

[49] Gao, X. H., Qian, J., Zheng, S.Y., Changyi, Y.Z., Zhang, J.P., Ju, S.H., ... Li, C. Overcoming the blood-brain barrier for delivering drugs into the brain by using adenosine receptor nanoagonist. *ACS Nano*, **2014**, *8*(4), 3678–3689. Available from https://doi.org/10.1021/nn5003375.

[50] Wiley, D.T., Webster, P., Gale, A., & Davis, M.E. Transcytosis and brain uptake of transferrin containing nanoparticles by tuning avidity to transferrin receptor. *Proceedings of the National Academy of Sciences of the United States of America*, **2013**, *110*(21), 8662–8667. Available from https://doi.org/10.1073/ pnas.1307152110.

[51] Kong, S.D., Lee, J., Ramachandran, S., Eliceiri, B.P., Shubayev, V.I., Lal, R., & Jin, S. Magnetic targeting of nanoparticles across the intact blood-brain barrier. *Journal of Controlled Release*, **2012**, *164*(1), 49–57. Available from https://doi.org/10.1016/j.jconrel.2012.09.021.

[52] Koffie, R.M., Farrar, C.T., Saidi, L.J., William, C.M., Hyman, B.T., & Spires-Jones, T.L. Nanoparticles enhance brain delivery of blood-brain barrier-impermeable probes for *in vivo* optical and magnetic resonance imaging. *Proceedings of the National Academy of Sciences of the United States of America*, **2011**, *108*(46), 18837–18842. Available from https://doi.org/10.1073/pnas.1111405108.

[53] Song, Q. X., Huang, M., Yao, L., Wang, X.L., Gu, X., Chen, J., ... Gao, X.L. Lipoprotein-based nanoparticles rescue the memory loss of mice with Alzheimer's disease by accelerating the clearance of amyloid-beta. *Acs Nano*, **2014**, *8*(3), 2345–2359. Available from https://doi.org/10.1021/nn4058215.

[54] Hanada, S., Fujioka, K., Inoue, Y., Kanaya, F., Manome, Y., & Yamamoto, K. Cell-based *in vitro* blood-brain barrier model can rapidly evaluate nanoparticles' brain permeability in association with particle size and surface modification. *International Journal of Molecular Sciences*, **2014**, *15*(2), 1812–1825. Available from https://doi. org/10.3390/ijms15021812.

[55] Sonavane, G., Tomoda, K., & Makino, K. Biodistribution of colloidal gold nanoparticles after intravenous administration: Effect of particle size. *Colloids and Surfaces B-Biointerfaces*, **2008**, *66*(2), 274–280. Available from https://doi.org/10.1016/j.colsurfb.2008.07.004.

[56] Decuzzi, P., Godin, B., Tanaka, T., Lee, S.Y., Chiappini, C., Liu, X., & Ferrari, M. Size and shape effects in the biodistribution of intravascularly injected particles. *Journal of Controlled Release*, **2010**, *141*(3), 320–327. Available from https://doi.org/10.1016/j.jconrel.2009.10.014.

[57] Kolhar, P., Anselmo, A.C., Gupta, V., Pant, K., Prabhakarpandian, B., Ruoslahti, E., & Mitragotri, S. Using shape effects to target antibody-coated nanoparticles to lung and brain endothelium. *Proceedings of the National Academy of Sciences of the United States of America*, **2013**, *110*(26), 10753–10758. Available from https://doi.org/ 10.1073/pnas.1308345110.

[58] Bramini, M., Ye, D., Hallerbach, A., Raghnaill, M.N., Salvati, A., Aberg, C., & Dawson, K.A. Imaging approach to mechanistic study of nanoparticle interactions with the blood-brain barrier. *Acs Nano*, **2014**, *8*(5), 4304–4312. Available from https://doi.org/10.1021/nn5018523.

[59] Huang, X.L., Li, L.L., Liu, T.L., Hao, N.J., Liu, H.Y., Chen, D., & Tang, F.Q. The shape effect of mesoporous silica nanoparticles on biodistribution, clearance, and biocompatibility *in vivo*. *ACS Nano*, **2011**, *5*(7), 5390–5399. Available from https://doi.org/10.1021/nn200365a.

[60] Fathi, S., & Oyelere, A.K. Liposomal drug delivery systems for targeted cancer therapy: Is active targeting the best choice? *Future Medicinal Chemistry*, **2011**, *8*(17), 2091–2112. Available from https://doi.org/10.4155/fmc-2016-0135

[61] Vogg, A.T.J., Doczi, R., Szigeti, K., Horvath, I., Mathe, D., Roller, M., ... Varga, Z. Targeted liposomal drug delivery system for radionucleosides- a theranostic approach. *European Journal of Nuclear Medicine and Molecular Imaging*, **2016**, *43*, S468, S468.

[62] Craparo, E.F., Bondi, M.L., Pitarresi, G., & Cavallaro, G. Nanoparticulate systems for drug delivery and targeting to the central nervous system. *CNS Neuroscience & Therapeutics*, **2011**, *17*(6), 670–677. Available from https://doi.org/10.1111/j.1755-5949.2010.00199.x

[63] Kumari, A., Yadav, S.K., & Yadav, S.C. Biodegradable polymeric nanoparticles based drug delivery systems. *Colloids and Surfaces B-Biointerfaces*, **2010**, *75*(1), 1–18. Available from https://doi.org/10.1016/j. colsurfb.2009.09.001.

[64] Martins, S., Tho, I., Reimold, I., Fricker, G., Souto, E., Ferreira, D., & Brandl, M. Brain delivery of camptothecin by means of solid lipid nanoparticles: Formulation design, *in vitro* and *in vivo* studies. *International Journal of Pharmaceutics*, **2012**, *439*(1-2), 49–62. Available from https://doi.org/10.1016/j.ijpharm.2012.09.054

[65] Yusuf, M., Khan, M., Khan, R.A., & Ahmed, B. Preparation, characterization, *in vivo* and biochemical evaluation of brain targeted Piperine

solid lipid nanoparticles in an experimentally induced Alzheimer's disease model. *Journal of Drug Targeting*, **2013**, *21*(3), 300–311. Available from https://doi.org/10.3109/ 1061186x.2012.747529.

[66] Venishetty, V.K., Komuravelli, R., Kuncha, M., Sistla, R., & Diwan, P.V. Increased brain uptake of docetaxel and ketoconazole loaded folate-grafted solid lipid nanoparticles. *Nanomedicine-Nanotechnology Biology and Medicine*, **2013**, *9*(1), 111–121. Available from https://doi.org/10.1016/j.nano.2012.03.003.

[67] Jin, J., Bae, K.H., Yang, H., Lee, S.J., Kim, H., Kim, Y., ... Nam, D.H. *In vivo* specific delivery of c-Met siRNA to glioblastoma using cationic solid lipid nanoparticles. *Bioconjugate Chemistry*, **2011**, *22*(12), 2568–2572. Available from https://doi.org/10.1021/bc200406n.

[68] Kakkar, V., & Kaur, I.P. Evaluating potential of curcumin loaded solid lipid nanoparticles in aluminium induced behavioural, biochemical and histopathological alterations in mice brain. *Food and Chemical Toxicology*, **2011**, *49*(11), 2906–2913. Available from https://doi.org/10.1016/j.fct.2011.08.006

[69] Dhawan, S., Kapil, R., & Singh, B. Formulation development and systematic optimization of solid lipid nanoparticles of quercetin for improved brain delivery. *Journal of Pharmacy and Pharmacology*, **2011**, *63*(3), 342–351.Availablefromhttps://doi.org/10.1111/j.2042-7158.2010.01225.x

[70] Montenegro, L., Campisi, A., Sarpietro, M.G., Carbone, C., Acquaviva, R., Raciti, G., & Puglisi, G. *In vitro* evaluation of idebenone-loaded solid lipid nanoparticles for drug delivery to the brain. *Drug Development and Industrial Pharmacy*, **2011**, *37*(6), 737–746. Available from https://doi.org/10.3109/03639045.2010.539231

[71] Hsu, S.H., Wen, C.J., Al-Suwayeh, S.A., Chang, H.W., Yen, T.C., & Fang, J.Y. Physicochemical characterization and *in vivo* bioluminescence imaging of nanostructured lipid carriers for targeting the brain: Apomorphine as a model drug (vol 21, 405101, 2010). *Nanotechnology*, **2010**, *21*(49). Available from https://doi.org/ 10.1088/0957-4484/21/49/499802, Artn 499802.

[72] Patel, S., Chavhan, S., Soni, H., Babbar, A.K., Mathur, R., Mishra, A.K., & Sawant, K. Brain targeting of risperidone-loaded solid lipid nanoparticles by intranasal route. *Journal of Drug Targeting*, **2011**, *19*(6), 468–474. Available from https://doi.org/10.3109/1061186x.2010.523787.

[73] Gupta, Y., Jain, A., & Jain, S.K. Transferrin-conjugated solid lipid nanoparticles for enhanced delivery of quinine dihydrochloride to the brain. *Journal of Pharmacy and Pharmacology*, **2007**, *59*(7), 935–940. Available from https://doi.org/10.1211/jpp.59.7.0004.

[74] Souto, E.B. An overview on the design, development, characterization and applications of novel nanomedicines for brain targeting. *Current Nanoscience*, **2011**, *7*(1).

[75] Gromnicova, R., Davies, H.A., Sreekanthreddy, P., Romero, I.A., Lund, T., Roitt, I.M., ... Male, D.K. (2013). Glucose-coated gold nanoparticles transfer across human brain endothelium and enter astrocytes *in vitro*. PLoS One, 8(12). Available from https://doi.org/10.1371/journal.pone.0081043, ARTN e81043.

[76] Guerrero, S., Araya, E., Fiedler, J. L., Arias, J.I., Adura, C., Albericio, F., ... Kogan, M. J. Improving the brain delivery of gold nanoparticles by conjugation with an amphipathic peptide. *Nanomedicine*, **2010**, *5*(6), 897–913. Available from https://doi.org/10.2217/Nnm.10.74.

[77] Li, S.D., & Huang, L. Nanoparticles evading the reticuloendothelial system: Role of the supported bilayer. *Biochimica Et Biophysica Acta-Biomembranes*, **2009**, *1788*(10), 2259–2266. Available from https://doi.org/10.1016/j. bbamem.2009.06.022.

[78] Lee, S.Y., Ferrari, M., & Decuzzi, P. Shaping nano-/micro-particles for enhanced vascular interaction in laminar flows. *Nanotechnology*, **2009**, *20*(49). Available from https://doi.org/10.1088/0957-4484/20/49/495101, Artn 495101.

[79] Nance, E.A., Woodworth, G.F., Sailor, K.A., Shih, T.Y., Xu, Q.G., Swaminathan, G., ... Hanes, J. A dense poly(ethylene glycol) coating improves penetration of large polymeric nanoparticles within brain tissue. *Science Translational Medicine*, **2012**, *4*(149). Available from https://doi.org/10.1126/scitranslmed.3003594, ARTN 149ra119.

[80] Brambilla, D., Le Droumaguet, B., Nicolas, J., Hashemi, S.H., Wu, L.P., Moghimi, S.M., & Andrieux, K. Nanotechnologies for Alzheimer's disease: Diagnosis, therapy, and safety issues. *Nanomedicine*, **2011**, *7*(5), 521–540. Available from https://doi.org/10.1016/j.nano.2011.03.008.

[81] Crismon, M.L. Tacrine: First drug approved for Alzheimer's disease. *Annals of Pharmacotherapy*, **1994**, *28*(6), 744–751. Available from https://doi.org/10.1177/10600280940280061.2.

[82] Wilson, B., Samanta, M.K., Santhi, K., Kumar, K.P.S., Paramakrishnan, N., & Suresh, B. Poly(n-butylcyanoacrylate) nanoparticles coated with polysorbate 80 for the targeted delivery of rivastigmine into the brain to treat Alzheimer's disease. *Brain Research*, **2008**, *1200*, 159–168. Available from https://doi.org/10.1016/j. brainres.2008.01.039.

[83] Lockhart, I.A., Mitchell, S.A., & Kelly, S. Safety and tolerability of donepezil, rivastigmine and galantamine for patients with Alzheimer's disease: Systematic review of the 'real-world' evidence. *Dementia and*

Geriatric Cognitive Disorders, **2009**, *28*(5), 389–403. Available from https://doi.org/10.1159/000255578.

[84] Wavikar, P.R., & Vavia, P.R. Rivastigmine-loaded in situ gelling nano-structured lipid carriers for nose to brain delivery. *Journal of Liposome Research*, **2015**, *25*(2), 141–149. Available from https://doi.org/10.3109/08982104.2014.954129.

[85] Beitz, J.M. Parkinson's disease: A review. *In Schol (Ed.), Front Bioscience*, **2014**, *6*, 65–74.

[86] Serra, P.A., Esposito, G., Enrico, P., Mura, M.A., Migheli, R., Delogu, M.R., ... Miele, E. Manganese increases L-DOPA auto-oxidation in the striatum of the freely moving rat: Potential implications to L-DOPA long-term therapy of Parkinson's disease. *British Journal of Pharmacology*, **2000**, *130*(4), 937–945. Available from https://doi.org/10.1038/sj.bjp.0703379.

[87] Cortesi, R., Esposito, E., Drechsler, M., Pavoni, G., Cacciatore, I., Sguizzato, M., & Di Stefano, A. L-dopa co-drugs in nanostructured lipid carriers: A comparative study. *Materials Science and Engineering: C*, **2017**, *72*, 168–176. Available from https://doi.org/10.1016/j.msec.2016.11.060.

[88] Hawthorne, G.H., Bernuci, M.P., Bortolanza, M., Tumas, V., Issy, A.C., & Del-Bel, E. Nanomedicine to overcome current Parkinson's treatment liabilities: A systematic review. *Neurotoxicity Research*, **2016**, *30*(4), 715–729. Available from https://doi.org/10.1007/s12640-016-9663-z

[89] André, E.M., Passirani, C., Seijo, B., Sanchez, A., & Montero-Menei, C.N. Nano and microcarriers to improve stem cell behaviour for neuroregenerative medicine strategies: Application to Huntington's disease. *Biomaterials*, **2016**, *83*, 347–362. Available from https://doi.org/10.1016/j.biomaterials.2015.12.008.

[90] Andrew, S.E., Paul Goldberg, Y., Kremer, B., Telenius, H., Theilmann, J., Adam, S., ... Hayden, M.R. The relationship between trinucleotide (CAG) repeat length and clinical features of Huntington's disease. *Nat Genet*, **1993**, *4*(4), 398–403.

[91] Dayalu, P., & Albin, R.L. Huntington disease: Pathogenesis and treatment. *Neurologic Clinics*, **2015**, *33*(1), 101–114. Available from https://doi.org/10.1016/j.ncl.2014.09.003.

[92] Armstrong, M.J., & Miyasaki, J.M. Evidence-based guideline: Pharmacologic treatment of chorea in Huntington disease: Report of the Guideline Development Subcommittee of the American Academy of Neurology. *Neurology*, **2012**, *79*(6), 597–603. Available from https://doi.org/10.1212/WNL.0b013e318263c443.

[93] Zuccato, C., & Cattaneo, E. Brain-derived neurotrophic factor in neurodegenerative diseases. *Nature Reviews Neurology*, **2009**, *5*(6), 311–322

[94] Compston, A., & Coles, A. Multiple sclerosis. *Lancet*, **2008**, *372*, 1502–1517

[95] Tischner, D., & Reichardt, H.M. Glucocorticoids in the control of neuroinflammation. *Mol Cell Endocrinol*, **2007**, *275*(1-2), 62–70. Available from https://doi.org/10.1016/j.mce.2007.03.007.

[96] Schmidt, J., Metselaar, J.M., Wauben, M.H.M., Toyka, K.V., Storm, G., & Gold, R. Drug targeting by long-circulating liposomal glucocortico-steroids increases therapeutic efficacy in a model of multiple sclerosis. *Brain*, **2003**, *126*, 1895–1904.

[97] Linker, R.A., Weller, C., Luhder, A., Mohr, A., Schmidt, J., Knauth, M., ... Cold, R. Liposomal glucocorticosteroids in treatment of chronic auto-immune demyelination: Long-term protective effects and enhanced efficacy of methylprednisolone formulations. *Experimental Neurology*, **2008**, *211*, 397–406.

[98] Ferrante, R.J., Browne, S.E., Shinobu, L.A., Bowling, A.C., Baik, M.J., MacGarvey, U., ... Beal, M.F. Evidence of increased oxidative damage in both sporadic and familial amyotrophic lateral sclerosis. *Journal of Neurochemistry*, **1997**, *69*, 2064–2074.

[99] Kizelsztein, P., Ovadia, H., Garbuzenko, O., Sigal, A., & Barenholz, Y. Pegylated nanoliposomes remote-loaded with the antioxidant tem-pamine ameliorate experimental autoimmune encephalomyelitis. *Journal of Neurochemistry*, **2009**, *213*, 20–25.

[100] Turjeman, K., Bavli, Y., Kizelsztein, P., Schilt, Y., Allon, N., Katzir, T.B., ... Barenholz, Y. Nano-drugs based on nano sterically stabilized liposomes for the treatment of inflammatory neurodegen-erative diseases. *PLoS One*, **2015**, *10*(7), e0130442. Available from https://doi.org/10.1371/journal.pone.0130442.

[101] Heckman, K.L., DeCoteau, W., Estevez, A., Reed, K.J., Costanzo, W., Sanford, D., ... Erlichman, J.S. Custom cerium oxide nanoparticles protect against a free radical mediated autoimmune degenerative dis-ease in the brain. *ACS Nano*, **2013**, *7*(12), 10582–10596. Available from https://doi.org/10.1021/nn403743b.

[102] Severino, P., Szymanski, M., Favaro, M., Azzoni, A.R., Chaud, M.V., Santana, M.H.A., ... Souto, E.B. Development and characterization of a cationic lipid nanocarrier as non-viral vector for gene therapy. *European Journal of Pharmaceutical Sciences*, **2015**, *66*, 78–82. Available from https://doi.org/10.1016/j. ejps.2014.09.021.

[103] Lemos, H., Huang, L., Chandler, P.R., Mohamed, E., Souza, G.R., Li, L., ... Mellor, A.L. Activation of the STING adaptor attenuates experimental autoimmune encephalitis. *Journal of Immunology*, **2014**, *192*(12), 5571–5578. Available from https://doi.org/10.4049/jimmunol.1303258.

[104] Vijayanathan, V., Thomas, T., & Thomas, T.J. DNA nanoparticles and development of DNA delivery vehicles for gene therapy. *Biochemistry*, **2002**, *41*(48), 14085–14094

8

Challenges and Intellectual Property Rights Prospects Particular to Nanotechnology in Treating Brain Tumors

Abstract

The blood–brain barrier or BBB serves as a protective barrier and is essential for preserving the brain's delicate equilibrium, allowing only a limited number of molecules to pass through. Brain tumors are the second most common kind of tumor of the central nervous system and the second largest cause of cancer-related mortality. Finding effective therapies for brain cancers has proven to be difficult due to the BBB's poor permeability and its selective response to traditional anticancer medications. In the past two decades, innovative delivery strategies, such as nanotechnology-mediated targeted delivery systems, have emerged, offering hope for progress against brain cancer. This synopsis highlights some of the issues associated with employing nanotechnology-based brain-tumor-targeted delivery, along with safety concerns raised regarding this approach. Additionally, we explore the development of a patented nanomedicine specifically designed to treat aggressive brain cancers.

8.1 Introduction

According to the World Health Organization (WHO), cancer claimed the lives of 8.8 million people in 2015 [1]. Primary tumors of the brain and other malignancies of the central nervous system (CNS) are quite common, affecting individuals of all ages and accounting for 85%–90% of all CNS tumor diagnoses [2]. Among children and young adults (aged 0–19), the most prevalent solid tumor and the main reason for cancer-related fatalities in this age range is brain cancer [3, 4]. Furthermore, according to figures from 2016 [3, 4], brain tumors are the second leading cause of cancer-related death in those under the age of 39. According to their morphology, cytogenetics, molecular genetics, and immunologic markers, different kinds of brain cancer are categorized by the WHO [2]. The malignancy level of brain tumors is determined by their histology and rate of development, which can be slow or rapid [5]. The WHO's 2016 classification and grading system for brain tumors are summarized in Table 8.1 [6]. According to the American Cancer Society, in 2017, it was estimated that there would be almost 23,000 new instances of brain tumors and other nervous system malignancies in the United States, resulting in 16,700 fatalities. Glioblastoma is the most prevalent type of brain tumor and has a bad prognosis [3, 7]. The most frequent kinds of brain tumors are glioblastomas or anaplastic astrocytomas, which make up around 38% of all cases [2, 8, 9]. The second most frequent kind of brain cancer, meningiomas, and associated mesenchymal tumors account for 27% of all brain malignancies [2]. Fourth-grade astrocytoma, sometimes referred to as glioblastoma multiforme (GBM), is a highly vascularized, necrosis-prone, and mitotically active tumor [7]. Ionizing radiation, the Epstein–Barr virus, and the human immunodeficiency virus (HIV), among others, are the causes of brain tumors [2, 10–12]. Additionally, there is mounting proof that using a cell phone, being around radio waves, and being around electromagnetic fields (EMFs) all increase the chance of developing brain cancer [13–15].

Having asthma and other allergic reactions like hay fever, dermatitis, and food allergies was inversely correlated with the risk of getting brain cancer [16, 17]. Brain cancer incidence has been linked to the workplace and environmental dangers, albeit the precise mechanism by which this happens is not entirely understood [18]. The symptoms and warning signs depend greatly on the type of tumor and the location of the lesions inside the brain. The most frequent intracranial brain tumor is meningioma, which arises from the dura mater; the most frequent CNS intraparenchymal tumor is symptomatic GBM [19, 20]. Headache, nausea, convulsions, anorexia, vomiting, a loss of focus, mood swings, and loss of appetite are all common signs of a brain tumor [2, 19]. However, it is not always the case that a lesion in the frontal lobe will lead to mood changes, that a lesion in the temporal lobe will lead to aphasia, or that a lesion in the cerebellum will lead to ataxia and walking issues [19]. For medications to reach tumor cells in the brain, they must first be able to pass through the body's protective barrier against foreign substances known as BBB [21]. Systems for delivering drugs using nanotechnology utilize nanoscale components and technologies for therapeutic and biological purposes [22–24]. Nanotechnology-based drugs can pass the blood–brain barrier (BBB) and interact with cells and tissues at the subcellular level. To find the best nanotechnology delivery systems, scientists

Table 8.1 WHO tumor grading system.

WHO level	Conditions
I	The tumor cell resembles normal cells and has a low capacity for reproduction.
	As compared to tumor cells of grades II, III, and IV, this one grows at a more leisurely pace.
	Surgical excision alone may be effective in curing the disease.
II	Increased proliferative potential and decreased mitotic activity compared to grade I tumor cells.
	The growth and spreading rates of tumor cells in grades III and IV are lower.
	It is more likely that grade II or III tumor cells will persist following surgery and grow again.
III	Tumor cells differ greatly in appearance from healthy cells and have a stronger proliferation capacity than those of grades I and II.
	Remarkable alterations in histopathology, including an uptick in mitotic activity and a strong tendency toward metastasis.
	Took severe adjuvant chemotherapy.
IV	Tumor cells have a strong capacity for further division, leading to disease progression and death after surgery.
	Cancer cells divide rapidly and die easily.
	Although vigorous adjuvant chemotherapy cannot cure grade IV cancers, it can significantly enhance the standard of living for a patient.

have long studied liposomes, dendrimers, solid lipid nanoparticles, and polymeric nanoparticles [25–29]. Following systemic (intravenous) therapy, the drugs can be administered to the brain tumor with minimal systemic side effects [21]. For effective medication administration due to the intricacy of brain tumors, a multidisciplinary team with experience in physiology, pharmacology, cell biology, engineering, chemistry, and medicine is required [30]. The blood–brain barrier is explored along with contemporary nanotechnologies for medicine delivery to brain malignancies.

8.2 Obstacles in Delivering Drugs to the Brain

At any given year, almost 1.5 billion people worldwide are affected by a disorder of the CNS [31]. Researchers face a significant obstacle in their pursuit of a solution to the expanding demand for safe and effective treatments:

the blood–brain barrier's inherent permeability. Since the population as a whole is becoming older, it is only natural that the number of persons suffering from CNS problems will rise as well. The number of people suffering from conditions affecting the CNS is expected to rise to almost 1.9 billion by 2020 if viable treatments are not developed quickly enough to fulfill the need [32]. Medications have a difficult time crossing the BBB and reaching their destination within the brain because of enzymes that break them down. Homeostasis in the brain depends on the selective admission of molecules, including drugs, via the blood–brain barrier and enzymes like those that break down drugs [33]. Because of protective barriers of BBB such as a biochemical and anatomical barrier, toxic substances cannot reach the brain. When compared to the microvasculature found in the rest of the body, the endothelial cells lining brain capillaries make much tighter connections with one another, are closely connected, have modest fenestrations, and are stuffed with pinocytic vesicles. Hydrophilic chemicals and macromolecules cannot enter the brain through TJ, also known as zonulae occlude. Tight junctions form a junctional complex, comprising proteins like claudins and occludins junctional adhesion molecules that keep the endothelial-cell junction stable [34–36]. The BBB is strengthened even further by the presence of astrocyte foot processes surrounding the endothelial cells. Because of the high likelihood of therapy failure for CNS diseases like brain tumors, Alzheimer's, Parkinson's, and mood disorders, researchers are trying to discover new and improved techniques for brain drug delivery. About 1% of the world's pharmaceutical corporations are currently investing in brain medication delivery programs, despite the urgent need for better treatment of brain-related illnesses [37]. Researchers can learn how to avoid the failure of effective brain drug delivery by studying the physiology of the BBB under normal/disease conditions and the nature of the numerous transport receptors at the BBB. Several mechanisms contribute to BBB breach and subsequent brain penetration [38]. The molecule's mass, the existence of functional groups, the presence of charged residues, lipophilicity, and enzymatic breakdown of a drug are all variables in its ability to cross the BBB [39, 40]. Catabolic enzymes in brain tissue render the medication inert, despite its entry into the brain and therapeutic availability [41, 42]. Another major obstacle to efficient medicine delivery in the brain is drug resistance [43]. Transport through the blood–brain barrier and subsequent access to brain targets depends on lipophilicity. Nonetheless, the BBB permeability of numerous lipophilic medicines has been substantially lower than expected [44]. Drug efflux transporters and the MDR1 and MDR2 families of proteins in the BBB have a high binding affinity for these medications [45–47]. High-lipophilicity anticancer medicines have a dismal track record of success in treating primary and metastatic brain cancers. These medications are less likely to be effective because they have a strong affinity for binding to multidrug ABC transporters including P-gp and MRP (Table 8.2) [48–51].

8.3 Perils of the Blood–Brain Barrier and Blood–Brain Tumor Barrier

The blood–brain barrier (BBB) tightly regulates the passage of substances into the brain, allowing only extremely small chemicals to cross its tight connections between epithelial cells and reach the brain tissue below. While the BBB is crucial for protecting the central nervous system (CNS) from damage, infection, and toxicity, its restrictive nature poses challenges in treating glioblastoma. The BBB is composed of brain microvascular endothelial cells (BMECs), along with other cellular and molecular components such as pericytes, astrocytes, the basement membrane, and chemokines that contribute to its structure and function [52]. Molecular components like efficient transporters and nutrient transporters play a role in regulating the influx and efflux through the BBB [53]. Tight junction formation and efflux transporters, including P-glycoprotein, help maintain the BBB and transport nutrients to the brain [54]. However, these same transporters can also pump potential therapies out of the CNS, making drug delivery challenging [55]. Pericytes surrounding BMECs contribute to BBB development and the polarization of astrocyte end feet through gene expression [56]. Astrocytes also sheathe the capillaries with their apical processes, assisting in maintaining the BBB by secreting various substances [57, 58]. The BBB plays a vital role in controlling and safeguarding the CNS.

Blood–brain tumor barriers (BBTBs), which gliomas can create, allow oxygen and nutrients to enter the developing tumor cells. Vascular endothelial growth factor (VEGF), which is generated in hypoxic areas of brain tumors, promotes capillary expansion and the development of the BBTB. The BBTB poses an additional barrier to delivering therapeutic drugs to brain tumors, as it expresses efflux transporters similar to the BBB [59]. BBTB permeability is influenced by both the population's kind of microvessels and their geographic distribution. Microvessels can be categorized into those with continuous fenestrations, those without, and those with interendothelial gaps, and the size of molecules that can pass through these microvessels varies [60]. The BBTB has notable differences compared to the BBB as it consists of aberrant capillaries rather than normal cells, presenting an opportunity, without altering the BBB, to target the BBTB [61]. Studies on drug transport

Table 8.2   Brain-expressed drug transporter associated with drug-resistance in brain tumors.

S. no.	Transporter	Summary	A drug used to treat cancer
1.	P-gp (MDR1; ABCB1)	A classic example of a multidrug-resistant transporter in cancer cells, which requires both energy and Na1 for its function. The ABCB1 gene, often known as MDR1, regulates P-glycoprotein expression (multidrug resistance 1).	Epirubicin, Etoposide, Idarubicin, Methotrexate, Mitoxantrone, Paclitaxel, Doxorubicin, and Daunorubicin
2.	MRP1 (ABCC1)	The human MRP1 protein is encoded by the ABCC1 gene. This is especially true for neuroblastoma, where the ABCC1 transporter protein is highly expressed.	Vinblastine, Vincristine, Vinblastine, Doxorubicin, Epirubicin, Etoposide, Melphalan, and Methotrexate
3.	MRP2 (ABCC2)	The ABCC2 gene, humans have a protein called canalicular multispecific organic anion transporter 1 (cMOAT), also known as multidrug resistance-associated protein 2 (MRP2).	Epirubicin, Etoposide, Flavopiridol, Methotrexate, Cisplatin, Doxorubicin, and Vincristine
4.	MRP3 (ABCC3)	The human ABCC3 gene codes for the ATP-binding cassette (ABC) transporter superfamily member known as multidrug resistance-associated protein 3 (MRP3).	Methotrexate, Teniposide, and Etoposide
5.	MRP4 (ABCC4)	MRP4 is a protein that is encoded by the ABCC4 gene in humans and has been associated with multidrug resistance.	6-Mercaptopurine, thioguanine, topotecan, and methotrexate
6.	MRP5 (ABCC5)	The human gene ABCC5 produces the protein 5 linked with multidrug resistance.	Thioguanine with 6-mercaptopurine
7.	MRP6 (ABCC6)	Multidrug resistance-associated protein 6 (MRP6), also known as multispecific organic anion transporter E, is a protein that is encoded for by the ABCC6 gene in humans.	Actinomycin D, Cisplatin, Daunorubicin, and Doxorubicin
8.	BCRP (ABCG2)	Second, the ATP-binding cassette transporter superfamily member big breast cancer resistance protein (BCRP) supports cell health (ABCG2). In humans, the ABCG2 gene controls its synthesis.	Methotrexate, Mitoxantrone, Topotecan, Bisantrene, and Irinotecan

across the BBB and BBTB, along with local intracranial trials, have yielded therapeutically effective levels of active medicines.

8.4 Overcoming BBB's Obstacles

8.4.1 Convection-enhanced delivery (CED)

Intracranial catheters have been employed to perform convection-enhanced delivery (CED), a technique that involves the local injection of fluid under positive pressure in an attempt to bypass the blood–brain barrier (BBB). CED was initially developed in 1994 by Bobo et al. [62], and it has subsequently been used to successfully deliver pharmaceutical molecules for ailments as diverse as AD, PD, and GB [63]. Several factors, such as the molecular weight of the molecule, the size of the tumor, the pace of infusion, the size and form of the cannula, and the volume of the infused fluid, can affect the administration and distribution of a solute through CED [64]. Insufficient medication administration has been reported by several CED patients, such as drug leakage into the subarachnoid space as a result of abnormal tumor vasculature, edema, air bubbles, and backflow [64]. Using CED, researchers were able to successfully deliver a medication several centimeters away from the injection site in a study with animals [62]. Drug delivery may and has been optimized further through the use of computational models and algorithms, the creation of redesigned catheters, the careful consideration of target tissue anatomy, and the implementation of new delivery techniques [65]. Several clinical experiments have investigated the viability and effectiveness of CED, with mixed outcomes [63]. In the PRECISE study, patients with recurrent GB were randomized to receive Gliadel® (a carmustine wafer) or CED of IL13-PE38QQR. A recombinant Pseudomonas exotoxin called IL13-PE38QQR targets the interleukin-13 receptor, which is highly expressed in GB. Those who received Gliadel® treatment outlived those who received CED of IL13-PE38QQR considerably more often [63]. The poor efficacy results were attributed to inadequate medication distribution as a result of catheter implantation [66, 67]. Patients with recurrent GB were studied by Lidar et al., who assessed CED-administered paclitaxel's clinical efficacy, neuroimaging analysis of distribution, and safety [68]. Some sort of anticancer reaction was seen with the CED of paclitaxel, but the treatment was linked with several adverse events. These included chemo- and infection-related side effects, as well as temporary neurologic impairment from increased peritumoral edema. Similar to this, Young et al. [69] present canine experimental glioma with polymeric magnetite nanoparticles containing temozolomide as a CED. Using magnetic resonance imaging (MRI), researchers were able to determine that only 70% of patients were effectively reached with the infusion, even when the catheters were placed in the most advantageous locations. Only 1 out of 10 mice showed a discernible decline in tumor volume. Zhang et al. [70] took use of the special diffusion properties of nanoparticles by using CED to transport cisplatin-loaded brain-penetrating nanoparticles. PEGylating the brain-penetrating particles improved their ability to penetrate and spread throughout the brain. Brain tumor growth was suppressed and median survival was significantly improved when cisplatin nanoparticles were administered though treatment with CED was more effective than with saline-treated controls, un-PEGylated cisplatin particles, and cisplatin alone. Although cisplatin and CED were given to all treatment groups, there was a considerable increase in survival in the PEGylated nanoparticle cisplatin delivery group, with 80% long-term survivors. Carboplatin's safety in treating GB has been studied in both human and animal research, and the results have been promising. Intracranial distribution of carboplatin in both rodent and pig brains was promising, and the drug was confirmed to remain in the brain after 24 hours after administration through CED in a rat model of GB [71]. Based on these findings, a Phase I study of carboplatin dosage escalation through CED for patients with recurrent GB was designed and conducted [72]. Due to its non-specific cytotoxicity and quick clearance from the brain after administration, encapsulation was developed as a means of administering carboplatin. Arshad et al. [73] developed an injectable form of carboplatin nanoparticles by coating them in a poly-lactic acid-glycolic acid copolymer (PLGA). Neuronal toxicity, distribution, and clearance were all found to increase after CED administration in rat and pig studies and cytotoxicity was confirmed in GB cell cultures. Carboplatin-encased liposomes were administered to GB animal models by Shi et al. [74] via CED, and they found conflicting outcomes. Evidenced by the fact that the treatment that performed best in actual patients was the one that had the worst track record in the lab, it is clear that the selection and use of proper animal models are crucial to this type of translational research. Additionally, despite general safety concerns [75–77], CED has been studied in preclinical models of GB for the administration of chemotherapeutic drugs via liposomes. Further research is needed to confirm that active and bioavailable compounds diffuse more readily at therapeutic concentrations, to modify or encapsulate the drug of choice, to select suitable animal models, and to ensure local delivery. The Cleveland Multiport Catheter, which is now being studied [78], and similar devices that use transcutaneous bone anchors for recurrent CED infusions [79] have both been developed as part of research into these problems. To ensure tumor cytotoxicity with the necessary specificity, CEDs must be infused without reflux, using an efficient infusion schedule. This requires advanced catheter technology [80].

8.4.2 Gene therapy and virotherapy

Using the abnormality in gene therapy, the gene expression found in GB cancers is currently under study as a possible treatment. Viable strategies for gene therapy include viral gene delivery, nanotechnology, and stem cell therapy. If oncolytic, these medicines can also provide options in gene therapy including antiangiogenic medicines, immunostimulating cytokines, and genes that kill tumors or immune cells. Given that the HSV can contain the HSV-TK suicide gene, which prevents DNA replication in rapidly proliferating cells, it is common using viruses as targets for gene therapy. Cancer stems cell therapies are unique in that they can actively migrate to the tumor site and even cross the BBB to get there. Tumor burden can be lowered with the use of neural and mesenchymal stem cell therapies by introducing immunostimulatory cytokines. Inducing apoptosis through the tumor necrosis factor family (TRAIL) is an important step [81]. In cancer, the p53 pathway is aberrant, allowing tumors to escape repression, promote tumor growth, and invade healthy tissue. As previously mentioned [82], cell proliferation, apoptosis, invasion, and motility are all thought to be influenced by the PI3K-PTEN-Akt-mTOR pathway. As part of innovative combination therapy, Nandhu et al. [83] propose inhibiting tumor-derived fibrillin-3. Many factors, including uneven access to gene therapy in some areas, poor transfer efficiency, host immunity, and GB's inherent unpredictability, contribute to such wide variation in clinical outcomes [84]. Using local delivery mechanisms to help target and distribute genes to tumor cells may be one solution to these problems [85–87]. *In vitro* studies have shown promise for using the oncolytic virus TG6002 to treat GB. With its high rate of replication in tumor cells, TG6002 targets only those that lack thymidine kinase and ribonucleotide reductase. TG6002 enhances the effects of 5-flucytosine (5-FC) by converting it into the cytotoxic metabolites 5-FU and 5-FUMP. The preliminary evidence in favor of continuing with a Phase 1 clinical investigation is the longer life after therapy with TG6002 and 5-FC in mice with orthotopic GB [88]. Insight into the oncolytic virus's clinical safety and efficacy will be gained through this trial.

8.4.3 The carmustine wafer

Intracranial medicine delivery has been created as an alternate strategy to avoid systemic distribution and instead target the brain due to the difficulties involved with bridging both the blood–brain barrier (BBB) and the blood–brain tumor barrier (BBTB). It has been demonstrated that several different polymer formulations can successfully transport chemotherapy drugs to the site of tumor excision. Carmustine has been used systemically for GB patients for quite some time [89, 90], and the FDA has given it approval. To identify the ideal mixture for distributing carmustine, a wide range of polymers were initially tried. The least toxic material was a biodegradable bis(p-carboxy phenoxy) polymers Sebacic acid with propane copolymer toxicity profile and therefore the optimum formulation for distribution in an intracranial implantation investigation. Many studies using rodents and monkeys [91, 92] confirmed this finding. Biodistribution investigations of 12 N in rabbits use autoradiography. Three weeks after implantation [93], the polymer-released carmustine disseminated throughout the parenchyma at therapeutically relevant levels, whereas the carmustine solution injected intravenously was discovered within 72 hours; this was not the case. Yang et al. [90] used a rat model to determine that the drug concentration was 40-fold higher in the hemisphere with the implant than in the contralateral hemisphere or the peripheral circulation. What's more, the polymer implanted hemisphere showed 100% bioactive carmustine for as long as nine days, but the contralateral hemisphere and peripheral circulation showed 0% bioactivity. After the first day, carmustine was discovered 5 mm from the site of implantation in non-human primates [91], and on days 3–14, it was detected 1 mm from the implantation site. The carmustine-loaded wafer is both safe and effective in a rodent model of gliosarcoma [88, 92, 93]. A Phase I–II study evaluating three loading doses of carmustine (1.93%, 3.85%, and 6.35%) was carried out in 21 patients with recurrent malignant glioma based on the conclusions of these rigorous preclinical investigations [94]. Using a dose of 3.85% in a later placebo-controlled randomized study was shown to be a doable and safe way to test the novel hypothesis. There were 222 patients and 27 cm of tumor in this prospective, placebo-controlled, double-blind, randomized investigation of recurrent malignant glioma [95]. One to eight BCNU wafers were inserted into the void left by the removed tumor as soon as possible after surgery. Researchers found that carmustine wafers significantly increased survival time in research including 112 patients, with a median survival duration of 31 weeks, while it was only 9 weeks for those who received placebo wafers. Once initial research was conducted on those who had experienced a recurrence of glioma, studies on patients with freshly diagnosed GB were conducted. For patients given carmustine, the overall survival time was 13.4 months versus 9.2 months for those fed placebo wafers ($p = 0.012$) [96]. Also, at 12 months, the carmustine group had a far higher overall survival rate. The median survival time for patients who were treated for GB after a recent diagnosis was 13.9 months, while the median survival time for those who were given a placebo was just 11.6 months [97]. Recurrent GB patients have had success with carmustine wafer implantation since 1996 [98]. As a follow-up to its first clearance in 2002, the FDA cleared the wafers for use in surgery on all malignant gliomas in 2003. Research by Pallud et al. [99], which comprised 787 patients with newly diagnosed GB, found that wafer implantation was associated with increased progression-free survival. Many meta-analyses [100, 101] have looked at the benefits of locally implanted wafers. The median survival duration for patients with newly diagnosed high-grade glioma rose from 13.1 months to 16.4 months after treatment with carmustine wafers. This increase in survival was established after Chowdhary et al. analyzed data from 60 studies including 4898 patients. The total survival rate at two years increased from 15% to 26% while using the wafer. Carmustine wafers made from biodegradable materials have shown promise as a therapy for both newly diagnosed and recurring GB. Patients' outcomes have improved significantly but only somewhat thanks to these wafers, suggesting the need for more research into and development of locally targeted therapy. It is possible to translate highly effective chemotherapeutics, new small compounds that cannot withstand systemic delivery, and combination therapies into clinical practice by employing local delivery techniques [100].

8.4.4 Ultrasound and brain tumors

The term "ultrasound" is used to refer to sonic waves with a frequency greater than 20 kilohertz, and while it is most commonly used in the clinical setting for diagnosis, it is increasingly being used for therapy; especially by incorporating MRI guidance technology, focused ultrasound can be performed with pinpoint accuracy (MRgFUS) [101, 102]. In addition to being studied as a treatment for a wide range of illnesses, the FDA has approved MRgFUS for the treatment of essential tremors associated with Parkinson's disease including CSF rerouting, epilepsy surgery, depression treatment, and the removal of tumors from the brain [102]. It is possible to target specific areas for thermal ablation of tissues and malignancies with the use of ultrasonic energy when it is guided by resonance magnetic, as in "ultrasound guided by magnetic resonance imaging" (MRgFUS) [103]. The unusually low complication risk of MRgFUS has been attributed to its lack of effect on non-target organs [104]. Using high-intensity focused ultrasound, ultrasound power densities over 1000 W/cm^2 are delivered through the skull, making the procedure both safe and noninvasive [105]. For the concentrated ultrasound to be evaluated and tracked in real time [106], MRI guiding technology's thermometric cap capabilities are a great asset. Focused ultrasound's benefits are not only temporary; they add up over time. Tissue thermal ablation has direct therapeutic promise for glioblastoma multiforme (GB) and other brain tumors [107]. In the following section, we discuss how focused ultrasound can be utilized to boost the penetration of chemotherapy by using sonic cavitation to cause indirect and, at lower doses, non-thermal damage to the BBB [108]. Drugs used to treat gliomas have trouble crossing the BBB. The BBB separates the brain's vascular system from the brain's extracellular fluid and is made up of densely linked endothelial cells [109]. In the name of N. EL DEMERDASH et al. P-glycoprotein actively pumps out possible neurotoxins, making it difficult to provide treatment for glioma, whereas glucose and amino acids are passively transported. Yet, it has been found that the use of focused ultrasound in conjunction with microbubbles (MBs) can increase the effectiveness of medicine administration by crossing the blood–brain barrier in mouse models of glioma [109]. Cavitation is caused by the use of concentrated ultrasound, which causes vibrations in the microbubbles [110]. Microbubbles, or gas-filled microspheres, are extremely echogenic due to their small size. The diameter of the microbubbles used in the treatment has a negative correlation with the time it takes for the BBB to open and close; therefore, larger microbubbles have shorter opening windows. Membrane tearing/puncturing and epithelial cell separation are induced by focused ultrasound, and the BBB is compromised as a result [111]. Microbubble oscillations must be maintained at steady oscillations, free of inertial cavitation and transitory bubble collapse, to breach the BBB. Focused ultrasound with microbubbles can cause damage to healthy brain tissues; however, this danger can be mitigated using passive cavitation detection (PCD) monitoring [112]. Studies like this suggest targeted ultrasound's potential utility in this situation even if the FDA has not yet licensed it for treating brain tumors. Focused ultrasound may be utilized to break up the BBB, according to several Phase I/II clinical trials that are currently being conducted [111]. Current animal studies show that polysorbate-80 modified pacli taxel-loaded PLGA nanoparticles may be readily transported over the BBB by focused ultrasound. The blood–brain barrier (BBB) collapse has been linked to damage to tight junctions, decreased P-glycoprotein expression, and APOE-dependent polysorbate-80 permeability [113]. In a rat model of glioma, researchers found that systemic injection of cisplatin-loaded brain-penetrating nanoparticles with MRgFUS reduced tumor development and invasiveness and marginally improved survival [109]. It has been demonstrated that the antiangiogenic monoclonal antibody bevacizumab may successfully cross the BBB in a mouse model of malignant glioma [114]. In a rat glioma model, targeted ultrasound with microbubbles was used to successfully deliver trypan blue and liposomal doxorubicin over the BBB while monitoring for PCD [112]. When the BBB is transiently disrupted using MRI-monitored focused ultrasound with microbubbles, Wei et al. [115] found that an increased CSF:plasma temozolomide concentration ratio was observed. Recently, it was reported that the first patients to receive MRgFUS treatment in a clinical environment were five people with malignant high-grade glioma. Transdermal administration of liposomal doxorubicin and temozolomide was shown to be both possible and safe in this investigation [108]. These developments in MRI-guided focused ultrasound indicate that the technology may one day be used to treat gliomas locally, but further research is needed.

8.5 Laws Protecting the Use of Nanomedicine to Treat Brain Tumors as a Protected Invention

Table 8.3 provides a summary of various patents describing nanomedicine to cure cancerous brain tumors.

8.6 Conclusion

There has been a substantial rise during the past two decades in investigations exploring the success of various therapeutic approaches for the administration of glioblastoma (GB). If successful, these solutions could improve upon the state of the art in treatment. Effective medication therapy has been hampered by the BBB's and BBTB's complicated hurdles.

Biodegradable wafers have been around for almost a decade, and with good reason: they are safer and more effective than previous methods of localized treatment. In light of the translation of preclinical research, it is time for clinical studies to show the therapeutic potential of alternative medicines such as targeted nanoparticle therapy, focused ultrasound, and immunotherapy. The next major medical advance may come from ongoing and future research aimed at perfecting the targeted administration of therapeutic agents.

Table 8.3 Various formulation patents for brain targeted delivery of drug.

Authorized patent title	Summary	Founders	Patent registration no.	Reference
Treatment for brain tumors	Liposomes containing a topoisomerase inhibitor are the subject of this invention, which details a technique for their manufacture.	Zamboni William Engbers Charles, Yu Ning, Tonda Margaret, and Stewart Barbara	US 20070254019	[116]
Targeting liposomes	Crossing the blood–brain barrier with temozolomide-loaded cationic liposomes that are also conjugated to an antibody fragment to eradicate brain tumors is described in this invention.	Chang Esther H., Kim Sangsoo, and Rait Antonina	US 20140120157	[117]
Invasive tumor therapy with nanocarriers	Preparing sub-200 nm liposomes containing imipramine blue to combat malignant tumors that have spread throughout the brain.	Jennifer M. Munson, Ravi V. Bellamkonda, and Jack L. Arbiser	WO 2010124004 A2	[118]
Polymeric nanoparticle-based intranasal medicinal formulations	Methotrexate-loaded PLGA/PLA nanoparticles are described for intranasal administration to treat glioblastoma multiforme (GBM)	Darshana S. Jain and Amrita N. Bajaj	WO 2015087083 A1	[119]
O6-benzyl guanine nanoparticles for delivery to malignant gliomas in the brain	Preparation of O6-benzyl guanine-coupled cross-linked chitosanpolyethylene oxide nanoparticles for this invention relates to the distribution of temozolomide for the treatment of brain tumors.	Miqin Zhang, Richard G. Ellenbogen, Forrest Kievit, John R. Silber, Zachary Stephen, and Omid Veiseh	US 20140286872 A1	[120]

Title	Description	Authors	Patent number	Reference
Formulas of temozolomide composed of polymeric particles	In order to cure cancerous brain tumors, a biodegradable PLGA nanoparticle formulation containing temozolomide is described, along with its composition and production process.	Ekaterina Vasilenko, Evgeny Vorontsov, Evgenij Severin, Victor Gulenko, Maxim Mitrokhin, and Maksim Iurchenko	WO2014091078 A1	[121]
Nanoparticles of fotemustine solid lipid and their preparation	Fotemustine solid lipid nanoparticles, as described in this invention, are effective either ingested or administered intravenously in the treatment of malignant glioma.	Li Yaping, Chen Lingli, and Gu Wangwen	CN101606907 B	[122]
Targeted administration of dendrimers to brain tumors	This patent describes the production of PAMAM-hydroxyl-terminated dendrimers and their distinctive ability to cure brain tumors.	Antonella Mangraviti, Panagiotis Mastorakos, Manoj K. Mishra, Kannan Rangaramanujam, Betty M. Tyler, and Fan Zhang	WO 2016025741 A1	[123]
Anti-tumor activity of sn-38-loaded micelles	This finding explains how convection-enhanced transport of sn-38-loaded micelles can selectively target brain tumors across the blood–brain barrier (BBB).	Ryuta Saito and Teiji Tominaga	WO 2016030748 A1	[124]
Structure and technique of preparing a micelle-based nanopreparation for use in cancer diagnostics and therapy	The goal of this invention is to comprehend how sub-12 nm polymeric micelles loaded with hypericin can penetrate the blood–brain barrier (BBB) and treat glioblastoma.	Chulhee Choi, Kyuha Chong, and Jiho Park	US 9393308 B2	[125]

References

[1] Ferlay, J., Soerjomataram, I., Ervik, M., Dikshit, R., Eser, S., Mathers, C., Bray, F. Cancer incidence and mortality worldwide: IARC Cancer Base No. 11 GLOBOCAN 2012v1. 0. *Lyon: International Agency for Research on Cancer*, **2013**.

[2] Mehta, M., Vogelbaum, M. A., Chang, S., & Patel, N. Neoplasms of the central nervous system. In V. T. DeVita, Jr, T. S. Lawrence, & S. A. Rosenberg (Eds.), *Cancer: Principles and Practice of Oncology*, **2011**, 17001749. PA: Lippincott Williams & Wilkins

[3] Adams, S., Braidy, N., Bessesde, A., Brew, B. J., Grant, R., Teo, C., & Guillemin, G. J. The kynurenine pathway in brain tumor pathogenesis. *Cancer Research*, **2012**, *72*(22), 56495657

[4] Siegel, R. L., Miller, K. D., & Jemal, A. Cancer statistics, 2016. *CA: A Cancer Journal for Clinicians*, **2016**, *66*(1), 730.

[5] Kleihues, P., Burger, P. C., & Scheithauer, B. W. The new WHO classification of brain tumors. *Brain pathology*, **1993**, *3*(3), 255268.

[6] Louis, D. N., Perry, A., Reifenberger, G., von Deimling, A., Figarella-Branger, D., Cavenee, W. K., ... Ellison, D. W. The 2016 World Health Organization classification of tumors of the central nervous system: A summary. *Acta Neuropathologica*, **2016**, *131*(6), 803820.

[7] Ellor, S. V., Pagano-Young, T. A., & Avgeropoulos, N. G. Glioblastoma: Background, standard treatment paradigms, and supportive care considerations. *SAGE Publications Sage. CA: Los Angeles, CA*, **2014**, 171–182.

[8] Nagane, M. Neuro-oncology: Continuing multidisciplinary progress. *The Lancet Neurology*, **2011**, *10*(1), 18.

[9] Tzeng, S. Y., & Green, J. J. Therapeutic nanomedicine for brain cancer. *Therapeutic Delivery*, **2013**, *4*(6), 687704.

[10] Perkins, M., & Liu, G. Primary brain tumors in adults: Diagnosis and treatment. *American Family Physician*, **2016**, *93*(3), 211217

[11] McNeill, K. A. Epidemiology of brain tumors. *Neurologic Clinics*, **2016**, *34*(4), 981998.

[12] Schabet, M. Epidemiology of primary CNS lymphoma. *Journal of Neuro-Oncology*, **1999**, *43*(3), 199201.

[13] Group, I. S. Brain tumor risk in relation to mobile telephone use: Results of the INTERPHONE international casecontrol study. *International Journal of Epidemiology*, **2010**, dyq07

[14] Kheifets, L. I., Sussman, S. S., & Preston-Martin, S. Childhood brain tumors and residential electromagnetic fields (EMF). *Reviews of environmental contamination and toxicology*, **1999**, 111129. Springer

[15] Schüz, J., Jacobsen, R., Olsen, J. H., Boice, J. D., McLaughlin, J. K., & Johansen, C. Cellular telephone use and cancer risk: Update of a nation-wide Danish cohort. *Journal of the National Cancer Institute*, **2006**, *98*(23), 17071713.

[16] Amirian, E. S., Zhou, R., Wrensch, M. R., Olson, S. H., Scheurer, M. E., Il'Yasova, D., Lau, C. C. Approaching a scientific consensus on the association between allergies and glioma risk: A report from the glioma international case-control study. *Cancer Epidemiology and Prevention Biomarkers*, **2016**, *25*(2), 282290

[17] Wigertz, A., Lönn, S., Schwartzbaum, J., Hall, P., Auvinen, A., Christensen, H. C., Schoemaker, M. J. Allergic conditions and brain tumor risk. *American Journal of Epidemiology*, **2007**, *166*(8), 941950.4

[18] da Silva, J. DNA damage induced by occupational and environmental exposure to miscellaneous chemicals. *Mutation Research/Reviews in Mutation Research*, **2016**, *770*, 170182.

[19] Aizer, A., & Alexander, B. Brain tumors—epidemiology. *Pathology and Epidemiology of Cancer*, **2017**, 279290, Springer.

[20] Vernooij, M. W., Ikram, M. A., Tanghe, H. L., Vincent, A. J., Hofman, A., Krestin, G. P., van der Lugt, A. Incidental findings on brain MRI in the general population. *New England Journal of Medicine*, **2007**, *357*(18), 18211828.

[21] Crawford, L., Rosch, J., & Putnam, D. Concepts, technologies, and practices for drug delivery past the blood-brain barrier to the central nervous system. *Journal of Controlled Release*, **2016**, *240*, 251266.

[22] Lalu, L., Tambe, V., Pradhan, D., Nayak, K., Bagchi, S., Maheshwari, R., Tekade, R. K. Novel nanosystems for the treatment of ocular inflam-mation: Current paradigms and future research directions. *Journal Controlled Release*, **2017**, *268*, 1939

[23] Tekade, R.K., Maheshwari, R., Soni, N., Tekade, M. and Chougule, M.B. Nanotechnology for the development of nanomedicine. In *Nanotechnology-based approaches for targeting and delivery of drugs and genes*, **2017a**, 3–61. Academic Press.

[24] Tekade, R.K., Maheshwari, R., Soni, N. and Tekade, M. Carbon nano-tubes in targeting and delivery of drugs. In *Nanotechnology-based approaches for targeting and delivery of drugs and genes*, **2017**, 389–426. Academic Press.

[25] Maheshwari, R. G., Tekade, R. K., Sharma, P. A., Darwhekar, G., Tyagi, A., Patel, R. P., & Jain, D. K. Ethosomes and ultradeformable liposomes for transdermal delivery of clotrimazole: A comparative assessment. *Saudi Pharm J*, **2012**, *20*(2), 161170.

[26] Maheshwari, R., Tekade, M., Sharma, P. A., & Kumar Tekade, R. Nanocarriers assisted siRNA gene therapy for the management of cardiovascular disorders. *Current Pharmaceutical Design*, **2015b**, *21*(30), 44274440.

[27] Soni, N., Soni, N., Pandey, H., Maheshwari, R., Kesharwani, P., & Tekade, R. K. Augmented delivery of gemcitabine in lung cancer cells exploring mannose anchored solid lipid nanoparticles. *J Colloid Interface Sci*, **2016b**, *481*, 107116.

[28] Soni, N., Tekade, M., Kesharwani, P., Bhattacharya, P., Maheshwari, R., Dua, K., Hansbro, P. M., & Tekade, R. K. Recent Advances in Oncological Submissions of Dendrimer. *Curr Pharm Des*, **2017**, *23*(21), 30843098.

[29] Tekade, R.K., Maheshwari, R., Tekade, M. and Chougule, M.B. Solid lipid nanoparticles for targeting and delivery of drugs and genes. In *Nanotechnology-based approaches for targeting and delivery of drugs and genes*, **2017c**, 256–286. Academic Press.

[30] Silva, G. A. Nanotechnology approaches for drug and small molecule delivery across the blood-brain barrier. *Surgical Neurology*, **2007**, *67*(2), 113116.

[31] Brasnjevic, I., Steinbusch, H. W., Schmitz, C., Martinez-Martinez, P., & Initiative, E. N. R. Delivery of peptide and protein drugs over the blood-brain barrier. *Progress in Neurobiology*, **2009**, *87*(4), 212251.

[32] Pardridge, W.M. *Brain drug targeting: the future of brain drug development*. Cambridge University Press, **2001**.

[33] Pablo Rigalli, J., Ciriaci, N., Domingo Mottino, A., Alicia Catania, V., & Laura Ruiz, M. modulation of expression and activity of ABC transporters by the phytoestrogen genistein. Impact on Drug Disposition. *Current Medicinal Chemistry*, **2016**, *23*(13), 13701389.

[34] Agarwal, S., Sane, R., Oberoi, R., Ohlfest, J. R., & Elmquist, W. F. Delivery of molecularly targeted therapy to malignant glioma, a disease of the whole brain. *Expert Reviews in Molecular Medicine*, **2011**, *13*, e17.

[35] Ballabh, P., Braun, A., & Nedergaard, M. The blood-brain barrier: An overview: Structure, regulation, and clinical implications. *Neurobiology of Disease*, **2004**, *16*(1), 113.

[36] Vartanian, A., Singh, S. K., Agnihotri, S., Jalali, S., Burrell, K., Aldape, K. D., & Zadeh, G. GBM's multifaceted landscape: Highlighting regional and microenvironmental heterogeneity. *Neuro-Oncology*, **2014**, *16*(9), 11671175

[37] Pardridge, W.M. The blood-brain barrier: bottleneck in brain drug development. *NeuroRx*, **2005**, *2*, 3–14.

[38] Upadhyay, R. K. Drug delivery systems, CNS protection, and the blood-brain barrier. BioMed Research International, 2014. *NeuroRx*, **2014**, 2(1), 314

[39] Huttunen, K. M., & Rautio, J. Prodrugs-an efficient way to breach delivery and targeting barriers. *Current Topics in Medicinal Chemistry*, **2011**, *11*(18), 22652287.

[40] Schaddelee, M. P., Voorwinden, H. L., Groenendaal, D., Hersey, A., Ijzerman, A. P., Danhof, M., & De Boer, A. G. Blood-brain barrier transport of synthetic adenosine A 1 receptor agonists in vitro: Structure transport relationships. *European journal of Pharmaceutical Sciences*, **2003**, *20*(3), 347356.

[41] Foti, R. S., Tyndale, R. F., Garcia, K. L., Sweet, D. H., Nagar, S., Sharan, S., & Rock, D. A. "Target-site" drug metabolism and transport. *Drug Metabolism and Disposition*, **2015**, *43*(8), 11561168

[42] Tamai, I., & Tsuji, A. Drug delivery through the blood-brain barrier. *Advanced Drug Delivery Reviews*, **1996**, *19*(3), 401424.

[43] Löscher, W., & Potschka, H. Drug resistance in brain diseases and the role of drug efflux transporters. *Nature Reviews Neuroscience*, **2005b**, *6*(8), 591602.

[44] Begley, D. J. ABC transporters and the blood-brain barrier. *Current Pharmaceutical Design*, **2004**, *10*(12), 12951312.

[45] de Lange, E. C. Potential role of ABC transporters as a detoxification system at the blood-CSF barrier. *Advanced Drug Delivery Reviews*, **2004**, *56*(12), 17931809.

[46] Lingineni, K., Belekar, V., Tangadpalliwar, S. R., & Garg, P. The role of multidrug resistance protein (MRP-1) as an active efflux transporter on blood-brain barrier (BBB) permeability. *Molecular Diversity*, **2017**, 111.

[47] Sun, H., Dai, H., Shaik, N., & Elmquist, W. F. Drug efflux transporters in the CNS. *Advanced Drug Delivery Reviews*, **2003**, *55*(1), 83105.

[48] Bart, J., Groen, H., Hendrikse, N., van der Graaf, W., Vaalburg, W., & de Vries, E. The blood-brain barrier and oncology: New insights into function and modulation. *Cancer Treatment Reviews*, **2000**, *26*(6), 449462

[49] Kemper, E. M., Boogerd, W., Thuis, I., Beijnen, J. H., & van Tellingen, O. Modulation of the blood-brain barrier in oncology: Therapeutic opportunities for the treatment of brain tumors? *Cancer Treatment Reviews*, **2004**, *30*(5), 415423.

[50] Oberoi, R. K., Parrish, K. E., Sio, T. T., Mittapalli, R. K., Elmquist, W. F., & Sarkaria, J. N. Strategies to improve the delivery of anticancer drugs across the blood-brain barrier to treat glioblastoma. *Neuro-Oncology*, **2016**, *18*(1), 2736.

[51] Wardill, H. R., Mander, K. A., Van Sebille, Y. Z., Gibson, R. J., Logan, R. M., Bowen, J. M., & Sonis, S. T. Cytokine-mediated blood-brain barrier disruption as a conduit for cancer/chemotherapy-associated neurotoxicity and cognitive dysfunction. *International Journal of Cancer*, **2016**, *139*(12), 26352645.

[52] Almutairi MM Gong, C, Xu, YG, et al. Factors controlling permeability of the blood-brain barrier. *Cell Mol Life Sci.*, **2016**, *73*(1), 57–77.

[53] Tamai I, Tsuji A. Transporter-mediated permeation of drugs across the blood-brain barrier. *J Pharm Sci.*, **2000**, *89*(11), 1371–1388.

[54] Bhowmik A, Khan R, Ghosh MK. Blood-brain barrier: a challenge for effectual therapy of brain tumors. *Biomed Res Int.*, **2015**, *2015*, 320941.

[55] Begley DJ. ABC transporters and the blood-brain barrier. *Curr Pharm Des.*, **2004**, *10*(12), 1295–1312.

[56] Armulik A, Genové G, Mäe M, et al. Pericytes regulate the blood-brain barrier. *Nature*, **2010**, *468*(7323), 557–561.

[57] Abbott NJ, Ronnback L, Hansson E. Astrocyte-endothelial interactions at the blood-brain barrier. *Nat Rev Neurosci.*, **2006**, *7*(1), 41–53.

[58] Daneman R, Prat A. The blood-brain barrier. *Cold Spring Harb Perspect Biol.*, **2015**, *7*(1), a020412.

[59] Groothuis DR. The blood-brain and blood-tumor barriers: a review of strategies for increasing drug delivery. *Neuro Oncol.*, **2000**, *2*(1), 45–59.

[60] van Tellingen O, Yetkin-Arik B, de Gooijer MC, et al. Overcoming the blood-brain tumor barrier for effective glioblastoma treatment. *Drug Resist Updat.*, **2015**, *19*, 1–12.

[61] Zhou W, Chen C, Shi Y, et al. Targeting glioma stem cell-derived pericytes disrupts the blood-tumor barrier and improves chemotherapeutic efficacy. *Cell Stem Cell*, **2017**, *21*(5), 591–603.e4.

[62] Bobo RH, Laske DW, Akbasak A, et al. Convection-enhanced delivery of macromolecules in the brain. *Proc Natl Acad Sci USA*, **1994**, *91*(6), 2076–2080.

[63] Mehta AM, Sonabend AM, Bruce JN. Convection-enhanced delivery. *Neurotherapeutics*, **2017**, *14*(2), 358–371.

[64] Raghavan R, Brady ML, Rodríguez-Ponce MI, et al. Convectionenhanced delivery of therapeutics for brain disease, and its optimization. *Neurosurg Focus*, **2006**, *20*(4), E12. 18 N. EL DEMERDASH ET AL.

[65] Sampson JH, Brady ML, Petry NA, et al. Intracerebral infusate distribution by convection-enhanced delivery in humans with malignant gliomas: descriptive effects of target anatomy and catheter positioning. *Neurosurgery*, **2007**, *60*(1), ONS89–98.

[66] Sampson JH, Akabani G, Archer GE, et al. Intracerebral infusion of an EGFR-targeted toxin in recurrent malignant brain tumors. *Neuro Oncol.*, **2008**, *10*(3), 320–329.

[67] Sampson JH, Archer G, Pedain C, et al. Poor drug distribution as a possible explanation for the results of the PRECISE trial. *J Neurosurg.*, **2010**, *113*(2), 301–309.

[68] Lidar Z, Mardor Y, Jonas T, et al. Convection-enhanced delivery of paclitaxel for the treatment of recurrent malignant glioma: a phase I/II clinical study. *J Neurosurg.*, **2004**, *100*(3), 472–479.

[69] Young JS, Bernal G, Polster SP, et al. Convection-enhanced delivery of polymeric nanoparticles encapsulating chemotherapy in canines with spontaneous supratentorial tumors. *World Neurosurg.*, **2018**, *117*, e698–e704.

[70] Zhang C, Nance EA, Mastorakos P, et al. Convection enhanced delivery of cisplatin-loaded brain penetrating nanoparticles cures malignant glioma in rats. *J Control Release*, **2017**, *263*, 112–119.

[71] White E, Bienemann A, Pugh J, et al. An evaluation of the safety and feasibility of convection-enhanced delivery of carboplatin into the white matter as a potential treatment for high-grade glioma. *J Neurooncol.*, **2012**, *108*(1), 77–88.

[72] White E, Bienemann A, Taylor H, et al. A phase I trial of carboplatin administered by convection-enhanced delivery to patients with recurrent/progressive glioblastoma multiforme. *Contemp Clin Trials*, **2012**, *33*(2), 320–331.

[73] Arshad A, Yang B, Bienemann AS, et al. Convection-enhanced delivery of carboplatin PLGA nanoparticles for the treatment of glioblastoma. *PLoS One*, **2015**, *10*(7), e0132266.

[74] Shi M, Anantha M, Wehbe M, et al. Liposomal formulations of carboplatin injected by convection-enhanced delivery increases the median survival time of F98 glioma bearing rats. *J Nanobiotechnology*, **2018**, *16*(1), 77.

[75] Huo T, Barth RF, Yang W, et al. Preparation, biodistribution, and neurotoxicity of liposomal cisplatin following convection enhanced delivery in normal and F98 glioma bearing rats. *PLoS One*, **2012**, *7*(11), e48752.

[76] Nordling-David MM, Yaffe R, Guez D, et al. Liposomal temozolomide drug delivery using convection enhanced delivery. *J Control Release*, **2017**, *261*, 138–146.

[77] Sewing ACP, Lagerweij T, van Vuurden DG, et al. Preclinical evaluation of convection-enhanced delivery of liposomal doxorubicin to treat

pediatric diffuse intrinsic pontine glioma and thalamic high-grade glioma. *J Neurosurg Pediatr.*, **2017**, *19*(5), 518–530.

[78] Barua NU, Hopkins K, Woolley M, et al. A novel implantable catheter system with transcutaneous port for intermittent convection-enhanced delivery of carboplatin for recurrent glioblastoma. *Drug Deliv.*, **2016**, *23*(1), 167–173.

[79] Vogelbaum MA, Brewer C, Barnett GH, et al. First-in-human evaluation of the cleveland multiport catheter for convection-enhanced delivery of topotecan in recurrent high-grade glioma: results of pilot trial 1. *J Neurosurg*, **2018**, 1–10.

[80] Barua NU, Gill SS, Love S. Convection-enhanced drug delivery to the brain: therapeutic potential and neuropathological considerations. *Brain Pathol.*, **2014**, *24*(2), 117–127

[81] Kwiatkowska A, Nandhu MS, Behera P, et al. Strategies in gene therapy for glioblastoma. *Cancers* (Basel), **2013**, *5*(4), 1271–1305.

[82] Mao H, Lebrun DG, Yang J, et al. Deregulated signaling pathways in glioblastoma multiforme: molecular mechanisms and therapeutic targets. *Cancer Invest*, **2012**, *30*(1), 48–56.

[83] Nandhu MS, Kwiatkowska A, Bhaskaran V, et al. Tumor-derived fibulin-3 activates pro-invasive NF-kappaB signaling in glioblastoma cells and their microenvironment. *Oncogene*, **2017**, *36*(34), 4875–4886.

[84] Tobias A, Ahmed A, Moon K-S, et al. The art of gene therapy for glioma: a review of the challenging road to the bedside. *J Neurol Neurosurg Psychiatry*, **2013**, *84*(2), 213–222.

[85] Guerrero-Cazares H, Tzeng SY, Young NP, et al. Biodegradable polymeric nanoparticles show high efficacy and specificity at DNA delivery to human glioblastoma *in vitro* and *in vivo*. *ACS Nano*, **2014**, *8*(5), 5141–5153.

[86] Lynn DM, Anderson DG, Putnam D, et al. Accelerated discovery of synthetic transfection vectors: parallel synthesis and screening of a degradable polymer library. *J Am Chem Soc*, **2001**, *123*(33), 8155–8156.

[87] Tzeng SY, Higgins LJ, Pomper MG, et al. Student award winner in the Ph.D. category for the 2013 society for biomaterials annual meeting and exposition, april 10–13,2013, Boston, Massachusetts: biomaterial-mediated cancer-specific DNA delivery to liver cell cultures using synthetic poly(beta-amino ester)s. *J Biomed Mater Res A*, **2013**, *101*(7), 1837–1845.

[88] Idbaih A, Erbs P, Foloppe J, et al. TG6002: A novel oncolytic and vectorized gene pro-drug therapy approach to treat glioblastoma. *J Clin Oncol*, **2017**, *35*(15), e13510–e13510.

[89] Tamargo RJ, Myseros JS, Epstein JI, et al. Interstitial chemotherapy of the 9L gliosarcoma: controlled release polymers for drug delivery in the brain. *Cancer Res*, **1993**, *53*(2), 329–333.

[90] Yang MB, Tamargo RJ, Brem H. Controlled delivery of 1,3-bis (2-chloroethyl)-1-nitrosourea from ethylene-vinyl acetate copolymer. *Cancer Res*. **1989**, *49*(18), 5103–5107.

[91] Fung LK, Shin M, Tyler B, et al. Chemotherapeutic drugs released from polymers: distribution of 1,3-bis(2-chloroethyl)-1-nitrosourea in the rat brain. *Pharm Res*, **1996**, 13(5), 671–682.

[92] Sipos EP, Tyler B, Piantadosi S, et al. Optimizing interstitial delivery of BCNU from controlled release polymers for the treatment of brain tumors. *Cancer Chemother Pharmacol*, **1997**, *39*(5):383–389.

[93] Grossman SA, Reinhard C, Colvin OM, et al. The intracerebral distribution of BCNU delivered by surgically implanted biodegradable polymers. *J Neurosurg*, **1992**, *76*(4), 640–647.

[94] Brem H, Mahaley MS, Vick NA, et al. Interstitial chemotherapy with drug polymer implants for the treatment of recurrent gliomas. *J Neurosurg*. **1991**, *74*(3), 441–446.

[95] Brem H, Piantadosi S, Burger PC, et al. Placebo-controlled trial of safety and efficacy of intraoperative controlled delivery by biodegradable polymers of chemotherapy for recurrent gliomas. The polymer-brain tumor treatment group. *Lancet*, **1995**, *345*(8956), 1008–1012.

[96] Valtonen S, Timonen U, Toivanen P, et al. Interstitial chemotherapy with carmustine-loaded polymers for high-grade gliomas: a randomized double-blind study. *Neurosurgery*, **1997**, *41*(1), 44–48.

[97] Westphal M, Hilt DC, Bortey E, et al. A phase 3 trial of local chemotherapy with biodegradable carmustine (BCNU) wafers (Gliadel wafers) in patients with primary malignant glioma. *Neuro Oncol*. **2003**, *5*(2), 79–88.

[98] Mangraviti A, Tyler B, Brem H. Interstitial chemotherapy for malignant glioma: future prospects in the era of multimodal therapy. *Surg Neurol Int*., **2015**, *6*(1): S78–84.

[99] Pallud J, Audureau E, Noel G, et al. Long-term results of carmustine wafer implantation for newly diagnosed glioblastomas: a controlled propensity-matched analysis of a French multicenter cohort. *Neuro Oncol*., **2015**, *17*(12), 1609–1619.

[100] Chowdhary SA, Ryken T, Newton HB. Survival outcomes and safety of carmustine wafers in the treatment of high-grade gliomas: a meta-analysis. J Neurooncol. 2015;122(2):367–382.

[101] Xing WK, Shao C, Qi Z-Y, et al. The role of Gliadel wafers in the treatment of newly diagnosed GBM: a meta-analysis. *Drug Des Devel Ther*. **2015**, *9*, 3341–3348

[102] Hersh DS, Kim AJ, Winkles JA, et al. Emerging applications of therapeutic ultrasound in neuro-oncology: moving beyond tumor ablation. *Neurosurgery*, **2016**, *79*(5), 643–654.

[103] Lee EJ, Fomenko A, Lozano AM. Magnetic resonance-guided focused ultrasound: current status and future perspectives in thermal ablation and blood-brain barrier opening. *J Korean Neurosurg Soc*. **2019**, *62*(1),10–26.

[104] Hijnen NM, Heijman E, Köhler MO, et al. Tumour hyperthermia and ablation in rats using a clinical MR-HIFU system equipped with a dedicated small animal set-up. *Int J Hyperthermia*, **2012**, *28*(2), 141–155.

[105] Jenne JW, Preusser T, Gunther M. High-intensity focused ultrasound: principles, therapy guidance, simulations and applications. *Z Med Phys*. **2012**, *22*(4), 311–322.

[106] Ries M, de Senneville BD, Roujol S, et al. Real-time 3D target tracking in MRI guided focused ultrasound ablations in moving tissues. *Magn Reson Med*, **2010**, *64*(6), 1704–1712.

[107] Colen RR, Sahnoune I, Weinberg JS. Neurosurgical applications of high-intensity focused ultrasound with magnetic resonance thermometry. *Neurosurg Clin N Am*, **2017**, *28*(4), 559–567.

[108] Mainprize T, Lipsman N, Huang Y, et al. Blood-brain barrier opening in primary brain tumors with non-invasive MR-guided focused ultrasound: a clinical safety and feasibility study. *Sci Rep*, **2019**, *9*(1), 321.

[109] Timbie KF, Afzal U, Date A, et al. MR image-guided delivery of cisplatin-loaded brain-penetrating nanoparticles to invasive glioma with focused ultrasound. *J Control Release*, **2017**, *263*, 120–131.

[110] Dong Q, He L, Chen L, et al. Opening the blood-brain barrier and improving the efficacy of temozolomide treatments of glioblastoma using pulsed, focused ultrasound with a microbubble contrast agent. *Biomed Res Int.*, **2018**, *2018*, 6501508.

[111] Poon C, McMahon D, Hynynen K. Noninvasive and targeted delivery of therapeutics to the brain using focused ultrasound. *Neuropharmacology*, **2017**, *120*, 20–37.

[112] Sun T, Zhang Y, Power C, et al. Closed-loop control of targeted ultrasound drug delivery across the blood-brain/tumor barriers in a rat glioma model. *Proc Natl Acad Sci USA*, **2017**, *114*(48), E10281–e10290.

[113] Li Y, Wu M, Zhang N, et al. Mechanisms of enhanced antiglioma efficacy of polysorbate 80-modified paclitaxel-loaded PLGA

nanoparticles by focused ultrasound. *J Cell Mol Med*, **2018**, *22*(9), 4171–4182

[114] Liu H-L, Hsu P-H, Lin C-Y, et al. Focused ultrasound enhances central nervous system delivery of bevacizumab for malignant glioma treatment. *Radiology*, **2016**, *281*(1), 99–108.

[115] Wei KC, Chu P-C, Wang H-YJ, et al. Focused ultrasound-induced blood-brain barrier opening to enhance temozolomide delivery for glioblastoma treatment: a preclinical study. *PLoS One*, **2013**, *8*(3), e58995.

[116] Zamboni W, Engbers C, Yu N, Tonda M, Stewart B. Method for treating brain cancer. US20070254019, **2007**.

[117] Chang EH, Kim S, Rait A. Targeted liposomes. US20140120157, **2014**.

[118] Jennifer M. Munson, Ravi V. Bellamkonda, Jack L. Arbiser. Nanocarriers for therapy of invasive tumors. WO2010124004 A2, **2010**.

[119] Jain SD, Bajaj AN. Intranasal pharmaceutical compositions of polymeric nanoparticles. WO 2015087083 A1, **2015**.

[120] Miqin Z, Richard GE, Forrest K, John RS, Zachary S, Omid V. Nanoparticles for targeting brain tumors and delivery of O6 - benzylguanine. US20140286872 A1, **2014**.

[121] Ekaterina V, Evgeny V, Evgenij S, Victor G, Maxim M, Maksim I. WO2014091078 A1, **2014**.

[122] Li Yaping, Chen Lingli, Gu Wangwen. Fotemustine solid lipid nanoparticles and prepration method thereof. CN101606907 B, **2011**.

[123] Antonella M, Panagiotis M, Manoj KM, Kannan R, Betty MT, Fan Z. Selective dendrimer delivery to brain tumors. WO 2016025741 A1, **2016**.

[124] Ryuta S, Teiji T. Ced of sn-38-loaded micelles against brain tumor. WO2016030748 A1, **2016**

[125] Chulhee C, Kyuha C, Jiho P. Micelle structure of nanopreparation for diagnosis or treatment of cancer disease and preparation method thereof. US9393308 B2, **2016**.

Index

A

ABCG2 55, 106, 177
Absorptive endocytosis 107
Adherent junctions 53, 173
Alzheimer's disease 181–182
Angiogenesis 13, 19, 27–38, 92,
    109, 138, 146
ANGPT2 27
Anorexia 150, 198
Antibodies 38, 59, 61, 64, 77,
    79, 87–91, 93, 110, 149, 157,
    178–179
Anticancer 19, 28, 37–38, 57,
    83–85, 88–89, 106, 108–109,
    117, 124, 146, 157, 177, 197,
    200, 203
Aptamers 77, 79
Astrocytes 3–4, 13, 28, 33, 35, 52,
    54, 57–58, 62, 93, 106, 109, 146,
    173, 201
AUC 108
Axons 2, 4, 28

B

Basement membrane 29, 34, 37, 52,
    53, 201
Basic fibroblast growth factor 31,
    109
BCRP 106, 177

Blood–brain barrier 3, 12–13, 30,
    33, 38, 51–53, 56–58, 60–64,
    77–78, 83, 85–88, 91, 95, 105,
    108–109, 123, 125, 137–138,
    140, 154, 171–173, 176, 178,
    180, 184–185, 197–201, 203,
    206, 208
Blood vessels 7, 13, 18, 27–28,
    30–31, 34–37, 52–54, 58, 60,
    91–92, 105, 109, 154, 173
Bone marrow 138

C

Cancer 1–2, 4, 14– 20, 27, 29,
    30–31, 33–38, 51, 55, 77–78,
    83–88, 91, 93, 95, 105–106, 109,
    124, 138 139, 145, 147–149,
    154, 157, 197–198, 205
Capillaries 13, 51–54, 62, 106, 109,
    114, 116, 200–201
Carrier-mediated transport 58,
    107–108
Chemotherapy 15, 19–20, 33,
    77–78, 84–85, 87, 90, 93, 106,
    109, 124, 137, 145, 206, 208
Choroid plexus 4, 12–14, 52, 54,
    58, 62
Clinical studies 38, 62, 137, 157,
    209

CNS 1–5, 7, 12, 14–15, 18–21, 28,
    33, 36, 51–52, 54–56, 58, 60–61,
    64, 105–107, 109–110, 112,
    124–125, 171–173, 184,
    197–201
Convulsions 198
CSF 4–5, 12–16, 33, 51–52, 55,
    57–59, 207, 209
Cytokines 32, 60, 146, 184, 205

D
Degenerative diseases 171
Dendrimer 62–63, 148–150
Diffusion 12–13, 21, 33, 54–55, 59,
    64, 117, 139, 175–176, 204
DNA 19–20, 62, 93–94, 110, 146,
    150–151, 184, 205

E
Efficacy 84, 86, 88–89, 95, 118,
    137, 140, 148, 157, 178, 182,
    203, 205
Endocytotic 51, 59, 64
Endogenic substances 175
Endothelium 13, 52–55, 60, 109,
    138, 140, 171, 173, 175–176,
    178, 180
Ependymal cells 3–4, 15–16
Exosomes 140, 145–147
Extracellular vesicles 145

F
FDA 115, 145, 172, 181, 206–208
Fibronectin 29, 34, 52
Folic acid 77, 79, 86–87, 125, 145

G
Glial cells 1, 3, 16, 109
Glioblastoma 4, 16, 19, 27, 31–33,
    35–37, 83, 85, 88–91, 93,
    137–138, 142, 146, 149, 154,
    157, 198, 201, 208, 209
Glioblastoma multiforme 16, 19,
    36, 85, 93, 137, 142, 146, 198,
    208
Glycoprotein 55, 57, 83, 85, 89,
    106, 147, 175, 177, 201, 208

H
Headache 198
HIV 64, 198
Homeostasis 8, 13, 28, 34, 57, 60,
    64, 105, 175, 200
Hormones 32–33, 175
HSPG 52
Hybrid 83, 171
Hypoxia 21, 27, 30–33, 36–37, 92,
    152

I
Infarctions 27
Infections 4, 27, 51, 172

L
Lactoferrin 62, 79, 85–86
Laminin 52
Lipid 33, 52, 54–56, 85, 87–88,
    105, 107, 109, 111–119,
    121–123, 125, 140, 152, 171,
    175, 177–178, 182, 199
Liposomes 59, 61, 63, 83–84, 86,
    89, 95, 111, 113, 140–142, 145,
    177, 179–180, 183–184, 199, 204
Loss of appetite 198
Loss of focus 198

M
Macrophages 30, 52, 146, 149, 175,
    183
Malignancy 21, 146, 198

Markers 38, 77, 90, 109, 146, 198
Mediators 27, 29, 109, 175
Metabolites 54, 172, 175, 205
Micelles 83, 87–88, 94, 95, 152, 154, 177
Microglia 3–4, 52, 146, 149, 173, 175, 185
Microvesicles 145
Mood swings 198
MRP1 106

N
Nanocarriers 77, 86–87, 95, 105, 110, 147–149, 177–178, 180, 183–185
Nano-enabled 137
Nanoparticle 2, 5, 21, 77, 111, 115, 117–119, 121–122, 124, 138, 171, 179, 185, 204, 209
Nanotechnology 2, 77, 90, 124, 137, 171, 173, 181, 197–198, 205
Nausea 145, 198
Neuroglia 16, 53
Neurological system 2, 5, 28
Neuron 2–3, 28, 38, 53, 183
Neurotoxins 33, 171–172, 208
Noncoding microRNAs 146

O
Occludens 52, 108
Ocular neovascularization 28
Oligodendrocytes 3–4, 16

P
Paracellular 52, 106, 174–176
Parenchyma 12, 28, 30, 33, 60, 62, 78, 91–92, 110, 139, 140, 175, 181, 206
Parkinson's disease 58, 61–62, 182, 185, 207

Peptides 55, 57, 59, 62–64, 77, 79, 94–95, 123–124, 140, 149, 152, 154, 158, 175, 178, 181
P-gp 106–107, 175–177, 201
Pharmacokinetic 64, 108, 124, 147, 171
Polymeric 87–88, 91, 111, 113, 122, 140, 147–148, 171, 177–179, 199, 203

S
Safety 19, 137, 150, 182, 197, 203–205
Solid lipid nanoparticles 85, 88, 105, 112, 123, 177, 199
Solid tumor 149, 197
Surgery 15, 19–20, 77, 90, 147, 206–207

T
Targeted 60–61, 77–78, 83–84, 86–95, 105, 110, 112, 123–125, 138, 145, 147–148, 172, 184, 197, 207–209, 211
Therapeutics 64, 124, 137, 146
Therapy 2, 15, 18–21, 34, 38, 78, 84–85, 88–90, 92–94, 106–107, 109–110, 137, 140, 145, 147, 149, 172, 182–184, 199–200, 205, 207, 209
Thrombin growth factor 27
Tight junctions 13, 52, 55, 106, 108, 173–174, 200, 208
Transferrin 59–61, 77, 79, 83–85, 108, 125, 149, 178
Tumors 1–8, 11, 14–21, 27–33, 35–38, 59–60, 62, 77–79, 83–92, 94–96, 106–107, 109–110, 137–138, 140, 146, 148–149, 152, 154, 157, 176, 197–202, 205, 207–209

V

VEGF 19–20, 27, 30–38, 92–93,
    109, 152, 201
Vomiting 18, 145, 198

W

WHO 1, 16–17, 20, 109, 145,
    197–199, 203, 206–207

X

Xenobiotics 175

Z

Zonulae 106, 200

About the Editors

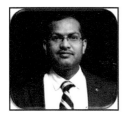

Rishabha Malviya received the B.Pharm. degree from Uttar Pradesh Technical University and the M.Pharm. (pharmaceutics) degree from Gautam Buddha Technical University, Lucknow Uttar Pradesh, India. His Ph.D. (pharmacy) work was in the area of novel formulation development techniques. He has 12 years of research experience and has been working as an Associate Professor with the Department of Pharmacy, School of Medical and Allied Sciences, Galgotias University since eight years. His area of research interest includes formulation optimization, nanoformulation, targeted drug delivery, localized drug delivery, and characterization of natural polymers as pharmaceutical excipients. He has authored more than 200 research/review papers for national/international journals of repute. He has 58 patents (19 grants, 38 published, and 1 filed) and publications in reputed national and international journals with a total of 191 cumulative impact factors. He has also received an Outstanding Reviewer Award from Elsevier. He has authored/edited/editing 46 books (Wiley, CRC Press/Taylor and Francis, Springer, River Publisher, IOP Publishing, and OMICS publication) and has authored 31 book chapters. His name has been included in word's top 2% scientist list for the year 2020 and 2021 by Elsevier BV and Stanford University. He is the Reviewer/Editor/Editorial Board member of more than 50 national and international journals of repute. Dr. Malviya has been invited as an author for "Atlas of Science" and pharma magazine dealing with industry (B2B) "Ingredient south Asia Magazines."

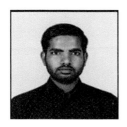

Arun Kumar Singh received the B.Pharm. and M.Pharm. degrees from Galgotias University, India. He has authored one book (ISBN No. 9780750358392, publication date, June 2023) with IOP Press and three of his authored books are in printing with Scrivener Publishing, Wiley, Apple Academic Press, and River Publisher. He has authored three book chapters and published manuscripts with reputed publishers, such as *Biochimica et Biophysica Acta (BBA) – Reviews on Cancer* (Impact factor 11.414), *Journal of Controlled Release* (Impact factor: 11.467), *Current Cancer Therapy Reviews* (Scopus), *Recent Advances in Food, Nutrition & Agriculture* (Scopus), *Recent Patents on Anti-Cancer Drug Discovery* (Impact factor: 3.038), and *Current Cancer Drug Targets* (Impact factor: 2.907).

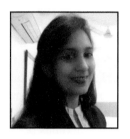

Sonali Sundram received the B.Pharm. and M.Pharm. (pharmacology) degrees from AKTU, Lucknow, India. She has worked as a Research Scientist in the project of ICMR in King George's Medical University, Lucknow, India. After that, she joined BBDNIIT, and she is currently working with Galgotias University, Greater Noida, India. Her Ph.D. (pharmacy) work was in the area of neurodegenera-tion and nanoformulation. Her areas of research interest are in neurodegen-eration, clinical research, and artificial intelligence. She has authored/edited/editing more than 15 books (Wiley, CRC Press/Taylor and Francis, IOP Publishing, Apple Academic Press/Taylor and Francis, Springer Nature, and River Publisher). She has attended as well as organized more than 15 national and international seminar/conferences/workshops. She has more than eight national and international patents to her credit. She has published six SCI indexed manuscripts (cumulative impact factor: 20.71) with reputed interna-tional publishers. Prof. Sundram has delivered oral presentation in interna-tional conferences organized in different European countries.

For Product Safety Concerns and Information please contact our EU representative GPSR@taylorandfrancis.com Taylor & Francis Verlag GmbH, Kaufingerstraße 24, 80331 München, Germany